Principles and Practice
of Child Psychiatry

Principles and Practice
of Child Psychiatry

Stella Chess, M.D.

and

Mahin Hassibi, M.D.
New York University Medical School
New York, New York

Plenum Press · New York and London

Library of Congress Cataloging in Publication Data

Chess, Stella.
  Principles and practice of child psychiatry.

  Includes index.
  1. Child psychiatry. I. Hassibi, Mahin, joint author. II. Title. [DNLM: 1. Child psychiatry.
WS350 C524pa]
RJ499.C473   618.9'28'9   78-1604
ISBN 0-306-31131-3

© 1978 Plenum Press, New York
A Division of Plenum Publishing Corporation
227 West 17th Street, New York, N.Y. 10011

Printed in the United States of America

Foreword

Stella Chess's many admirers throughout the world have long looked forward to the day when she would produce her own textbook of child psychiatry. They will not be disappointed in this thoughtful and perceptive account of the principles and practices of the subject, written in collaboration with Dr. Hassibi. It has all the hallmarks we have come to recognize as distinctive of the Chess approach to child psychiatry—gentle yet subtle and penetrating, always appreciative of the feelings and concerns of both the children and their parents, well informed and critically aware of research findings but far from overawed by the contributions of science, and above all immensely practical. Anyone who wants to know how one of the world's outstanding clinicians appraises what child psychiatry has to offer could do no better than to read this book.

Child psychiatry differs from general psychiatry in being concerned with a developing organism, and it is entirely appropriate that the book begins with an account of child development and of the principal theories put forward to explain it. Chess and Hassibi recognize the importance of theory in organizing ideas and in suggesting explanations, but they remain skeptical of how far existing theories do in fact account for the outstanding issues in development. They note the limitations of all theories in explaining *how* development takes place and *why* individual differences occur in the way they do. The sociological and psychological theories of delinquency are met with similar interest combined with doubt. In their discussion of development, Chess and Hassibi emphasize the reciprocity of parent–child interaction. Parenting is rightly seen as doing things *with* children, rather than imposing patterns on a passive and immature recipient. The crucial role of temperamental differences is discussed with the insight expected of one of the originators of the pioneering New York longitudinal study, which demonstrated just how important were the differences between children in behavioral style. Chess and Hassibi point out that personality development does not mean the unfolding of a predetermined set of temperamental characteristics. Instead, there is a vital and dynamic interplay between nature and nurture with the "mesh" between parent and child being particularly crucial.

The book provides a discriminating and thoughtful review of the various factors involved in the etiology of child psychiatric disorders. Genetic factors are largely discussed in terms of schizophrenia and manic-depressive psychosis in adults—a reflection perhaps of the current reluctance to invoke hereditary explanations for individual differences in personality functioning and intellectual level. Perinatal complications and postnatal diseases are given a somewhat more extended discussion, but the main focus is on temperamental differences and family influences. Sex differences in behavior are noted only very briefly in passing—clearly the authors are not strident feminists although they note the role of cultural sex typing. Sociocultural issues are also considered fully and carefully. But the one striking omission is any discussion of the influence of schooling. Of course, it is the given wisdom of the moment to doubt whether it has much impact, but in other respects Chess and Hassibi have not been afraid to question authoritative judgments. It would be curious if an environment in which children spent half their waking hours for a dozen years had no effect.

The bulk of the book consists of a smooth flowing description of presenting symptoms, the process of assessment, and the range of clinical problems extending from everyday eating and sleeping difficulties to the psychoses. This provides a distillation of Chess's great clinical experience and acumen, complemented by references to relevant research findings and illustrated by admirably succinct and pertinent case histories. There are sensitive descriptions of how to interview children and of the role of play. It is very much a psychiatrist's account in that not very much is said about the contributions of teachers, psychologists, and social workers although their value is explicitly recognized. Biological factors are discussed with both good sense and authoritative knowledge. The most helpful discussions of children's responses to physical illness, of the personality development of mentally retarded children, and of the problems of blind and of deaf young people draw well (but rather modestly) on Chess's rich research contributions in these fields as well as on her personal clinical experience.

Psychoanalytic, pharmacological, and behavioral approaches to treatment are specifically described in separate sections of the book, but it is clear from the earlier chapters that the authors' preferences are for an eclectic approach that relies mainly on counseling and psychotherapeutic skills. They are mildly doubtful of some of the more dogmatic claims of those who espouse one or the other of the specific therapeutic techniques that are said to be based on some all-encompassing theory.

All in all, the book is a delight to read. It is rich in clinical wisdom and makes good use of research findings, which is what we expect of authors who are scholars and researchers as well as practitioners. But the science does not get in the way of a sensitively written and insightful clinical account of immense value to both the student and the practicing clinician.

Michael Rutter, M.D., F.R.C.P., F.R.C. Psych.
Professor of Child Psychiatry
Institute of Psychiatry
University of London

Preface

In the many years since Dr. Leo Kanner wrote the first American textbook on child psychiatry, our field has undergone enormous growth. This development has occurred in all directions—theoretical formulations, research methodology and findings, practical clinical skill, programs of prevention and models for the delivery of services. At the same time, we have become aware of the inadequacies of previous simplistic explanations of etiology and unidimensional approaches to treatment and prevention. As our knowledge and experience expands, it is ever clearer how many basic questions are still unanswered, and how much more complex the answers will be than was expected in the past.

The proliferation of data, experience, and concepts in the field of child psychiatry makes the task of providing this information in one volume formidable indeed. This is especially true since the ground to be covered ranges from genetic, neurochemical, and psychophysiological issues, through developmental, behavioral, psychometric, and psychosocial approaches, to the sociological and even political arenas. Some authors of recent volumes have dealt with this problem by providing edited texts with multiple authorship by experts in various fields. Such compendia serve an important and necessary purpose. At the same time, there is a need for integrated textbooks to provide up-to-date reviews of theories and reports of research, as well as conceptualizations based on extensive clinical experience and commitments to interactionist views of normal and deviant development.

We have attempted in this volume to provide such an integrated text. In order to obtain critical reaction to our formulations, individual chapters were sent to a number of leading colleagues for their review: Roger Freeman, Melvin Lewis, Marcia Lowry, Frank Menolascino, Daniel Offer, and Peter Wolff. They all responded generously and thoughtfully. We are grateful for their careful comments, which helped us to sharpen a number of areas, and to be content with others. Special thanks must go to Michael Rutter and to Lynn Burkes, who both read the work as a whole. We are, of course, responsible for the content of the book in its entirety and for all the formulations in each chapter.

All books receive multiple nurturing, and this one is no exception. We wish to extend our thanks to Seymour Weingarten of Plenum Press, who first sought us out because he believed that such a book was necessary. To Ronnie Sandroff go our thanks for her patient and intelligent editing of the manuscript. Mrs. Marcia Gershovitz typed and retyped our drafts and final copy, a task which was much more than routine. Mrs. Marguerite Rosenberg lent her able assistance in proofreading the final version.

The designation of child psychiatrist is synonymous with the role of "child advocate." In attempting to fill such a function, we hope that this book will reflect our concern for the children whose problems and strengths we have become familiar with in the course of our professional lives. We will have achieved our purpose if this volume assists students in our field to become effective child advocates.

Stella Chess
Mahin Hassibi

New York

Contents

IV: Methods of Psychiatric Intervention

I
INTRODUCTION TO CHILD PSYCHIATRY

1

A Historical Overview

The observation that today's children will be tomorrow's adults has been made since the dawn of man. But it is only quite recently that serious, sophisticated attention has been paid to the factors involved in this transformation. The body of theory and practice we call child psychiatry has grown out of many diverse areas of study. As a subspecialty of general psychiatry, child psychiatry is a part of medicine. However, as a complex aggregate of knowledge and skills, it has borrowed freely from such fields as the moral and philosophical bases of child rearing, the study of child development, and education. Over the course of history, the underlying concepts, such as normalcy and deviation, have undergone many changes. The historic controversy over the primacy of nature versus nurture has just begun to be viewed as an error in conceptualizing the interdependent relationships between organisms and the environment. And, in recent times, there has been an awareness of the magnitude of our ignorance about the complex mechanisms of development.

The question of when and where child psychiatry had its beginnings is unsolvable. In time-honored fashion one can turn to Hippocrates in the fourth century B.C. and find some statement that seems to predicate the subject. Clearly, Pavlov's (1849–1936) experiments with conditioned reflexes, while technically within the province of physiology, were forerunners of learning theory and an important basis for behavior therapy. Another forerunner was Locke, the 17th-century philosopher and physician, who was an exponent of environmentalism predating Watson's and Freud's attention to environmental causality. Locke described the infant as a *tabula rasa* whose later character, abilities, motivations, and problems result from the experiences to which he is exposed. The opposite view is found vividly portrayed in Samuel Butler's novel *The Way of All Flesh* (1903), which captures his era's concept of innate childhood wickedness.

Concepts of Childhood

It is impossible to do justice to the history of child psychiatry without an awareness of the changing concepts of infancy and childhood. Perhaps the only "truth" that has endured from earliest recordings is the obligation of nurturing adults to turn their young into the kind of people capable of coping with, and considered normal for, the culture into which they have been born. How this is to be achieved, which persons are traditionally assigned to the task, and what is to be done with the misfits are the content of the history of childhood through the ages.

Each era and culture, in addressing itself to the task of continuing its social conventions from generation to generation, does so from a specific philosophical stance as to the nature of children. Following Van Leeuwenhoek's (1632–1723) microscopic observation of the head of the sperm, his era viewed children as homunculi with not only bodies but also characters preformed *in utero*. Only time was required for the preordained physical form and moral character to mature and unfold. In other areas, children were considered as animals possessing both instincts and latent abilities. These two ideas did not necessarily contradict each other. It was often considered the duty of the conscientious parent to train out, beat out, or otherwise defeat the animal in the child so as to permit the human preformed characteristics to emerge. However, it was not always assumed that the animal nature was bad and degenerate. Jean Jacques Rousseau's (1712–1778) concept of the nobility of the unspoiled aspects of nature, both in the landscape and in the human, as expounded in *Discours sur les Arts et Sciences* in 1750, was a powerful influence in its period.

Whether evil was born or bred was first a question in the province of moral philosophy. Later, the nature–nurture controversy had a lengthy, scholarly existence. The debate broadened to include such diverse areas as talents, intelligence, ability to learn specific skills, and an as yet unexhausted list of human attributes. While some changes in concepts of the immutability or plasticity of childhood have led to alterations in child-rearing practices and public policies regarding children, one should also be aware that at other times changes in theories have continued to appear to justify maintenance of the same public attitude. For example, the assumption that the poor have innately lower intelligence had led to early tracking of students into curricula whose ceiling was determined by intelligence tests given in the early or middle school years. Later researchers found the intellectual ability of children to be vastly influenced by environmental stimulation. It was further theorized that a critical period exists before which this stimulation must take place in order to be effective. Since children of the poor suffer from "cultural deprivation" during preschool years, they are still considered forever doomed to be inferior. This attitude justifies a public policy that is indifferent to the quality of education offered in ghetto-area schools.

Throughout most of history, children were the property of parents, to be sold, bartered, exposed to die, mutilated, apprenticed to learn trades, or cherished or pampered as whim, desire, or economic necessity dictated. One of the most recent questions that has been added to the concerns of child psychiatrists is that of the rights of children: the right to be protected from both physical and emotional abuse and to be permitted to live with the parent, or the psychological parent, of their deepest attachment. With this right has come the corollary of parental obligations to provide children with adequate physical and emotional environments. Clearly, for child psychiatrists to participate in these arenas they must have a knowledge of children's basic emotional needs, a clear way of defining normalcy without losing the concept of normal variability, and an ability to differentiate between momentary discomfiture and abiding unhappiness. They must be able to distinguish stressful events that will lead to growth and greater ability to cope from those stresses that are excessive for that particular child at a given time.

Observing Child Behavior

Copernicus (1473–1543) and Galileo (1564–1642) (who, interestingly, was a physician among other professional acquirements) looked at the movement of the heavenly bodies, compared what they saw with what accepted knowledge said they should see, and found the accepted knowledge lacking. Similarly, when individuals dealing with children began to observe the children themselves, they discovered many discrepancies between expectation and facts. The areas of behavior examined were determined by the particular interests of individuals and could not, of course, transcend the physical, biological, and medical knowledge of the time.

The observations could also not transcend social conditions, and the high mortality rate of children in previous centuries may have contributed to the lack of scientific interest in their development. In 17th-century Venice, for example, only 7 out of 1000 babies cared for in foundling homes lived to the age of 10 (Langmeier and Matejcek, 1975)!

As with all science, each new theory of child development was of necessity at least partially wrong and incomplete. But each attempt to fit all the known facts into a theoretical framework provided the basis for the next step. New facts thus came to light, and discrepancies were made evident that gave impetus to new discoveries. This process is by no means complete, and the search for further knowledge and more refined observation continues. Identification of behavioral abnormality in children did not await the mapping out of normal behavior. Cases of extreme deviation in physical, moral, and intellectual development were described even before normal behavior was under organized scrutiny.

The first English-speaking psychiatrist giving attention to children was the noted Henry Maudsley (1835–1918). In his book *The Physiology and Pathology of the Mind*, written in 1867, recognizable, clear descriptions of aberrant child behaviors directly observed by the author are found. His description of night terrors rings true today. He distinguished between hallucinations in children and in adults and noted the fact that if "hallucinatory" episodes had a direct and reversible environmental origin, they were not to be given pathological status. It is curious that side by side with these magnificent direct observations Maudsley included in his book several descriptions by colleagues that were assumed accurate without verification. Some may be quite accurate and attest to the fact that psychiatric problems of the childhood years were not unusual. However, it is surprising to read in the very same book a case history introduced by the words, "Crighton quotes from Greding a well known case of a child which, as he says, was raving mad as soon as it was born." Detailed description is given of this infant, at 4 days of age, having laughing fits without discernible reason, tearing clothes, and climbing walls. Why, then, did Maudsley include this unverified description of a case written up more than 100 years previously and passed through several sources before reaching him? Probably because it fit so well into his thesis that the mind is physiological in origin. By insisting that intentional actions and madness could be observed even in newborn infants, Maudsley was attempting to move psychiatry from the realm of metaphysics and the idea that madness was a divine retribution. He examined animals, idiots, and normal children as reasonable sources from which to derive a picture of sensorimotor (his term) reflex activity growing gradually into volition.

Sigmund Freud (1856–1939) constructed over many years a developmental concept of child reactivity to environmental events and the attitude of caretakers as determining many features of pathology, character structure, and unconscious elements of behavior. Although neither Melanie Klein nor Freud's daughter, Anna Freud, were physicians, their further development of Freud's concepts through direct work with children was an extension of psychoanalytic child psychiatry. It is of interest that to our knowledge, Freud himself treated only one child, and this treatment was done via paternal reports and Freud's instructions.

In the year 1911 the term *schizophrenia* was introduced by Eugen Bleuler (1857–1939), and his book on this topic was later translated into English as *Dementia Praecox or the Group of Schizophrenias*. His very important point, verified many times since, was that "With relatively accurate histories, one can trace back the illness to childhood, or even the first years of life in at least five percent of the cases." In 1925 Sante de Sanctis first described *dementia praecox* in adolescent children. The term dementia praecox had first arisen from the observations that a dementia resembling senility could occur in younger adults.

Leo Kanner was a pioneer who gave child psychiatry a structure of its own. Not only did he write the first American textbook on this subject, *Child Psychiatry* (1957), in 1935, but he also organized the first child psychiatry–pediatric liaison. The clinical entity bearing his name as Kanner's disease, which is more generally referred to as infantile autism, was first described by Kanner in 1949.

Lauretta Bender, who became director in 1934 of the first children's unit within a psychiatric hospital at New York's Bellevue Hospital, is best known for her concepts and long-term studies of schizophrenic children. However, her influence within the field of child psychiatry is even greater than her numerous published writings. She began training child psychiatrists in 1934. Her students have since trained many others. Bender's contribution to child psychiatry has been the introduction of concepts such as the relation between insufficient affective stability in early life and formation of psychopathic personality; the nature of behavioral pathologies arising out of organic diseases in children; and indications of an organic basis for some—if not all—schizophrenia in children. These and other ideas have been passed on through training to a greater extent than one would realize through reading only her published works.

In the development of the mental hygiene movement, the appearance of child guidance clinics and special interest in mental retardation, on the one hand, and juvenile delinquency, on the other, have intertwined to form the rich background of child psychiatry in this country.

Mental Deficiency and Psychiatry

Distinctions of degree of defect within mental retardation are a relatively recent phenomenon. *Idiocy*, *cretinism*, and *mental retardation* were used synonymously over the centuries. Leo Kanner (1949) described Gugenbueuller's attempts to demonstrate in his Swiss school that intellectually subnormal children could improve with care and training. In 1801 a French psychiatrist, Itard, reported his attempts to educate Victor, the "Wild Boy of Aveyron," in his book *De l'Education d'un Homme Sauvage*. Itard used some of the methods he had employed in educational work with the deaf in his five-year heroic attempt to raise the level of Victor's functioning. It is unclear whether this experiment truly involved a biologically normal child fostered by wild animals, as Itard supposed, or an organically defective child discovered in a wild state. Seguin, also a French psychiatrist involved with educating the deaf, was stimulated by Itard's report and began to work with mentally deficient children. In 1846 he presented his ideas in a book, *The Moral Treatment, Hygiene and Education of Idiots and Other Backward Children*. Samuel Howe, an American psychiatrist working in Boston, not only introduced Seguin's methods but was also instrumental in bringing Seguin himself to the United Stated in the mid-19th century. Howe became the director of the first state-supported school for the retarded in Boston, and Seguin continued establishing schools and residential centers for "idiots and other feebleminded persons" in the United States.

The beginnings of the movement for education and treatment of the retarded in the United States was primarily a psychiatric concern; indeed all the charter members of the American Association on Mental Deficiency, founded in 1876, were psychiatrists. Lightner Whitmer's psychologic clinic, founded in 1896 at the University of Pennsylvania, was primarily concerned with the study, treatment, and training of the feebleminded. This may properly be considered the birthplace of the child guidance movement. Since this early period, however, psychiatric interest in and feelings of responsibility for mentally retarded children has undergone a number of changes, and much of the research and activity has been carried out by psychologists. In 1906 a research laboratory was opened at the Vineland Training School in New Jersey, where H. H. Goddard began to work in 1914. The psychometric movement began in France in 1904, with the development of the Simon–Binet test. It was created in order to identify why some Parisian children failed to benefit as much as expected from their educational exposure. Modified in Stanford, California, its American version is now known as the Stanford–Binet Test. The Wechsler Intelligence Test was first devised at Bellevue Hospital in New York City, ushering in an era of discussion as to the degree to which nature and nurture were responsible for test scores. Cyril Burt, a British psychologist who died in 1972, published data purporting to establish the existence of a large genetic component underlying intelligence test scores. His ideas were largely responsible for the British tracking system in education. However, Burt's conclusions have recently come under serious question with the allegation that a good portion of his data were manufactured (Wade, 1976).

Psychiatric Facilities

The first formal child guidance clinic in the United States was a court-related project organized in 1909 in Chicago by William Healy for investigating the antecedents of juvenile delinquency (Healy and Bronnor, 1948). Here, the American effort preceded the European. In 1925 August Eichhorn (in a book published in Austria with an introduction by Sigmund Freud) reported upon his psychological approach to his work with adolescent delinquents in Vienna. The book was subsequently published in the United States in 1935 under the title *Wayward Youth*. Healy published *The Individual Delinquent*, a psychoanalytically oriented discussion, in the year 1915. The formal child guidance movement advanced relatively quickly from this time. The children's clinic in Boston's Psychopathic Hospital opened in 1912 and included psychologists and social workers. The Phipps Clinic in Baltimore followed a year later under the direction of Adolph Meyer. Both of these outpatient departments and that of Allentown State Hospital in Pennsylvania (1915) admitted youngsters with a variety of psychiatric disorders. The Yale Clinic of Child Development opened its doors under the direction of Arnold Gesell in 1911, followed by other child study centers.

The need for facilities for children with psychiatric disorders became dramatic after World War I when an epidemic of encephalitis lethargica resulted in large numbers of children with behavior disorders, some as immediate sequelae and others with delayed effects of the disease becoming evident only after 5–20 years. Creation of inpatient facilities for these children resulted in the opening of a children's unit at Bellevue Hospital in New York City and at the Franklin School in Philadelphia. Demonstration clinics were founded in many cities. Fellowships, provided largely by the Commonwealth Fund and the Rockefeller Foundation, made possible the training of psychiatrists, psychologists, and social workers for such clinics. Frederick Allen, founder and head of the Philadelphia Child Guidance Clinic until his death in 1964—and David Levy, in New York, who died in 1977—were two of those most intimately concerned with the establishment of these clinics. In 1937 a separate adolescent unit, the first of its kind, was established by Frank Curran at Bellevue Hospital in New

York and used for both service and teaching. Still later, departments of psychiatry developed divisions of child psychiatry. Currently accreditation regulations for training require some type of affiliation with a recognized medical center.

Professional Organizations

In 1924 the American Orthopsychiatric Association was founded. It acted as a clearinghouse for exchanging news of activities and set up unofficial standards for training. In 1946, the American Association of Psychiatric Clinics for Children became a standard-setting body, although without formal mandate. The National Mental Health Act of 1946 made federal funds available for advanced training and research in child psychiatry. Finally, the American Academy of Child Psychiatry was founded in 1952 as the official representative of child psychiatry in the United States and Canada. Its journal, initiated a few years later, has acted as an important outlet for clinical, research, and theoretical work in the field. Although the American Board of Psychiatry and Neurology was incorporated in 1934, it was not until 1959 that the creation of examinations in child psychiatry as a subspecialty of psychiatry with a separate certification established child psychiatry as an official field in itself. The International Association for Child Psychiatry and Allied Professions was founded in 1948 and had its first official meeting in Paris. Its first president was Frederick Allen, from the United States.

Research in Child Psychiatry

So far our discussion has focused on the birth of child psychiatry as an independent field. However, those engaged in the practice of child psychiatry also began systematic investigation and observation of the behavioral patterns of their patients in order to check in an organized fashion the validity of their own impressions and the usefulness of their consequent intervention. As the clinical field matured and differentiated over time, so also did the research inquiry into etiology of normal and abnormal development and the effects of various interventions.

Scientific studies can be broadly divided into two categories: (1) Exploratory research in which data are collected by systematic observation and organized into clusters, patterns are noted, and finally explanatory hypotheses are formed. Theoretical principles deduced from such studies are ideally coherent, logical, and consistent with all the known facts and have some degree of predictive value. (2) Confirmatory studies in which theoretical principles and specific hypotheses are tested by controlling various dependent and independent variables.

Most researches in behavioral sciences are of an exploratory nature because of the multiplicity of determinants of any segment of human behavior and the difficulties in defining, controlling, and manipulating various factors. Furthermore, experiments on people under laboratory conditions for the purpose of isolating or influencing some parameter of their behavior are not always desirable or necessarily fruitful.

The earliest systematic studies reported in psychiatric literature are clinical descriptions and classifications of deviant behavior with or without some hypotheses regarding the possible etiology and prognosis of the natural course of the illness. Most of these early observations have remained valid, although incorrect conclusions have been made on the basis of generalizations of the behavior of unrepresentative samples or the predominant cultural and intellectual beliefs of the period. For example, the notion of "masturbatory insanity" or the pessimistic prognosis of dementia praecox reflected the characteristics of chronic patients in insane asylums; and the belief in harmfulness of excess of all kinds gave indiscriminate etiological significance to factors such as excessive use of alcohol, sexual activity, and academic pursuits. However, most current concepts, such as genetic predisposition, constitutional at-risk factors, and environmental stress, were mentioned in these early writings, although the possibility of the cumulative impact of environmental stress and the interaction among various pathogenic factors was commonly ignored. Behavior disorders of children and the continuity of behavioral abnormality between childhood and adult life received scanty attention except in cases of mental subnormality.

The mental hygiene movement in the early years of the 20th century sponsored the idea of prevention of mental disorders; thus the search for determinants of abnormal behavior was focused on childhood years. Although in 1909 William Healy established a court-related clinic in Chicago for the evaluation and treatment of juvenile delinquents, it was not until 1920 that a survey conducted by the National Committee for Mental Hygiene among schoolchildren discovered various mild and moderate degrees of behavior disorders among the nonretarded school-age population. Since then studies in child psychiatry and child development have become increasingly sophisticated and scientifically rigorous. The search for normative data on development has become more systematic, and observations in natural settings have begun shortly after birth. Longitudinal studies of children into adolescence have provided information regarding normal growth, which, in turn, has been tested in the less time-consuming and less expensive cross-sectional evaluations of various populations. Design and standardization of different developmental scales are now based on more accurate observations, and this has improved their evaluatory and predictive usefulness. Awareness of the multiplicity of operative factors in the development and maintenance of behavioral patterns is reflected in a more careful selection of samples, better description of the context within which observed behavior occurs, and more cautious and parsimonious generalization. Replications in different settings and across socioeconomic and cultural backgrounds are attempted in order to define the limits of generalization and whether universality can be assigned to any set of conclusions.

Studies of deviant behavior in child psychiatry, as in adult psychiatry, are hampered by semantic confusion and inconsistent definition of clinical entities (Group for Advancement of Psychiatry, 1957). Most investigations of the prevalence and incidence of behavior disorders have attempted to discover the distribution of a particular symptom or cluster of symptoms among various populations and to identify factors that may contribute to a differential rate of prevalence among various groups. Furthermore, by comparison of the prevailing rate of any deviant behavior in various age groups within a designated area, some light is shed on the natural evolution of a particular symptom, and a global measure of prediction and prognostication is achieved.

Problems of Method

The search for the etiology of behavioral disorders has thus far yielded few solid results. Etiological investigations have been relatively nonproductive because of the inconsistency of diagnostic criteria, the absence of an acceptable measure for degree of severity, and the lack of quantifiable biochemical or neurophysiological concomitants for various behavioral abnormalities. The issue is further complicated by the fact that various causative factors may result in similar behavioral manifestations.

Studies of causative links between patterns of behavior and organismic and environmental factors are thus, by necessity, correlational in nature. Differences between the population under study and a control group that is matched for all variables except the one under investigation are subjected to statistical analysis. Whenever such differences cannot be assigned to a chance occurrence of less than 5 times out of 100, the results are considered statistically significant. The underlying hypothesis in such correlational studies (null hypothesis) is that if the likelihood of occurrence of two sets of variables can be explained by chance, no consistent relationship can be assumed to exist between the two. However, it must be noted that statistically significant correlation does not imply a causative link; the two parameters may be manifestations of a third factor, or they may be a response to one another. For example, when correlations are found to exist between behavioral pathology in children and their parents, it is as valid to assume that parental attitudes are responses to the child's behavior as it is to say that parents play a causative role. Statistically significant but inappropriate correlations may also result from methodology and the nature of the subject matter. For example, control groups may be matched for irrelevant parameters, or all the relevant factors may not be known, and thus the similarities and dissimilarities between the two groups, although real, may be independent of the behavior deviation. Or the sample under study may not be representative of all children with a particular problem, and conclusions are therefore of limited value. If the definition and conceptualization of the issues are overly simplistic, the results may not allow further elaboration and appropriate generalization.

Collaborative studies in various centers and randomized study samples are efforts to assure a more representative group for investigatory purposes. Phenomenological descriptions and operational definitions promise to produce more uniform criteria for inclusion in any research project. On the other hand, the choice of relevant and irrelevant factors remain bound by psychiatric opinion and knowledge at the time of investigation and the personal experiences and professional orientation of the investigators. Similar factors limit the interpretation of any correlational findings. Some studies are faulted on the ground that an important known fact has not received appropriate attention. For example, while a good portion of genetic theorizing of the etiology of mental disorders is based on the comparisons of concordance and discordance rates between dizygotic and monozygotic twins, the fact that monozygotic twins as a group are at risk of more obstetrical complications, lower birth weight, and more frequent signs of neurological damage has been ignored (Campion and Tucker, 1975). However, genetic theories have given impetus to longitudinal studies of infants of schizophrenic parents, epidemiological surveys of normal children raised in foster homes with schizophrenic members, and progeny of schizophrenics reared in normal foster homes. It is thus hoped that while no single study has provided a conceptual frame that accounts for all the known facts about schizophrenia, the outcome of different investigations helps in the construction of a more explanatory theory.

Research projects dealing with the effectiveness of various therapeutic interventions are among the least illuminating ones in child psychiatry (Eysenck, 1952; Rie, 1971; Anthony, 1974). Uncertainties about the natural course of childhood behavior disorders, vagueness of diagnostic criteria, and lack of a uniformly acceptable definition and measure of change are compounded by an absence of a clear description of psychotherapy and an ignorance about the site, mode of action, and biochemical effects of psychopharmacological agents. The majority of large-scale studies of the effectiveness of various kinds of psychotherapies have failed to show a statistically significant correlation between the outcome among disturbed children who have and have not received psychotherapy. Clinical impressions of practitioners and even reports of beneficial effects by patients and their families and teachers do not reach a higher level of significance than would be expected by chance occurrence.

In drug studies, the design of the research protocols have become increasingly sophisticated and detailed. In a sample for a pilot study, usually children who have failed to respond to more conventional treatment modalities are chosen. To circumvent the problem of a matched control group, subjects are used as their own control. Furthermore, because it is known that psychological factors are operative in response to any medication in medical practice, the placebo effect is included as a parameter to be studied. Children are thus given an initial period of placebo "washout" and then placed on an alternate predetermined course of active agent and placebo. Because neither patients and their caretakers nor the investigator are aware at the time if the patient is receiving an active agent or a placebo, these are called *double-blind studies*. The child's behavior is periodically observed and rated on scales of severity during the course of investigation. Changes in behavior taking place during administration of the pharmacological substance as compared to placebo period are assumed to be due to the effects of medication. Aside from the methodological limitations inherent in pharmacological researches, most studies have so far failed to find any drug with more than a symptom suppression quality. However, when deviant behavior interferes with the child's ability to function in interpersonal and learning situations, any amelioration of the disruptive behavior and its consequences is an important therapeutic step, provided that the long-term disadvantages of drugs do not outweigh their temporary benefits.

Investigations of the course of cognitive, emotional, and social development in childhood may be expected to provide important information about factors involved in personality organization and behavior disorders in children as well as the antecedents of adult mental illness (Wolff, 1970). On the other hand, neurophysiological and bio-chemical studies are more likely to be initiated among well-defined clinical entities in adults, and only positive findings are likely to be replicated in children. A single exception is the study of the biological concomitants of mental retardation, where important discoveries have been made by research studies in young patients. Animal studies and ethological researches (Sechzer *et al.*, 1973) have provided confirma-tory evidence for some clinical impressions in child psychiatry and many new concepts regarding the evolution of behavior.

2

Normal Child Development

Disorders of behavior, learning, and physical growth must be studied in relation to normal child development. Historically, interest in the exceptional child predated studies in normal development, but the invention of objective measures of growth and change for normal children has sharpened our understanding of abnormality. A knowledge of the mechanisms through which children learn, for example, helps the psychiatrist in his quest to understand why a particular child is not learning. Similarly, a grasp of the process through which children are socialized to control aggression broadens our understanding of the delinquent child.

The development of children results from a dynamic interaction between nature and nurture or biology and the environment. While nature and nurture can be separated linguistically, in reality they are always overlapping and interacting. Chronological growth is the result of simultaneous changes and interactions in the overlapping areas of nature and nurture. Environmental factors may trigger the unfolding of some functions and regulate and control the rate and direction of development. Conversely, organismic peculiarities may block, weaken, or heighten the impact of environmental stimuli, or they may impose an idiosyncratic structure upon them.

Scientific observations of child development have involved descriptions and measurements of such objective indices as height, weight, language acquisition, motor capacity, and intellectual performance, as well as the more subjective changes in feelings, attitudes, and perceptions. The term *developmental status* is used to express the sum total of all the various measures and functional levels at any given point in a child's life. It is a more inclusive concept than chronological age, which is only one among the many variables that influence developmental status.

Theories of child development strive to find the lawful relationships among various aspects of development and the mechanisms through which changes emerge. Until recently, there was great controversy over whether genetic endowment or experience was primarily responsible for various aspects of human behavior. Modern theories recognize that attempts to isolate genetic and environmental influences may be futile for many areas of development. Even before birth, the infant's constitution develops through the interaction of his inborn characteristics and the uterine environment. And, too, the child's later environment is produced by his individual impact on others as well as their influence on him. While the child's sex, ordinal position, and style of activity and reactivity are his initial contributions to the atmosphere that surrounds him, this ambience is in a constant state of flux. New patterns of behavior exhibited by the child will require modifications and accommodations from the environment, and the child will, in turn, be influenced by the new reactions of others. Parental personalities, states of physical and psychological health, and social class memberships are important variables in creating the environment that constitutes the child's early reality and presents a unique combination of interactional opportunities. Thus far, studies have failed to find significant correlations between measureable indices of environmental qualities—such as child-rearing practices and social class—and identifiable patterns of development and personality types. However, the relationship between extremely distorted experiental backgrounds and deviant personality development has been well established. Furthermore, experimental manipulation of environmental variables in animals has caused disturbances in the social, cognitive, and affective development of animal infants analogous to pictures of abnormal behavior in humans. Although such observations do not explain the totality of human development, they indicate that the quality and nature of experience plays an important role in the developmental process (Sameroff, 1975; Bell, 1968).

Genetic and Constitutional Factors

The unique psychology of each individual is underpinned by a particular anatomical, physiological, and biochemical makeup determined, in part, by the genes. The number of possible genotypes is far greater, even by conservative estimate, than is the number of all of the people who have thus far lived on the earth. Except for identical twins, each individual's genetic makeup is dissimilar from all others.

The constitutional composition of the newborn infant is a result not only of genetic inheritance but of the biochemical environment of the intrauterine milieu, which exerts differential influences upon the fetus at various stages of growth. Genetic influences are persistent throughout the life of the organism; and genetic potentialities become evident whenever the necessary combination of genetic predisposition and environmental factors reaches the critical level for occurrence.

There is evidence of individuality in the size, number, structure, and arrangement of neurons in the central nervous system. These differences, however, have not been related to differences in behavior in human infants. Researchers of animal behavior have managed to enhance or suppress some behavioral characteristics, such as learning ability or aggression, by planned breeding in certain animals. Human variations in blood composition, enzyme levels, and the size and activity of the endocrine glands have been reported. However, only extreme deviations have thus far been shown to result in clinically identifiable differences in behavior. This heterogeneity in constitutional endowment must be recognized as the foundation of the infinite number of personality structures that develop as the result of dissimilar interactional opportunities with the environment.

Motor Development

In neonates, most motor behavior consists of uncontrolled, uncoordinated responses to general stimuli, except for the organized reflexes, such as sucking, grasping, and stepping, which are present shortly after birth. However, while initially any gustatory or olfactory stimulation elicits the sucking reflex, later on the response becomes specifically associated with stimulation of the buccal membrane, cheeks, chin, and upper lips. The organization of motor movements is reflected in an increased threshold of excitation and tendency toward segmented and particularized activities. Postural control precedes voluntary locomotion, and the direction of motor development follows a cephalocaudal axis.

For the majority of children, motor development is a sequence of orderly stages, which begins with postural control of the neck at about 3–4 weeks and ends in independent walking by about 18 months. Shirley (1931) described five stages in motor development according to the kind of postural and locomotive skills acquired: control of the neck, sitting alone, crawling, standing, and walking. By 6 months of age, the majority of normal children are capable of lifting and holding their heads up in both prone and supine positions. This skill requires control over the muscles of the neck, chest, and shoulders. As early as 5 months of age, some children are able to sit unsupported; by 12 months more than 90% of infants are able to do so. Crawling precedes the infant's early attempts at standing. Coordinated movements of the lower limbs are first reflected in the child's ability to walk when led and to pull himself up to a standing position by holding on to furniture.

Motor maturation does not follow a rigid time sequence; for example, unsupported sitting does not always precede creeping. Every baby seems to follow his own line of development so that there is an overlapping of various stages and time variations for the mastery of particular skills. Practice is of questionable value in advancing motor development. Pikler (1971) reported that with self-induced movement children achieve the motor landmarks at about the same time as those who have been coached. The relationship between intellectual ability and the speed of motor development is not very clear. Even severely retarded children achieve locomotion, though motor landmarks may be delayed. Conversely, intellectually gifted children may not show precocious motor development.

While disturbances in the neuromuscular system may be associated with mental retardation, not all children with motor handicaps show intellectual deficiencies. While the importance of motor activity in the general scheme of development should not be minimized, it should be noted that the influence of motor behavior on emotional and intellectual growth has not been clarified.

Fine Motor Coordination. The gaining of control of the muscles in each part of the body proceeds from the proximal to the distal sections. At birth, tactile stimulation of the palm elicits a grasping response, but there is no intentional prehension until the infant begins to reach for an object in his line of vision. At about 24 weeks of age, most infants try to scoop up objects with the aid of all fingers and the palm. By 9 months of age, the thumb and forefingers are used for holding. At this time, finer control over the wrist, forearm, and shoulder gives the child the ability for more voluntary precision in the use of his hands.

Fine motor coordination, involving control over the distal muscles, is a prerequisite for the development of self-care skills. As the child begins to imitate and follow directions, various self-care skills become possible. The child learns such activities as dressing and undressing, washing and combing, and eating with utensils, all of which require various degrees of fine motor coordination. Infant intelligence tests include many items that are dependent upon fine motor coordination, and the infant's developmental quotient is largely a reflection of his ability to engage in purposeful activities requiring control and coordination of his muscular system.

The majority of the so-called soft neurological signs are examples of poor performance in various tasks involving fine motor coordination. Control and coordination of the lower extremities is reflected in the child's ability to climb stairs, stand on one foot, and skip on one or alternating feet. The development of the vocal-motor system is a prerequisite of expressive language and clear articulation. Children with dysphasia with apraxia are unable to imitate various movements. When the disturbance involves the face muscles, the child cannot imitate movements such as frowning or whistling and may have defects in articulation.

Preference for the left or right side of the body develops slowly. The young child tends to use both hands indiscriminately and alternately. Although a majority of children are right-preferred by about 6 years of age, a significant minority show a mixture of right and left preferences in usage of various parts of the body. They may be right-handed but use their left foot to start walking or their left eye to look through a hole. The exact cause of lateral dominance and the implications of mixed dominance are not fully understood, though some authors have reported a high correlation between mixed dominance and disorders of spoken and written language (Clements, 1966).

Differences in motor development have been reported for various ethnic groups and geographical locations. The development of locomotions appears to be largely independent of learning and stimulation, but the level of nutrition and general health does influence the time of appearance and rate of progression of motor landmarks. Fine motor coordination, however, is more affected by practice. Some skills, such as skating or bicycle riding, must be taught. Others, such as handwriting, show continuous improvement with practice.

Perception

The processing of sensory information into meaningful wholes by the central nervous system is called *perception*. Accurate perception depends on the type of stimulus, the intactness of the sense organs, and the integrity of the central nervous system. Perception is also influenced by the motivation and intelligence of the individual through the mechanism of selective attention to various stimuli (Bruner, 1973). The functioning of the subject's perceptual processes is inferred from his verbal or motoric responses. Failure at a set of tasks designed to assess perception in children must be considered a reflection of impairment of the cognitive–motivational, motor, and perceptual systems. The following sections divide psychological functioning in early infancy for purposes of discussion rather than to assert the independence of these processes.

Visual Perception. The environmental stimulus for vision is direct or reflected light received by the eye and transmitted to the occipital lobes of the brain for central processing. The eye movements necessary for visual scanning are under the control of the frontal lobes, so coordination between the occipital and frontal lobes is also necessary for accurate visual perception. The retina is sensitive to light at birth, and by 2 months of age the reflexive accommodation of the pupils to light is well established. Around four weeks after birth, most infants follow a moving light by moving their eyes and head. Shortly after that, coordinated movements of the two eyes make binocular vision possible, and visual scanning becomes purposeful. By studying the amount of time that infants focus on particular visual stimuli, researchers have discovered that infants show a preference for various visual patterns as early as 48 hours after birth (Berlyne, 1960). Among patterns of equal complexity, the human face seems to hold infants' attention for the longest period of time. This ability to discriminate between visual patterns and to recognize fine details increases with age, so that smiling in response to the human face becomes more frequent when the face is that of a familiar caretaker (Fantz and Fagan, 1975).

Some time before 6 months of age, most infants begin to reach for objects and bring objects placed in their hands toward their eyes. This hand–eye coordination is another stage of integration between perception and motor development, providing the child with expanded sensory information. The sensations received from touching objects are integrated with visual stimuli to give the child a clearer picture of the object. While body orientation and the perception of spatial relationships are among the earliest visual processing tasks of an infant, tests that can assess these functions are not yet available. In older children, identification of left and right on their own body and their mirror image and tasks requiring the construction of patterns and figures from wooden blocks give some indication of the child's ability in this area.

Discrimination based on a dominant feature of an object, such as shape, form, or color, requires both visual sensitivity to the feature and the storing and retrieval of visual impressions (visual memory). Fitting three-dimensional forms into appropriate holes (Gesell form board), choosing similar and dissimilar patterns, finding a figure embedded in a distracting background, and identifying an incomplete object are all tasks designed to assess visual discrimination. The inability to perform tasks that require attentive visual scanning, design reproduction, or discrimination of like and unlike designs may be a contributing factor in reading difficulties.

Auditory Perception. While the findings of research into the reaction of fetuses to sound are equivocal, there is little doubt that newborn infants have a functioning hearing apparatus. Investigating the soothing effects of sounds during the first four days of life, Birns *et al.* (1965) concluded that neonates respond differentially to various tones. The responses depend on the baby's state of arousal and the frequency and duration of the sounds. During a low state of arousal, newborn infants become excited following high-intensity sounds, while low-frequency sounds have a calming effect on excited neonates. By about 8 months of age, most infants show an active preference for particular sounds by looking for their source. Hardy (1960) found that 60% of infants who did not show this orienting behavior were diagnosed as having hearing dysfunctions in later years.

Auditory perception is the ability to select and organize pertinent auditory stimuli. It depends on both the presence of a functioning auditory apparatus and an intact auditory cortex localized in the temporal lobes. Impaired hearing may reflect a dysfunction in the sound-conducting system, while disturbances in discriminative hearing stem from problems in the analysis and synthesis carried on in the auditory cortex. Assessing hearing in very young children is difficult because of such interferences as inattentiveness, distractibility, hyperactivity, and emotional withdrawal. While a variety of signals can be used to discover whether the child differentiates between sound and no sound, the child must be able to use some form of communicative language in order to respond to tests of auditory cortex functioning. Through behavior observation one can draw some inferences about the child's ability to discriminate sounds of varying pitch or rhythm. However, the most important function of auditory perception—the analysis and synthesis of speech sounds—remains difficult to test in a nonspeaking child.

The development of receptive language requires adequate hearing and the ability to listen, discriminate between various phonemes, attribute meaning to sounds, and compare and store sound patterns in their unique sequential order for later retrieval and recognition. Some children fail to attend to sounds, while others do not recognize or remember recurring patterns. The outcome is a total or partial inadequacy in speech comprehension. In the partial inadequacy, for example, the child may understand the meaning of a key word but fail to appreciate the modifying implications of the sentence in which the particular word is used.

The production of speech comes later than speech comprehension. In children with intact vocal-motor systems, their random movements produce sounds that, through autofeedback and differential reinforcement, gradually approach the phonemic structure of the language used in their environment. A sequence of vocal movements is associated with the auditory impression of the created sound and is then stored for future use (Todd and Palmer, 1968).

Like their hearing peers, deaf children produce random vocalizations, but because their babbling is not accompanied by auditory stimuli, they lose interest in it. Another type of speech defect—namely, misarticulation—reflects a disturbance in the cycle of auditory perception and motor reproduction of speech. The majority of speech defects improve with age, but the roles played by experience and maturation of the vocal motor apparatus and/or the central nervous system in this improvement are not clear. With age, there are an increase in auditory acuity and some indications of differential sensitivity to low and high tones among the sexes. In aphasia-like disorders, the child is unable to remember the name of various configurations, although he may pick the correct words from a series of words or give the accurate name on some occasions. Other children are unable to reproduce the motor–kinesthetic sequence they want and substitute a word bearing a phonetic or semantic resemblance or one associated with the object. For example, a child may say "fireplace" when asked to name a picture of a snow-capped mountain or "scary bone" as a replacement for skeleton. In other children, language acquisition is age-appropriate, but the decoding of written language presents a special difficulty. Many researchers believe the fault lies in a failure of visual–auditory integration: the child is unable to translate written symbols into their auditory equivalents and vice versa.

Most studies regarding auditory perception are based on the disturbances that follow structural damage to the brain in adults. The inferences made about functional deficiencies and developmental lags are therefore necessarily hypothetical conclusions arrived at by analogy. In adults who have sustained brain damage, tissue destruction in the temporal area of the left hemisphere is frequently associated with disturbances in language, even in the majority of left-handed patients. However, young children with damage to the left brain manage to acquire speech, even though it may be at a somewhat later age. This had led to the inference that cerebral specialization and dominance are not fully developed before 2 or 3 years of age; therefore mixed dominance may be considered a contributing factor in language disorders only after the child has reached school age.

Haptic Perception. Touch, pain, temperature, and the sensation of muscle movement comprise the haptic system. This sensory information is received from both the body itself and the environment. The qualitites of shape, form, size, texture, consistency, hardness, and temperature are important attributes of the objective world. Orientation in space, pressure on the joints, and the angles and location of various parts of the body are necessary data for survival.

The questions of how haptic sensations are processed centrally and develop over time have not yet received much research attention. It is known, however, that blind children extensively use the haptic system and that at least some neurologically damaged children have impaired integration of visual and haptic sensations. There is some experimental evidence that suggests that tactile recognition (tested by single-point localization and multiple-point discrimination on the body) is a maturational process that is fully achieved around 7 years of age.

During the first 48 hours of life, infants respond to painful stimuli; at first their reaction is more pronounced to a pinprick on the face than on the legs. Even in the older infant, more frequent or stronger stimuli are necessary to produce the same degree of response from the legs as from the upper body. Even when the baby is asleep, cold stimuli produce discomfort, while heat is better tolerated unless it is markedly higher than the body temperature. Congenital absence of pain and temperature sensitivity has been identified in some children without any behavioral problems. Also, some cases of self-mutilating behavior raise the question of pain agnosia. Disturbances of kinesthetic sensation are postulated as underlying difficulties in articulation, depth perception, and other behavioral peculiarities of children with early psychosis.

Little is known about olfactory and gustatory sensations and their implications for psychological development. Some children with eating problems do exhibit idiosyncratic reactions to particular categories of nutrients.

Multiple-Stimulus Integration. For the individual to obtain a full picture of the object world, not only must each sensory system be intact, but the information received from the senses must be related and synthesized. There is little information regarding the nature and maturation of the integrative functioning of the central nervous system. It is known, however, that children whose sensory modalities are normal may have difficulty processing the information received from two or more systems. This condition is particularly relevant to neurologically damaged and intellectually deficient children whose learning difficulties may be related to a failure to synthesize multiple stimuli and correct impressions from one sense with information obtained from other channels.

Self-Perception. The mental picture of the body perceived by each individual is called *body image*. External and internal sensations and motor activities are the raw material out of which a sense of self-perception is constructed. This image, in turn, acts as an integrative core for the individual, assigning meaning and significance to his experience.

Observations of infants' behavior reveal the newborn's lack of differentiation between parts of his body an other objects in the environment. The infant is as intent in watching his own hands or grasping his own foot as he is when reaching for a toy. But through self-initiated and imposed activities, the child's body is touched by others. His spheres of vision and hearing are changed through both his own movements and those of his caretakers. The coordination and integration of these experiences result in a differentiated sense of self. Maturation influences this development, because as the child grows he has an expanding experience. However, the affective and emotional aspects of body image are mainly dependent upon the child's interactions with people around him. The caretakers' affective attitudes and judgments about the child's body, bodily functions, and activities become intertwined and incorporated into his self-perception (Schilder, 1938; Simmel, 1966). Children look at their reflection in a mirror with interest at about 1 year of age and search for the source of the image behind the mirror. Later on, they become aware that their motions are duplicated in the mirror.

Based on human figure drawings, Schilder (1938) postulated that different parts of the body gain prominence in the child's mind at various developmental stages; for example, 4- or 5-year-old children in their drawings include the mouth and eyes, but the ears are usually left out until 8 or 9 years of age. Children with deformities in various organs may represent these features prominently or leave them out of their drawings. Disturbances of body image have been noted in the figure drawings of neurologically damaged, neglected, and depressed youngsters and in the verbal reports of psychotic children with bodily delusions, adolescents with anorexia nervosa, and amputees who perceive a phantom limb.

Language Acquisition

During the past few decades, the process of language acquisition has attracted considerable attention from various schools of psychology. The proponents of different theories of psycholinguistics all agree that language acquisition depends on the interplay between biological and cultural factors. However, they disagree as to the mechanism through which this development takes place and the relative importance of organismic and social factors in the initiation and completion of the process.

For learning theorists, language is learned by gradual imitation and social reinforcement, and as for all higher-level skills, an intact central nervous system is the necessary substrate for the accumulation of information and the establishment of associations. For these theorists, the observation that the vocabulary, intonations, and accents of children resemble those of their parents, and that an increase in the sentence length of the caretakers leads to a similar increase in children, is convincing evidence of the primacy of environmental factors in language acquisition.

Developmental psychologists, on the other hand, maintain that learning by imitation does not account for the rapidity of language development. They also note that the early utterances of children are not copies of adult speech but are organized around the child's own grammar. Regardless of the language milieu surrounding the child, the acquisition of language seems to follow the same operating principles or strategies (Brown and Bellugi, 1964). According to Lenneberg (1967), a child must first abstract the laws and principles underlying the relationship between words and their referents. Only later will he become aware of the relationships among various types of words and learn the semantic structure of the language. Equipped with these two sets of principles, the child is able to generate his own language and employ words and sentences to express his opinions, feelings, and needs. In the earliest stage, the child's language consists of names, locations of objects, and desires for action. Statements about feelings and social relations are absent from the telegraphic utterances of the young child, and prepositions, adjectives, and adverbs are hardly used. When longer sentences are used, the child usually resists exceptions to the rules and special arrangements of various parts of speech. For example, an English-speaking child will say, "I can go?" rather than "Can I go?" or "I comed" instead of "I came."

Chomsky (1957) expressed the position of the developmental psycholinguists when he remarked, "Knowledge of the language results from the interplay of initially given structure of the mind, maturational processes and interaction with the environment." According to Chomsky, learning the rules of grammar and principles for transformation of the intended meaning (deep structure) into the spoken word (surface structure) is the developmental task for language production.

Receptive Language. Although language comprehension is the first step in the acquisition of language, the development of receptive language has not received as much attention from researchers as the production of communicative speech. Friedlander (1971) has shown that 8- to 15-month-old infants are able to differentiate and respond preferentially to samples of language consisting of forward and backward speech, high and low redundancy in segments of stories, and familiar and unfamiliar narrator voices. More recent studies (Cairns and Butterfield, 1975) have revealed that newborn infants are capable of discriminative responses to auditory stimuli; their attentiveness increases with age, so that as they grow older they spend a larger portion of their waking life in listening activities.

The infant must be able to analyze and synthesize a mass of auditory stimuli into meaningful information. The language environment of the infant is a mixture of half-truncated sentences, ambiguous and highly personalized communications among family members, and a considerable amount of background noise that may sometimes contain samples of spoken words. According to Piaget (1926), receptive language—like other kinds of perception—is at first a global impression: the child first understands the overall meaning of a verbal message and then begins to discover the exact meaning of each word and its special significance in the sentence (MacNamara, 1972). During the early years, receptive language is more advanced than expressive speech. Most children comprehend simple directions long before they can verbalize their own wishes. Even children who exhibit defects in language acquisition respond appropriately to simple commands and instructions. The role of motivation and attention span in the development of receptive language has not been fully clarified, although some authors have hypothesized that the apparent lack of speech comprehension in autistic children may be a psychological defense pattern.

Expressive Language. By about 4 weeks of age, infants produce a variety of sounds. During the prelingual stage, their cooings and gurglings become more diversified with the passage of time, so that sounds resembling the vowels and consonants of all languages are reproduced (Ingram, 1976). Like all other self-initiated activities, sound production seems to have a pleasurable quality for the baby and is essentially an exercise of functional capacity. By about 6–8 months of age, babbling becomes more socialized: it is more frequently associated with the presence of other people and is reinforced and rewarded by their attention and mutual imitation. The pitch and inflection of babbling slowly approaches the qualities of the language of the community, although individual words are not as yet recognizable. The first indentifiable word uttered by an infant is usually applied to a group of objects rather than to a single thing. When children try to imitate a polysyllabic word they have heard, they frequently repeat the ending: "fee" for "coffee," for example. This tendency is also apparent in echolalia, in which the last part of the sentence is usually the part that is echoed.

In a study of a large group of infants, Morely (1965) found that by their first birthday the majority of children in her sample were able to produce a few recognizable words and used them extensively to signify events and objects whose functional or objective resemblance was not always easy to fathom. The rate of progression from single words to short phrases and full sentences seems to be highly individualized. Some parents report a very short duration, while other children take a longer time for the transition. Gesell and Amatruda (1964) reported that by the second year of life the majority of children in their sample had a vocabulary of about 270 words and used phrases consisting of a noun and a verb. By the time children are 5 years old, their vocabulary has increased 10-fold, their sentences are longer, their grammatical mistakes are negligible, and they can engage in complete conversations relating events and feelings and expressing age-adequate impressions and thoughts. Lenneberg (1967) believes that the acquisition of speech is related to such indications of brain maturation as increase in weight, density of neuronal connections in the cortex, and changes in proportions of gray and white substance.

The lack of desire and/or need to communicate has been considered a factor in the underdevelopment of speech among children with early psychosis or those whose caretakers are quick to anticipate and fulfill their wants. However, the role of the parent–child relationship in the development of communicative skill remains hypothetical. On the other hand, it has been noted that the child's clarity of articulation, complexity of speech, and size of vocabulary are influenced by such environmental variables as parental education and the amount of verbal interaction between family members and the child. The impoverished language of disadvantaged children is reflected in the limited vocabulary and the short, simple sentences used by the lowest socioeconomic class. Some critics have pointed out that these children may indeed have a large vocabulary of words, but not necessarily those which are included in standardized tests of language proficiency.

The relationship between cognitive and language development is a complex one. Both receptive and expressive language are limited in mentally retarded children; in cases of severe retardation speech remains undeveloped. On the other hand, in children with severe hearing loss, the inability to receive and produce oral speech is not invariably accompanied by a cognitive deficiency. Vygotsky (1962) considers language a distinct aspect of cognitive functioning and not identical with it. He believes that verbal thought is born at the point that a child begins to realize that the name of an object is not another of its properties, such as shape and color, but rather a symbol standing in place of the object. The child then learns to abstract the common attributes of the symbols and their relationships to one another. Once the significative function of words is grasped, language plays an important role in further intellectual development and concept formation. At this point, words supplied by the common language become the cornerstones of the child's thinking, allowing him to build a structure of reality that is consensually validated and to discover the communal principles of logic. Although certain concepts may be equally or more efficiently conveyed by other symbol systems, such as mathematical formulas or musical notations, the fact remains that verbal symbols are the primary vehicle for the organization and expression of our thinking processes. The quality of verbalization is a reasonably reliable measure of the level of cognitive sophistication, and disturbances in the thinking processes are commonly detected from peculiarities of expressive language.

For the child's language to communicate efficiently, there must be an establishment of a mutual understanding of word meanings between the child and his human environment. Word meanings that are highly personalized and idiosyncratic may inhibit communication and delay the child's socialization and acculturation. Even though parents may understand the child's purpose despite his peculiar language use, the child will be unable to establish the relationships with his peers and other adults that are necessary for normal development. According to Vygotsky, there is a difference between "word sense" and "word meaning." The sense of a word is a dynamic and fluid complex that is "the sum of all the psychological events aroused in our consciousness by a word." Word meaning, on the other hand, is the stable core of the word sense complex, the area of shared understanding among members of a language community. While word sense may be used as a unit of inner speech, language meant for others must be constructed out of shared word meanings or it will not be understood. In some children, speech is of no, or poor, communicative value. This difficulty may be due to delay in the maturation of, or defect in, the central nervous system. On the other hand, the language of schizophrenic children seems to reflect a dysfunction in communication that arises from the idiosyncratic use of language: a failure to differentiate between common word meanings and highly personalized word sense.

The exchange of ideas, declarations of intent, and the expression of feelings and impressions are only part of the function of speech. Children soon learn that language can be used to affect changes in their social environment and obtain desired responses from the people around them. Name calling, teasing, expressions of helplessness, and accusations of various sorts are verbal activities intended to attain affective reactions and to regulate the emotional distance between the child and others. Thus an overprotected child who declares "I hate you" to his mother may not be expressing his true feelings but attempting to create some temporary emotional distance. The ability to be affected and moved by language is an important aspect of social interaction. The pleasure at hearing words of praise and hurt feelings following verbal disapproval are regulating agents of socialization and a fundamental principle of psychotherapeutic methodology.

Self-direction is another important function of language. Young children may be heard talking to themselves while engaged in activity. At times this running commentary precedes each step of an action; at other times it runs parallel to it. This self-directed, self-motivated speech is called *egocentric speech* by Piaget, who believes it is a reflection of the child's lack of differentiation between himself and others, which is extinguished as the child becomes more socialized. A contrary view is held by Vygotsky, who considers egocentric speech as the fore-runner of inner speech, which becomes soundless as the child grows older. The role of egocentric speech in learning various skills is not yet clear. However, inner speech is known to have an important function in the organization of perceptions, abstraction of common properties, and generalization of principles.

Concept Formation

Concepts are the essential links between the individual and the external world. The ability to abstract unifying principles and form articulate generalizations out of scattered impressions and unrelated perceptions is a developmental process. The competence of each person in solving problems, understanding reality, and interacting with his surroundings depends upon the level of cognitive maturity he has achieved.

In early infancy, the baby's internal and external perceptions and activities form a global, unarticulated mental image without any discernible laws or principles. As the child grows older, primitive generalizations are formed on the basis of similarities in color, shape, proximity in space, or some other concrete aspect of objects. But abstractions are highly unlikely because at this stage fundamental relationships are ignored. Later on, similarities of impressions or other functional qualities serve as the foundation for generalizations, and a new, higher level of conceptualization is attained. As the child approaches adolescence, the synthesis of abstract traits and relationships leads to the discovery of the principles of logic, which he is able to employ as the main instrument in his thinking.

Sensory data and language acquisition play an important part in the development of concepts. The maturation of the sensory modalities and central nervous system are decisive factors in the reception and organization of perceptions, while verbal definitions enable the child to analyze and synthesize his perceptual experiences. The role of formal instruction in concept formation is not fully understood. However, the child's environment and sociocultural value system may inhibit or accelerate his acquisition of certain concepts. While the development of some concepts must await the attainment of more fundamental notions, this sequential order is not strictly related to chronological age, so that children in some cultures show precocity or retardation when compared with their peers in another society. Concepts relating to social relationships and motivations are influenced by the socializing experiences of the child as well as his relatedness to people. The discovery of physical laws presupposes a certain level of brain maturation. The most complete and cohesive theory of cognitive development is Piaget's system, although not all of his empirical studies or basic assumptions have gone unchallenged.

The discovery of the laws and principles of the physical world begins with an awareness of the existence and permanence of objects. Infants at first receive and then actively seek visual stimuli emanating from various objects in the environment. By about 4 months of age, the object seen is also reached for and grasped if possible. At this stage, the infant's behavior seems to indicate either a lack of interest in or an absence of the notion of permanency, since when the object is removed from his visual field he does not search for it. As the child grows older, searching behavior is at first seen in random attempts to locate the object. Still later, searching is a well-focused and purposeful investigation of the area in which the object was previously encountered. This searching behavior is an indication that sensory data have left memory traces and that the infant has some primitive concept of space as a container of all objects (Piaget, 1937). Independent locomotion expands the child's reach, and objects are pulled, pushed, and hidden under or placed over each other, and the child accumulates further experiences with space and spatial relationships. However, while children of 3–4 years of age are able to distinguish between such topographical characteristics as under, over, inside, near, and far, it is not easy for them to differentiate their own vantage point from that of an observer standing in a different place and looking from a different direction.

Awareness of shape and visual configuration has been tested by measuring the amount of time that neonates spend looking at various designs. Infants as young as 6 months have been conditioned to respond to blocks of certain shapes. Children of 3–4 years recognize geometrical shapes even when they are in a different position, such as a diamond lying on its side. They can place blocks of different shapes in their corresponding holes. Attributes of forms such as roundness, flatness, and angularity are abstracted by school age: children can give examples of roundness, such as eggs, apples, and round tables, and describe flat and bumpy surfaces. Color is an intrinsic attribute of objects that attracts children's attention early in life. Color discrimination and matching precede correct labeling, which is commonly noted by about 4–5 years of age. Categorizing by color may remain the preferred method of grouping for some children, even though they have attained form concepts. Some investigators consider such a preference an indicator of intense emotionality and view "color reactors" as a distinct personality type. Response to color is one element in the interpretation of tests such as Rorschach inkblots, while form recognition and categorization are part of preschool intelligence tests.

Size, mass, weight, and volume are also physical attributes of objects in the child's surroundings. However, young children disregard these properties in favor of visual configurations and only slowly learn to distinguish gradual increments in size and recognize that mass remains the same when an object is broken into parts. The integration of haptic and visual perceptions is a prerequisite for learning that objects with equal mass may differ in weight. Sensory discrimination must be developed before comparisons between gradations of weight can be made. This process, like all other developmental ones, requires the maturation of the central nervous system and the accumulation of experience by interacting with the environment.

Only when the concepts of weight, length, and volume have been securely mastered can the child's verbal knowledge of measuring systems be applied to understanding and constructing aspects of physical reality. Before this cognitive development is complete, the child's use of measuring terms may not actually reflect the attainment of the concepts. Young children may learn to count by rote. But analyzing and abstracting the relationship between the ordinal positions of numbers and their cardinal value or the principles governing arithmetic require an understanding of the nature of number systems and the ability to perform logical deductions. The accurate use of verbal labels signifying time, such as *today, tomorrow,* and *yesterday,* appears during early childhood. According to some authors, this practical understanding is based on the child's own sequences of activities, which are related to the notions of morning and night. However, the concept of time as a dimension of physical reality with past, present, and an everchanging future is a cognitively advanced acquisition. Although children may learn to tell time by the clock or identify their sibs as younger or older than themselves, only when the notion of duration is grasped can the system of timekeeping and historical sequencing be comprehended.

At each stage of development, the concept of causality provides a central element in the child's view of the external world. As the infant begins to make a clear differentiation between himself and his surroundings, he must make certain assumptions regarding the forces that shape and maintain his environment. The notion that people and things around him obey different laws is alien as long as he can effect change by crying, smiling, and other actions. When the infant begins to notice the limits of his own influence on others, he assumes that all animate and inanimate objects possess a will of their own. He blames the chair for making him fall or stamps on a toy for having injured him. Later this universal animism is given up in favor of a partial and more discriminate one. During this period only moving objects are held responsible for their own motions, while nonmoving objects are considered the passive recipients of the activities of others. During the preschool years, children search for the motivations behind various occurrences. In answer to their numerous questions as to the "why" of every event, they expect to learn of a moving force or justification rather than a cause. Similarly their "because" is not a preface to a causal explanation but is usually followed by "I want to" or "he wants to." The earliest cause-and-effect relationships are based on the continuity of two phenomena in space or time: rain is caused by clouds, and fire by wood. The logical connections between occurrence and the immutable physical laws regulating the behavior of objects are understood slowly and piecemeal. The mature notion of "chance" as responsible only for "random occurrences" is not achieved before the principle of causality is fully understood.

The relationships between level of conceptualization and the child's emotional maturity and personality organization remain uncharted. While some authors, such as Bruner *et al.* (1966), believe that instruction can accelerate the rate of concept formation, others consider such attempts useless until the child has reached the state of preparedness for the attainment of various concepts. The influence of different levels of concrete or abstract notions on the behavioral pathology and symptoms exhibited by the child is not known. The mental age or intelligence quotient is viewed as a central issue only in mental retardation, even though the child's understanding of the world around him cannot help but affect his manner of relating to it.

Once concepts relating to physical reality are attained, they cannot be ignored. But awareness and understanding of concepts regarding social interactions do not guarantee that the individual will abide by them. Psychopathic individuals may be indeed well acquainted with the principles involved in social relationships, but this understanding does not impose a certain type of behavior on them.

Differences in problem-solving and thinking styles are due to the highly individual manner in which people organize the various components of their experience. Imagination, originality, and creativity can be viewed as only partly related to, or totally independent of, intelligence as measured by available tests. Children's fantasy products and artistic expressions differ in their flexibility in using materials and concepts and the inventiveness in finding new functions for objects. Although the developmental course of creativity and imagination has not been systematically studied, it is known that they are shaped and inhibited by cultural and educational factors. Highly imaginative children are usually well liked by their peers and teachers during the early school years. But as they grow older, they become the subjects of group criticism, are called wild daydreamers, and are openly ridiculed for their nonconformity (Arasteh, 1968). The contribution to normal and abnormal development of such individual differences as originality of perception, creative organization of experience, and high or low preference for novel stimuli is not known. This question is worth exploring since in some psychiatric disorders, like obsessive neurosis, inflexibility and rigidity of thinking are important components of the clinical picture, and in some highly imaginative children with disturbed emotions, bizarre and uncommon associations are made between simple items of experience and sensory data.

Socialization

The capacity to become aware of and seek contact with other people may be noted shortly after birth in human infants. The first observable indication of this interest is the visual behavior of the newborn. Evidence of eye contact is reported as early as the fourth week of postnatal existence. Fantz and Nevis (1967) believe that perceptual attraction to the human face is an unlearned and primary phenomenon in neonates. Rheingold (1966) considers visual contact as "the basis of human sociability." By about the second month of life, the early smile of the newborn appears, and although at first it is a reflexive and indiscriminate act, it soon accompanies the infant's sight of a human face, reinforcing the interactional value of the child's behavior (Emde and Harmon, 1972). Since the infant's visual contact and smile commonly elicit similar behavior from the caretakers, a reciprocal system of human interaction is established. As the baby grows older, the people who spend more time with him become more powerful stimuli for the social responses of smiling, looking, and anticipatory movements. Shortly thereafter, hearing the voice of the caretaker occasions the same joyful response from the baby, indicating a more discriminatory responsiveness. By about 6 months of age, the number of smiles directed at strangers decreases, and in some infants between 10 and 12 months, contact with strangers is avoided and their company is cause for distress.

Along with visual attention and expressions of pleasure, infants use the strategies of vocalization, clinging, and physical demonstrativeness to initiate and maintain the interactional processes with their caretakers. The reciprocal activities of the caretakers strengthen the system and provide the basis of attachment behavior on the part of the infant. Some authors—Bowlby (1969), for example—postulate an innate capacity for the development of attachment behavior, citing examples of similar behavior observed among primates to prove this hypothesis. Others are content to observe and record the course of sociability and the establishment of the attachment bond, without speculating as to whether social conventions or species-specific tendencies account for the nurturing of the young and the reinforcement of their social responsiveness. Most researchers believe that the interpersonal activities of the early years are among the most crucial elements for future cognitive and emotional development. However, whether the intensity of a single emotional bond or a variety of contacts is optimal for the development of interpersonal relationships is a matter of conjecture. The multiple mothering prevalent in some cultures has produced children who do not seem to suffer any psychological harm from the lack of one strong, exclusive attachment. But the intensity of affectional ties (symbiotic relationships) in some mother–child dyads is considered a hindrance to the individuation of the infant. What appears to be of special importance in the process of bond formation is the degree of adaptation and accommodation that both the mother and the infant are able to make to each other's style of reactivity, mode of expressiveness, and other temperamental and personality characteristics.

The ultimate goal of bond formation is to prepare the child for inclusion in the social network. The first step in this direction involves the imposition of socially acceptable patterns on the infant's biological behavior (Wolff, 1966). In most cultures, the mechanisms and methods of socialization are the outcome of the collective experiences of the group, rather than the individual temperamental and constitutional qualities of the child. The community's ideas about the most effective and desirable way of raising children are derived from its values, consensually validated information, views of human nature, and opinions. In the more diversified cultures, where a number of alternative techniques are available to the parents, the choice of child-rearing practices is influenced by factors such as the parents' social class standing, educational backgrounds, and aspirations and expectations for their child and themselves. The effectiveness of any method depends on the baby's adaptability, the compatibility of the child-rearing technique with his unique style, and the parents' pattern of reinforcement, devaluation, and/or prohibition. Studies of specific aspects of child rearing have so far failed to reveal any consistent relationships between childhood behavior, patterns of child rearing, and resultant adult personality types. It appears that the relevant, interdependent variables are simply too numerous to yield any correlation among the factors being studied.

Eating and sleeping behaviors are among the earliest targeted for regulatory intervention by the parents. Even when the infant is on a self-demand feeding schedule, the parents expect the schedule slowly to approximate the family's life cycle. Further, new foods are not introduced on the infant's demand but according to the nutritional philosophy and food supply of the community. In some cultures, the nutritional and health value of mother's milk is so highly regarded that children are encouraged to nurse even when they are capable of partaking of solid food. In areas with low food supply, mother's milk may be the sole source of infant nutrition or may supplement an inadequate diet. The daytime sleeping of newborns is at first accepted and later on merely tolerated. However, night wakefulness is disruptive and undesirable in most families. In addition, the cycle of nocturnal sleep and diurnal wakefulness is prerequisite for the maximum stimulation of the infant, increasing his opportunities to participate in the normal experiences of daily family life.

The regulation of the eliminatory functions is less urgent during the first year of postnatal life than when the baby acquires the skills of locomotion and his unregulated biological activities clash with the standards of cleanliness. At first, sphincter control training relies on the accurate timing and anticipation of the caretakers, who encourage the baby to communicate his needs. Later on, the regulation of functions is strongly demanded and even coercively imposed.

Postural control and locomotion, by all evidence, seem to be achieved without any necessary coaching, but most parents and their babies find these teaching exercises pleasurable and use them as opportunities for parent–child interaction. Fine motor coordination is extensively stressed by teaching the child such skills as dressing and undressing, using drinking and eating utensils, and other adaptive abilities.

Cultural values and safety standards require the family to set limits on the child's behavior. For example, the child's manipulation of his own body and exhibition of the genitals are discouraged in accordance with societal injunctions, while ingesting nonnutritious material, assaulting others, destroying objects, and self-injury are forbidden as safety precautions.

The definition of proper social conduct, and the encouragement and direction of interaction with other adults and children, at first begins at home with frequent visitors, relatives, and babysitters. Later on the child comes into contact with people outside of his home territory and is expected to learn to say hello and good-bye. During the first 2 to 3 years of life, a child's interaction with his own age group is minimal. Hitting, pushing, and fighting over possessions may be the only indications that the children are aware of each other's presence. Although they may watch and even imitate each other's activities, they do not play together. Even in a group, children may be observed playing alongside of each other, talking about their own activities, and engaging in parallel monologues. As the child becomes more interested in interactions with his peers, solitary games and individualistic, subjective play give way to more collective activities. An assigned role in a group game may at first be accepted at the suggestion of an adult, but later on mutual agreement with peers is necessary. At this stage, children are sensitive to each other's opinions, make comments about and criticize other children's performance and appearance, and show preference for a particular playmate. However, peer relationships during middle childhood are usually transient, even though children choose each other as partners in various games and feel justified in fighting to support their friends. When attitudes, likes, and dislikes are more crystallized, children may form small groups and exclude nonmembers from their activities. During adolescence, group membership may become particularly important; and the sense of belonging and prestige associated with popularity among members of one's own or the opposite sex are of paramount significance. At times, group formation may be based on the collective need to defy adult standards of behavior. On other occasions, the group serves as a source of psychological support and orientation during the crucial stage of transition between adolescent and adult identity and role assumption.

The ease and skill with which a child can interact with his peers and initiate and maintain friendly relationships play a significant part in his sense of adequacy and security. Anxious children, and those who find any novel situation trying, tend to avoid interactions with other youngsters and/or make prematurely exclusive relationships that are not always reciprocated by their friends. The natural shifting of companionship thus becomes a source of further insecurity and increases the child's hesitancy to initiate new friendships. Some children tend to dominate their peers, while others find the role of follower more congenial. The majority of children, however, are willing to experiment with various roles and are flexible enough to follow or dominate in the same and different relationships. Experiences within nursery school and kindergarten groups have not been shown to statistically influence the timing or the number of preferential peer relationships in children. However, early socializing opportunities, emotional responsiveness, and freedom from anxiety are necessary elements for the development of successful patterns of interaction with others.

Compared to relationships with nonrelated children, interactions with sibs present many unique aspects (Bank and Kahn, 1976). Sibs may be older or younger, and the child's expected role in relating to them varies accordingly. Brothers or sisters who are much older at times function in parental roles, nurturing, protecting, and disciplining the younger sibling. Younger sibs may be viewed as usurpers of the privileges that a child has come to call his own. Although some degree of competition and conflict is inevitable among children living in close quarters and sharing the attention and love of the same parents, parental preference for the sex, appearance, or qualities of one child may create extreme rivalry and jealousy among sibs. In some families, an unfavorable comparison with a brother or sister is used frequently to modify behavior and encourage conformity with family expectations. In other families, children are assigned various subsidiary parts in the disharmonious relationship among the adults. Such children become enmeshed in a network of conflictual relationships with each other that is not of their own making. The parents may view this situation as the normal or abnormal rivalry among the brothers and sisters. Some children's attitudes become so distorted and generalized that they cannot relate to their peers without recreating the conflictual pattern of their relationship with their siblings.

Affective Development

The distress of a newborn infant is communicated by his crying, and contentment by a calm appearance or absence of distress signals. Patterns of emotional demonstrativeness are established when the infant's smile, vocalizations, and body movements become associated with pleasurable interactions with people and reciprocal smiling, imitative vocalizations, and other expressions of pleasure are directed at the child (Brazelton *et al.*, 1974). As the child grows older, his style of affective expression is modified to approximate the age-appropriate manners determined by his culture. The subjective emotional states, on the other hand, are differentiated and organized in relation to the child's experiential opportunities, physical integrity, and cognitive capacity. While it is assumed that the child's ability for affective relationships is fostered or hampered by the kind of parenting he has experienced, this hypothesis is based on clinical impressions of disturbed children and common sense assumptions rather than on longitudinal observations and objective research.

Joy and Sadness. A child's ability to experience pleasure is dependent both on his own sense of mastery and feelings of being accepted and on the approval of his caretakers and other significant individuals (Sroufe and Wunsch, 1972). Dependence on adult approval is a powerful factor in the socialization and acculturation of the child. However, overdependence on the praise and attention of others may inhibit the establishment of a sense of self-gratification and restrain activities that, though pleasurable in themselves, do not have significance for the parents. Such children are unable to enjoy their own company, cannot amuse themselves, and are not task-oriented. While they can engage adults' attention and satisfy themselves with frequent changes of activity in early childhood, they tend to become bored and restless as they grow older and are expected to complete tasks without constant social reinforcement.

The feelings of physical and emotional distress are expressed by crying, disrupted sleep, apathy, and loss of appetite in infancy. As the child grows older and learns to speak, verbal indications of hurt feelings and sad mood accompany the nonverbal signals. The differentiation of such nuances of distress as sadness, loneliness, missing one's parents, or feeling rejected are learned through imitation, direct teaching, and the labels applied by adults to what they assume underlies the child's nonverbal signals. More cognitively sophisticated children are able to give an approximate account of their own feelings by applying the abstract terms to the circumstances of their own lives. Such introspection is only possible once the child has managed to develop a well-defined concept of himself, integrate his subjective experiences, and verbalize his feelings. The feeling of genuine sympathy appears when the child is able to understand the nature of another person's pain and distress. However, children learn the socially appropriate expressions of sympathy long before they can be expected to have any comprehension of the similarity between their own unpleasant experiences and the distress suffered by others.

Anger. Anger is a frequent reaction to frustration, which in one way or another is an inevitable part of any child's growth. As the infant grows older and the scope of his behavior widens, demands that he organize and control his self-initiated activities are intensified. The amount and intensity of frustration experienced by the child depend on the strength of his desire to continue a forbidden activity, the ease with which he learns new patterns, and the appropriateness of the environmental demands. On the other hand, the mode by which the child expresses his anger is determined by his overall capacity to cope with intense emotions, his distractibility or perseverance, and his verbal and nonverbal communicative skills (Kramer and Rosenblum, 1970). As in all other forms of behavior, parental reaction may encourage and reinforce a particular manner of expressiveness, and the child may model his expression of anger after the actions of other people in his environment. Temper tantrums, verbal or physical aggression toward others, autoaggression, destruction of objects, tearful outbursts, and withdrawal are among the prevalent expressions of frustration in childhood. Depending upon various environmental contingencies, the more primitive forms of temper tantrums may be carried over into the school years; however, under normal circumstances the frequency and intensity of tantrums diminish with age. Other forms of coping with frustrating situations are developed; the expression of anger and frustration becomes more stylized and socially acceptable. In most societies, children are expected to show their anger through verbalization and to resort to physical violence only in extreme situations. However, aggressive acts and verbal attacks against adults are usually frowned upon in all situations.

Chronic, unrelieved frustration leads to the formation of hostile attitudes. Further disappointments come to be expected and an offensive stance is adopted in most interpersonal encounters. At times, the source of the frustration lies within the child himself as, for example, in a child with a realistic or unrealistic sense of inadequacy. The child may be demoralized and withdrawn, blame others for his difficulties, exhibit extreme irritability, and have temper outbursts with very little provocation. These verbal and nonverbal expressions of anger give no more than temporary relief to the child, create more ill will and alienation toward him, and make it less likely for him to experience any conflict-free interactions. When the expression of anger leads to retaliation from the environment, fear becomes associated with anger. Even if this inhibits further expressions of aggressive feelings by the child, his discomfort is intensified. When the child begins to assume the blame for his inability to function in interpersonal situations, he becomes angry at himself. Usually quarrels and conflicts among children are short-lived, self-terminated, and easily forgotten. But for a hostile child, each fight represents another failed effort. Most children who cannot get along with others are deeply dissatisfied with themselves.

Fear and Anxiety. Infants are startled and distressed by any sudden stimulus of high intensity. However, fear as an emotional response cannot be said to exist before a child is able to perceive and interpret the environmental stimuli as threatening to his safety (Sroufe *et al.*, 1974). Learning plays an important part in the child's ability to identify and avoid danger. At first, children are expected to obey safety rules even though they are not convinced or afraid of the seriousness of the implied danger. At this stage, the child's trust in parental wisdom and care for him is the guiding principle of his life, and only occasional attempts to "find out for myself" may be expected. Some children appear fearless and engage in activities termed dangerous by their parents. This may be an indication of their profound mistrust of parental statements or lack of conviction about parental love and care. Or these youngsters may have been insufficiently warned or may not understand the scope of the danger and their own vulnerability.

Anxiety is a discomfort similar to fear that is experienced in response to ambiguous, anticipated threats to an individual's safety and security. Some authors maintain that what differentiates anxiety from fear is that fear is felt in the face of concrete, communally accepted danger signals, while anxiety is evoked by abstract symbols of individual significance associated with the person's experiential history and may be incomprehensible to others. Furthermore, while fear-inducing situations may be fled from or fought and one can expect to draw on external help in combating them, coping with anxiety is the lonely task of the individual himself, although the reassuring presence or statements of others may afford some temporary comfort. Strategies for combating anxiety are predominantly psychological in nature. Since the avoidance of anxiety-provoking situations is not always possible, nor are these circumstances always identifiable in advance, the individual engages in various mental maneuvers either to insulate himself against anxiety or to cope with it when it is aroused. The intensity of the anxiety, the extent of anxiety-provoking situations, and the success or failure of psychological defenses are important factors in an individual's freedom from discomfort and unpleasant feelings. Some children are chronically anxious, because of either their experiential background or their failure to develop coping strategies. Other children manage to deal with their anxieties by employing defenses that are maladaptive in other ways. For the majority of children, however, the experience of anxiety is infrequent and easily manageable. Although the manifestations and consequences of anxiety occupy a central position in modern psychiatric theories, its genesis, development, and relation to various environmental variables are only vaguely understood. While philosophical and psychological theorizing abounds, naturalistic studies and etiological research comprise a very small portion of the literature on anxiety.

Identity

The adoption of the values, attitudes, personality traits, or behavior of a valued model is called *identification*. Although learning by imitation plays a part in this process, it is the child's perception of the model's behavior and his understanding of the forces that motivate his actions that form the core of his identification. Parents are naturally the first models that a child encounters. However, the youngster's perception of parental behavior may be quite different from the one that parents intend or hope to convey. Furthermore, the affective quality of the parent–child relationship, the child's level of cognitive sophistication, and the child's view of himself are interrelating factors that decide the nature and degree of his identification with his parents. A child may find only some aspects of his parents' personalities congruent with his perception of himself or his temperamental qualities, and thus he may reject parts of a favored parent's attitudes. Or, conversely, he may incorporate some of the basic values of a less liked, or even despised, parent into his own personality structure. The process of identification, and the more complicated restructuring of the self-image, continues throughout the formative years and is not limited to parental models. Congruous elements of various people—teachers, acquaintances, family members, and public personalities of the past or present—are continuously incorporated into the self-concept. However, the adoption of a particular set of values, and the resultant personality transformation at each stage, increasingly excludes the acceptance of other attitudes, gradually limiting the types of potential models available for identification.

Sexual identity is the outcome of a complex interplay among biological, psychological, interpersonal, and social forces. The absence of the same-sex parent may delay the imitative learning of the culturally designated feminine or masculine behavior, but it does not, in itself, create confusion as to gender identity or disturb sexual orientation.

Moral Development

The process of moral development involves learning and internalizing a set of culturally determined prohibitions and obligations that, for the most part, purport to regulate the individual's relationships with his fellow men and women. Truthfulness, honesty, refraining from taking other people's property, and sharing with a selected group are among the earliest moral dicta imposed by parents on the young child. The consistency with which the parents enforce a moral dictum, the quality of their relationship with the child, and the degree to which their own behavior exemplifies their moral stance are factors that influence the development of a sense of morality in the child. Furthermore, at each stage of development, the child's cognitive level, his ability to make generalizations, and his understanding of the nuances involved in the exercise of moral judgments are significant components of his behavior. For example, a child who has accepted in principle that he should not take toys or money belonging to other children may nevertheless consider his own family and objects within the home exempt from such rules. Thus hiding a sibling's favorite toy or taking money from his mother's purse is not viewed as stealing, though the parental reaction that follows may be as strong as or stronger than when the forbidden behavior occurs outside the home.

Situational factors play an important role in the ability of young children to resist temptation and obey rules. Some youngsters are unwilling to take the risk of being detected by adults; others find the courage to do so when in the company of peers who engage in prohibited activities. At times, the parents misperceive or misunderstand the child's behavior, which confuses him and hinders his moral development. For example, when a child is unable to adhere to reality and gives a mixed account of his own fantasies and what actually happened, he may be accused of lying and may be reprimanded without having a clear idea as to what he did to displease his parents. Some adults react to a child's protective lying so vehemently that the child becomes even more frightened and less capable of acknowledging his misdeeds.

As the child grows older, his concept of right and wrong becomes more abstract; self-criticism and guilt, rather than fear of detection and punishment, are the deterrent mechanisms that regulate his behavior. The avoidance of the internal distress engendered by guilt provides the basis of self-control and the impetus for acting according to moral principles. Parallel to this development, the child's concept of morality undergoes changes from the rigid absolutism of the early years to a more realistic stance in which not only actions but intentions are taken into consideration (Kohlberg and Turiel, 1971). Even violations of moral dicta that are not detected and punished are considered wrong. Repentance or restitution becomes an acceptable price to pay for the infractions of moral principles (Piaget, 1932).

While a child's verbal knowledge of moral principles may reflect his general fund of information, the degree to which his behavior corresponds to the moral dicta is the outcome of his emotional maturity, experiential background, and view of himself and others. A child cannot be morally accountable for his behavior unless he is free from such distressful feelings as anxiety, hostility, and depression. An anxious child may lie indiscriminately because he is unable to tolerate any disapproval, whether real or fancied. A lonely youngster may steal in order to become a member of a group or to buy friendship. A hostile child expects to be rejected and frustrated; his world view does not afford him the luxury of benevolence and sympathy toward others. Another hindrance to moral development is parents who vehemently espouse certain mores that they fail to follow, leaving their disillusioned children with the task of reconciling the basic contradiction.

3

Theories of Child Development

Theories of child development and personality formation have their roots in the shared beliefs of Western man—those tacit assumptions and simple explanations of human behavior that are as old as recorded history. The systematic attempt to build, and scientifically verify, sets of explanatory hypotheses is, however, less than a century old. The formulation of the principles of what Heider (1958) called naive psychology and their critical examination and elaboration have given rise to various schools of psychology. Even a cursory glance at the history of any science reveals that with the passage of time and long struggle, untidy hypotheses are replaced by more rigorously scientific ones, and initially vague concepts and definitions are sharpened and clarified. In psychology, scientific formulations and concepts are still in the developing stage, so that no single theory has managed to make the rival theories obsolete.

The body of knowledge that comprises our present understanding of personality development is not yet so scientifically coherent that a unified presentation of tenets and principles can be made. The following discussion is therefore divided into a consideration of three schools in psychology—namely, psychoanalytic theory, the developmental theory of Jean Piaget, and learning theory. The presentation is not exhaustive, nor does it provide an exposition of all the significant developments within each theory. The theories were selected for this chapter because they are currently the most influential hypothetical frameworks within which new formulations and observations of child development are continuously being made.

Psychoanalytic Theory

Sigmund Freud's psychoanalytic theory has its roots in his training in neurology and his clinical experiences with hysteric patients.
However, his postulates are not strictly based on the observation and
collection of raw clinical data but rather employ such diversified
sources as introspection, dreams, slips of the tongue, literary myths,
and free associations by psychoanalytic patients. Freud's models of
mental functioning and motivational principles were constructed over
several decades, and he showed little interest in integrating his earlier
propositions with his later hypotheses. Consequently, the Freudian
legacy to psychology includes several sets of postulates, some of which
are contradictory in their implications.

Freud did not set out to construct a theory of child development,
but theoretical assumptions about child development have emerged
from the successive reformulation and expansion of his basic concepts.
It must be noted that because Freud was more interested in the nature
of motivational forces behind behavioral phenomena, his theory for the
most part ignores such issues in developmental psychology as the
mechanisms involved in learning, cognitive growth, and language acquisition (Baldwin, 1968).

The central concepts of psychoanalytic theory can be described as
follows: all behavior, thoughts, feelings, acts, dreams, and fantasies—
whether normal or pathological, rational or accidental—are motivated
and meaningful, even though the motivation may be obscure and the
meaning not easily discerned. The ultimate motivating forces in all behavioral phenomena are the instinctual drives. Because the immediate
and direct gratification of these drives is incompatible with the social
existence of man, the individual must develop indirect means and
compromises to adapt to external reality and find acceptable ways of
gratification. Conflict is therefore the inevitable component of the intrapsychic life of the individual.

The most important instinctual drive in psychoanalytic theory is
sexuality (libido). Aggression is postulated as another basic instinct,
but it has not received the elaboration or the status of the libido. Sexuality is conceived as rooted in biology, but the biological substrate for
aggression is not identified. The existence of drives relating to self-
preservation (ego instincts) is also acknowledged. But Freud did not
view such drives as hunger or thirst as playing a dynamic role in personality formulation (S. Freud, 1923/1961). Instinctual drives are viewed
as possessing energy. Although nonquantifiable, this energy is like
an electrical charge that propels every aspect of behavior (S. Freud,
1940/1964). The intervening mechanism between the instinctual

drives and psychological functioning is called *cathexis*. Cathexis is the investment of emotional significance in an activity, object, or idea. The instinctual drives cathect an idea or object in the external world into the individual's consciousness and thus provide the motivation for behavior.

Freud's Topographic System

The topographic system is the earliest of the several theoretical models of psychoanalysis. The set of propositions regarding this system was first presented in 1900 in *The Interpretation of Dreams*. However, the data derived from Freud's experience with hypnotized hysterics and study of accidental phenomena such as slips of the tongue, as well as dream material, were incorporated into his formulations.

Freud divided the mind into three distinct compartments: the unconscious, the preconscious, and the conscious systems. The unconscious system is said to include all those psychological processes that are unavailable to consciousness, while the preconscious sytem contains mental activities that, although momentarily out of awareness, can become conscious when the individual's attention is focused on them. Freud believed that an active censoring agent is responsible for keeping the unconscious material from gaining entrance into the preconscious and conscious systems. However, when the censor is weakened, such as during sleep, the mental activities and energy of the unconscious system strive for expression and discharge. These mental activities are presented as dream imageries. Freud further postulated that the mode of mental functioning in the unconscious (primary process) is different from conscious mentation (secondary process thinking).

Primary process thinking and the unconscious system are ontogenetically the earliest and most primitive part of the mental apparatus. This type of mental process is said to operate on the pleasure principle, that is, to discharge psychological energy by the most direct, immediate route without concern for the demands of reality. This mode of thinking is not bound by the laws of logic and makes no distinction between past and present. The memory traces of this stage are for the most part nonverbal, and images are superimposed, condensed, and distorted by each other. The memory traces of this era, representing infantile wishes and libidinal gratifications, continue to form a part of the mental functioning and dynamic force behind adult behavior, even though they have their origin in childhood.

As the infant grows older, he is faced with the demands and prohibitions of reality. Immediate instinctual gratification becomes impossible. The preconscious, censoring system begins to control the unconscious, and a different mode of mental functioning develops. With the acquisition of language, memory traces are transformed into verbal forms. Words are now cathected with mental energy. Thinking and problem solving are in line with the reality principle. And secondary process thinking gains ascendancy over the more primitive primary process functioning. The task of the conscious mind is to control the individual's activities and scrutinize subjective experience and objective reality. The rational, goal-directed behavior of the conscious mind may be interrupted or distorted if the preconscious fails to repress the unconscious forces. Neurotic symptoms and slips of the tongue signal the enfeeblement or malfunctioning of the censoring agent.

Freud's Structural Theory

Freud's elaboration of his early thinking on neurotic symptoms and pathological anxiety, as well as his dissatisfaction with the explanatory usefulness of the topographic model, resulted in a new set of propositions. His formulations of the structural model were published in 1923 in *The Ego and the Id*. In this model, the mind is still divided into three components, but these are based on function rather than on the degree of accessibility to consciousness. Consciousness and unconsciousness were now viewed as qualitative terms that describe certain aspects of mental activities (Arlow and Brenner, 1964).

The Id. The id is the innate psychic structure containing mental representatives of the instinctual drives. The psychological energy of the two instincts—that is, aggression and the libido—is of a highly mobile nature and strives for prompt discharge and gratification. Reality is totally ignored, and wishing is the only form of mentation. The pleasure principle is the reigning axiom of the internal life.

The Ego. As the infant grows older, the maturing perceptual and motor functions bring in increased sensory stimuli and knowledge of the limits of reality. The part of the mind that represents these increased functions begins to differentiate itself from the id and forms the nucleus of a second structure: the ego. The task of the ego is to control the instinctual desires of the id. It neutralizes them by binding and channeling the instinctual energy into more acceptable avenues of discharge. At times, the instinctual drives are simply repressed by the ego, but more often the ego attempts to find compromises and solutions that allow for the discharge of mental energy within the possibilities and opportunities provided by external reality. Maturational factors, language acquisition, and learning by imitation and identification play significant roles in the development of the ego. Furthermore, anxiety begins to occupy an important role in compelling the ego into action. According to Freud's later formulation, anxiety is aroused whenever the instinctual drives threaten to overwhelm the ego, seeking immediate discharge. The ensuing conflict between the two agencies of the mind—the ego and the id—motivates the ego to shore up its defenses and to tighten its control over the id. Because such situations are a frequent accompaniment of every child's normal growth, the ego has ample opportunity to expand structurally and grow stronger. The individual's character traits, mode of functioning, and successful or unsuccessful defenses against anxiety are the result of conflicts between the ego and the id. Failed defensive maneuvers and strategies of the ego are manifested in neurotic symptoms.

The Superego. The superego is a specialized part of the ego that contains the cultural and moral aspirations and prohibitions that regulate the individual's life. According to Freud, the superego is developed as the result of the child's identification with the parental authority. At times, the superego may be in direct conflict with the ego and thus form an alliance with the id. More frequently, however, the superego approves and strengthens the ego's attempts to find socially acceptable manners of discharging the instinctual drives. Disharmonious relationships between the ego and the superego give rise to feelings of guilt and remorse, and the individual may be moved to make restitution or punish himself.

Every behavior is the final outcome of the interactions between the three structures of the mind and thus multiply determined. This is called *overdeterminism.*

Freud's Genetic Theory

Freud's theory of psychosexual development complements and parallels his structural model of personality formation. The structural theory is a description of the cognitive development and adaptational efforts of the growing child, while the stages of psychosexual transformation reflect the impact of social experiences on the direction and the object of instinctual drives. The neonate's primary source of pleasure and gratification is his mouth, which according to Freudian terminology is an "erotogenic zone." Freud thus called the first period of psychosexual development the "oral stage."

The Oral Stage. Although Freud acknowledged that feeding and sucking activities are necessary for the survival and self-preservation of the infant, he pointed out that infants engage in nonnutritive suckings, such as sucking their own hands or mouthing various objects.

Because such activities have a calming effect on the restless infant, he assumed that the activity is pleasurable in itself and "for that reason may and should be termed sexual" (S. Freud, 1940/1964). Manifestations of the destructive instinct during this phase are noticed when the infant begins to teethe and finds pleasure in biting the breast or other objects. During the oral phase, the infant is in a passive–dependent position and, for the most part, unaware of the differences between his own wishes and environmental reality. His mental energy is cathected in himself and his own body, and his aim is to incorporate the objects of his desires. Accordingly, Freudian theory postulates a stage of "primary narcissism" as the central characteristic of this phase. Behaviors and character traits of later years that, on a more abstract level, can be designated as dependent and self-centered are said to originate from the oral stage.

The Anal Phase. During the second phase of sexual development, the anal area becomes the prominent erotogenic zone, and activities associated with elimination become the focus of the child's attention and mental energy. Freud considered this shift to be maturational in origin, although parental attitudes toward toilet training, their demands for regularity of function, and the prohibitions surrounding such activities are also important contributing factors. Experiences during this period may lead to such character traits as preoccupation with cleanliness, equation of the possession of impersonal objects with love and security, and a tendency to receive sexual pleasure from the anal region.

The Phallic Phase. The child's curiosity and attempts to obtain sexual pleasure gradually shift from the anal zone to the genital area. Anatomical differences between the two sexes are discovered. Boys find sexual pleasure from manipulating their penises, while girls are interested in examining and experimenting with their own external genitals. Furthermore, because of the importance placed on the penis by the male child and his parents, boys become extremely concerned about threats of harm and castration, while girls find the absence of a penis a source of sadness and become envious of the male genitals.

The relationships between children and their parents undergo significant changes at this stage. Boys become enamored of their mothers and jealous of their fathers, while girls develop a desire to possess their fathers and view their mothers as rivals. Realistic limitations, fear of retaliation by the same-sex parent, and defensive maneuvers by the ego result in the child's denunciation of his or her sexual desire for the opposite-sex parent, and thus the oedipal complex is resolved. The child now tries to identify with the same-sex parent and receives instinctual gratification from such identification. Fixation on this stage and unresolved feelings toward the opposite-sex parent, as well as fears and anxieties regarding castration, result in future strains in interpersonal relationships and choice of a sexual partner and in the development of neurotic symptomatology.

The development of the superego coincides with the phallic phase and is to a large extent dependent upon the child's identification with the same-sex parent and his denunciation of the oedipal aim. Failure to resolve the oedipal complex may be reflected in a superego that is harshly punitive or underdeveloped.

The Latency Period. Freud believed that following the turmoil of the phallic phase, the child's mental energy becomes oriented toward the mastery of the adaptational tasks required by the culture. A stable truce is established between instinctual wishes, the ego, and the superego. Sexuality becomes dormant, and sublimation manages to dispose of the ever-present desire for instinctual gratification. This is the period that corresponds to the child's entrance to school and the expansion of his social horizons beyond his family.

Adolescence. Between 12 and 14 years of age, there is a reawakening of sexual interest and a reliving of the genital period because of the biological changes of puberty. However, during adolescence, the individual begins to choose sexual partners among his or her peers, and the intense relationship between parents and children gives way to other interpersonal activities and the preparation for future adult roles.

Freudian theory considers the child–parent relationship as the prototype of all significant relationships in adult life. The experiences of each stage of psychosexual development are considered important determinants of future personality traits, behavioral styles, and particular manifestations of psychopathology. Because each developmental stage is viewed as structurally more advanced than the earlier ones, it is postulated that adaptational failure at each stage reactivates previous modes of adjustment. Regression to earlier phases of development is used as an explanatory concept in the causation of various maladaptive and deviant behavior.

Freudian theory has been criticized on various accounts. The emphasis on thoughts and feelings and the lack of operational definitions present great obstacles in devising independent research designs and methodology to assess the basic assumptions and concepts of the theory. The psychoanalytic method of data collection is regarded as unsatisfactory since the nature of the data is influenced by the method and both, in turn, are dependent upon Freudian hypotheses (Baldwin, 1968). The relationships between certain character traits and early life experiences have not been proved by longitudinal studies, and cross-cultural researchers have cast doubts upon some aspects of childhood experiences that Freud had termed universal.

Ego Psychology

The concept of the ego as a separate structure of personality has received a great deal of attention and elaboration since Freud's original formulation. Hypotheses and investigations regarding the functional properties of the ego have become so numerous that a group of psychoanalysts have come to be known as *ego psychologists*. Hartmann (1939) defined ego psychology as the meeting ground between psychoanalytic theory and nonanalytic psychology because it has focused on those issues of psychological import that received scanty attention from Freud and his earlier followers.

The theory of ego psychology received special impetus from the work of those psychoanalysts who engaged in direct work with children. Anna Freud (1946b), in her book *The Psycho-Analytic Treatment of Children*, emphasized the importance of psychoanalytic formulations that result from observing children during their developmental stages, as compared to those hypotheses that were the outcome of reconstructing the childhood memories of adults. Her assertion that the observation of surface behavior complements the understanding derived from depth analysis and that the conscious part of the ego and of the superego are legitimate areas of study strengthened the new movement in psychoanalysis (A. Freud, 1965).

According to proponents of this school, some basic properties of the ego, such as sensory perception, motility, and memory, are parts of the individual's innate endowment. These functions develop along a given maturational line independent of the outcome of conflicts between the instinctual drives and demands of reality. However, since the ego is the main agent of adaptation, its functional properties, such as language, cognition, and motor activities, are all involved in mediating efforts between the id and the external world. In pathological states, all or some of these functions may be impaired.

Ego psychologists accept the two instinctual drives proposed by Freud and believe that aggressive energy, like the libido, may become neutralized, bound, or sublimated in the service of adaptation or may be displaced on the individual himself. While in the early stages of psychosexual development the same activities that discharge sexual drive also dispose of aggressive energy, later on a variety of nonspecific activities such as biting, kicking, muscle movement, teasing, and cursing provide outlets for aggression. The libido can act as an inhibiting factor on the aggressive drive; or, in simpler terms, the fact that the mother is loved by her child makes her an unlikely target for the youngster's hostility (Kris, 1950).

Ego psychologists agree with Freud's claim that his theoretical assumptions are universal. However, the explanation for this is no longer based on biological or phylogenetic factors. Instead, Hartmann (1939) suggested that "the average expectable environment . . . and the average expectable internal conflicts" can account for the universality of experiences. For example, while Freud postulated that the intensity of the unrealistic fear of castration could be explained only as originating from memory traces of the human race, Hartmann considered the castration anxiety to be a response to all forms of real or imagined threats of adult aggression that every child is bound to experience.

The average expectable environment, which includes the sociocultural milieu created by man, is viewed as basically supportive to the child in that it provides both necessities for his survival and opportunities for his instinctual gratification. This is in contrast with Freud's contention that civilization is a source of frustration and discontent and adaptation to reality an unpleasant necessity. Although the sequence of stages of psychosexual development remain acceptable to ego psychologists, the role played by environmental factors in the outcome of each phase is particularly emphasized. While a systematic list of functions attributed to the ego has not been compiled and clear operational definitions of some concepts are lacking, certain functions are frequently mentioned in the literature as ascribable to the ego. The most significant among them are sensory perception, affective expression, thinking, memory, language, consciousness, reality testing, control of motor activities, the binding of and mastery over instinctual drives, the sense of identity, and, finally, the capacity to regress to a more primitive level of functioning in order to maintain the psychological integrity of the individual.

The developmental disturbances of the ego are viewed as either caused by congenital or acquired organic deficits or due to distorting experiential history. Two functions that have received special attention are the development of a sense of identity and the binding of instinctual drives through various defense mechanisms. Other functions, such as cognition, perception, locomotion, and learning, are considered autonomous apparatuses that develop within the "conflict free sphere" of the ego, and their exercise is a source of pleasure independent of the discharge of the instinctual tension.

Separation and individuation, or the process by which a sense of self is established, are the core of psychological development. At birth, the neonate lacks any concept of external reality, and his awareness of himself is limited to the sensations emanating from his own body. The restlessness and tension arising from hunger and the tranquility resulting from being fed are all experienced as coming from the same source. With the unavoidable delays in gratification and the impossibility of total indulgence, a dim awareness of external forces is gradually developed. During this phase, which covers the first six months of life, the infant does not differentiate between various caretakers and is totally dependent on his mother—a symbiotic relationship (Mahler, 1967). As the baby grows older, his ability to discriminate among sensory stimuli is enhanced, and the memory traces of previous experiences are accumulated, so that by the second half of the first year the primary caretaker is no longer interchangeable with substitutes. An attachment to the mother is formed and disruptions are now occasions for anxiety and distress. The child is actively engaged in reciprocal interaction with his mother and through her can relate and experiment with other aspects of his environment. The boundary between the self and others is gradually demarcated, and through the dual process of maturation and experience the child becomes aware of his own uniqueness. For example, when the child becomes capable of independent locomotion, he becomes aware of his own ability to leave and return to his mother. The process of individuation may be hampered or distorted by such factors as maternal deprivation, disruption of the attachment bond, or maternal overprotection and overindulgence. The consequences of such deviations may be manifested in various pathological stages, ranging from "symbiotic psychosis" to "affectionless personality" (Bowlby, 1946).

As a result of her work with children, Anna Freud has expanded her father's original concept of psychological defenses and has described 10 different mechanisms by which the ego attempts to control, neutralize, and channel the energy of instinctual drives (A. Freud, 1946). Although some defensive structures are said to be more primitive and to developmentally precede others, no chronological sequence is postulated. Repression marks the beginning of demarcation between the id and the ego and is the simplest form of resistance against instinctual drives, while sublimation and intellectualization require a more advanced level of cognitive growth. Identification is responsible for the acculturation of the child and the formation of the superego.

Although every individual has the capacity to use a variety of defenses to maintain a balance between internal conflicts and external demands, the success or failure of adaptation and the psychological health or pathology are marked by the predominance of certain defensive strategies. During the childhood years and crises of adult life, regression to a lower level of functioning may be employed in order to allow the ego to consolidate its resources and to prepare for a higher stage of integration or reintegration. Such regression is a normal feature of childhood development, while in adults it may serve such varied functions as receptivity to an aesthetic experience or the reestablishment of a sense of psychological integrity following the appearance of psychosis.

Longitudinal studies initiated under the impetus of ego psychology have yielded a great quantity of observational data regarding normal development. Hartmann considered such information to be superior to that collected by phenomenologists, in that data gathered by the ego psychologists are explanatory while other infant observations are merely descriptive. However, the explanatory quality of the theory is inextricably related to Freud's basic assumptions, and neither the analysis of children nor the longitudinal studies have provided independent empirical evidence for those theoretical formulations.

Erickson's Theory of Psychosocial Development

Erik Erikson's introduction to psychoanalysis was under the tutelage of Anna Freud. His theoretical assumptions are different from ego psychology only to the extent that he has attempted to incorporate a social dimension into the core of psychoanalytic formulations.

Erikson contends that man's life cycle and his social institutions have evolved together and that each stage of human development is influenced and directed by some basic elements in society. Psychological states, normal or pathological, are dependent upon the individual's relation to society as much as they are caused by conflicts among the structures of the mind. A sense of societal meaning and belongingness is necessary for adaptation and inner security throughout the individual's life. In each successive stage of development, the ratio between the positive and negative social interactions determines the psychological health of the person and his future adaptation (Erikson, 1963).

The interactions between the individual and the environment have three aspects: first, the ways of experiencing that are accessible to the individual's consciousness and that affect his view of himself and his life; second, the modes of behaving that are observable by others and determine the nature of the feedback that a person receives; and, third, the individual's inner dynamic state, which is unconscious, plays a significant motivational role, and can be revealed through psychoanalysis.

As the individual develops, he faces major turning points in his life that necessitate changes in his patterns of social interactions. Erikson views these turning points as crisis situations that are common to all men in all cultures. He has listed a succession of eight major adaptational steps from infancy to old age. The sequence of these stages is predetermined: biologically and psychologically the individual is ready to move on to a new level of interaction with his human environment. At the same time, society and culture are so constituted that they encourage and support the unfolding of these potentialities.

Because Erikson accepts the Freudian outline of instinctual transformation and the genetic stages of psychosexual development, he defines the sequence of psychosocial steps as epigenetic. However, only the first five stages on Erikson's epigenetic chart have their corresponding phases in Freudian theory. The last three stages of adult life are elaborations that transcend the original psychoanalytic system. Although the impact of the parents' attitudes during their own various phases of adaptation is not specifically described, it is clear that the effects of the interactional processes on the child's personality are dependent upon the interplay between parental influences and child behavior.

Basic Trust versus Mistrust. This stage corresponds to the oral phase of psychoanalytic theory. In the infant's state of total dependency and receptivity, parental consistency and acceptance of the baby's biological needs and functions are the factors that determine the degree of self-acceptance and social trust the infant develops. He may come to view himself or parts of himself as essentially bad, or he may consider his environment as unworthy of trust, malevolent, and noncaring. Such attitudes may receive further reinforcement in future interactions with others or may be corrected through other experiences. Examples of deep-seated social mistrust are found in schizophrenia of childhood and schizoid and depressive states in adults. However, it must be noted that patterns of trust or mistrust are not achievements that can be secured once and for all. Rather, they must be reestablished and renewed within the new crises and conflicts of every developmental stage.

Autonomy versus Shame and Doubt. In the anal phase, maturation and independent locomotion allow the child to experiment with different modes of interaction with his environment. He can now explore beyond the reach of his previous surroundings and exercise some degree of control over his own biological functions. Environmental reactions to this level of interaction may be supportive and encouraging of the child's autonomy, or they may stimulate a sense of shame and doubt. Excessive doubt and shame may paralyze the child and block his future exercise of free choice. When unmodified, such attitudes find expression in paranoic fears during the adult years.

The absence or loss of social trust may aggravate the failings of this stage; a previous sense of mistrust may, in turn, be solidified by personal doubts and social shame.

Initiative versus Guilt. The child's cognitive growth during the genital phase enables him to initiate, contemplate, and express his aspirations for new roles within his family. The limit-setting function of the family is, however, calculated to control and repress the unacceptable aspects of such behavior. As long as such control measures are protective and supportive, the child can maintain a feeling of self-esteem and a continued desire for initiating interactions with others. However, prohibitions and injunctions may be so excessive and indiscriminate that they create a sense of guilt, inhibiting the child's desire for independence and initiative. He may come to fear future responsibilities and commitments, and he may develop such pathological symptoms as hysterical paralysis or psychosomatic illnesses in order to avoid the guilt associated with the acknowledgment and assertion of his wishes.

Industry versus Inferiority. In every society, a child is expected gradually to prepare to assume a productive role and carve out a place for himself within the ranks of adults. Even in primitive communities where school as a separate institution does not exist, the fundamental technology of the culture must be transmitted to the young. By about 6–7 years of age, at the start of the latency period, the child's attention and his mental energy are focused on the task of learning; his major role is that of an apprentice. A child who can master the task of learning begins to develop a feeling of his own adequacy and ability, while a youngster who fails in this undertaking is left with a sense of incompetence and inferiority. Such failures, whether caused by the child's constitutional and experiential deficiencies or created by social prejudices and hindrance, have long-ranging consequences for the individual's future. Inability to achieve social competence as a potential productive member of the community colors the child's view of himself and deprives him of an important source of satisfaction and confidence.

Identity versus Role Confusion. According to Erikson, the biological changes and shifts in social expectations that occur during puberty produce a sense of discontinuity and bewilderment in the adolescent. Earlier doubts and uncertainties reemerge, conflicts reawaken, and the importance and relevance of old skills are questioned. Occupational prototypes are considered and rejected; moral obligations, social ideology, and relationships between the generations are reexamined. The established order is found wanting and defiance and rebelliousness justified, even though the need for a sense of belonging and group support may dictate blind adherence to certain codes of behavior sponsored by one's peers.

This crisis in identity is usually resolved successfully, a new level of integration and continuity is achieved, and the useful experiences of the past are incorporated into the new structure of the ego. The danger emanating from this stage is the failure of integration, with resultant diffusion of social and sexual roles and assumption of maladaptive patterns such as delinquency. Doubts about sexual identity may be reflected in disturbed relationships with peers of the same or the opposite sex, while a sense of social inferiority and inadequacy may block the adolescent's entrance into productive adult society.

Intimacy versus Isolation. The successful mastery of the tasks of the previous stage allows the youth to make personal and occupational commitments, to become a partner in intimate relationships, and to be prepared to make the necessary sacrifices and compromises involved in these affiliations. Conversely, role confusion and failure in reintegration leaves the individual with a sense of alienation from his community, and his fears of commitment reinforce his self-imposed isolation.

Generativity versus Stagnation. Erikson considers the need to be needed as the hallmark of emotional maturity and a desire for creativity and productivity as an important aspect of psychosocial development. Most mature adults also express their faith in the worth and future of the species by their willingness to procreate and provide for children. Failure in this stage results in a sense of futility and stagnation within a limited and impoverished psychological horizon.

Ego Integrity versus Despair. A life well lived provides the individual with a sense of inner peace and a conviction of his own personal significance, while a series of unsuccessful adaptations and unfinished tasks culminate in feelings of despair during old age. When the past is a continuous source of regret and the future holds no opportunities for compensation, the present becomes devoid of hope and meaning.

Erikson's theoretical formulations are based on his psychotherapeutic work with individual cases and his sociological and anthropological investigations. The lack of operational definitions and problems with designing appropriate methodology have prevented the application of his concepts in longitudinal studies of child development. Erikson is specifically against the construction of various scales to test the significant attitudinal changes of each development stage, arguing that his concepts are a dynamic process between opposing forces rather than static traits and functions established with age (Erikson, 1963).

PIAGET'S THEORY OF DEVELOPMENTAL PSYCHOLOGY

Jean Piaget's investigations into developmental psychology are the result of his lifelong interest in epistemology, specifically in genetic epistemology. The relation between knower and known and the mechanism by which man comes to construct an accurate image of the physical world are the subject matter of epistemology. According to Piaget, genetic epistemology can be defined as "the study of mechanisms whereby bodies of knowledge grow." The investigation of cognitive development is only one of the several methods by which Piaget has attempted to map the historical–developmental course of the acquisition and growth of knowledge. The theory of cognitive development, in turn, played an important part in Piaget's epistemological thinking. Applying the principles of developmental psychology, Piaget drew parallels between the evolutionary changes of scientific concepts in physics and the acquisition of concepts in the mind of a growing child. He demonstrated that the historical course of scientific evolution in various fields began with the observer's comprehension of the superficial characteristics of different phenomena and progressed to the state of delineation of the more complex relationships and principles underlying those characteristics. Piaget's concern with the growth of knowledge made the study of cognitive development the central issue of his psychological investigation.

In his attempt to explain cognitive development, Piaget rejects the assumptions of behavioral theorists and associationists, who, according to him, view the infant as a passive, though receptive, organism who builds a notion about external reality through successive environmental contacts and cumulative experiences. He is equally critical of those theorists who postulate an innate intellectual faculty that unfolds with age. For Piaget, intelligence is the outcome of active organismic adaptation to the external world. It can be viewed as originating within a biological substrate and evolving, through successive stages, from the interactions between the functional characteristics of the infant and the invariant properties of the environment.

Although the biological structures of the central nervous system and the sensory organs limit and condition the nature of the stimuli that we can perceive directly, cognition eventually transcends such limitations. For example, wave lengths that cannot be seen are conceptualized and known by their other properties. According to Piaget's theory, the biological endowment consists not only of the inborn neurophysiological structures but also of the mode of intellectual functioning or the manner in which transactions with the environment take place. Thus intellectual functioning is a special case of organismic adaptation to the external world. The process through which such adaptation is achieved can be conceptualized as analogous to other kinds of biological quests for adaptation and equilibrium. In fact, Piaget's terms are transposed from biology into psychology. The functional properties of intellectual activities are called assimilative and accommodative behavior, while the range of comprehensible stimuli at each stage is referred to as "aliments," or intellectual nourishment (Piaget, 1963). Stated differently, intelligence is a form of organization that structures the universe the same way that any biological organism structures its immediate environment. Adaptation is a transformation of the organism by the environment that results in an increased interchange between the two and thus preserves and perpetuates the organism.

Piaget further postulates the existence of a drive or motivational force for the cognitive structures to perpetuate themselves and integrate and organize more and more complex stimuli into their functional domain, so that even though at a particular period the child's behavior may be sufficiently adaptive to ensure his smooth transactions with the environment, his intrinsic need for the expansion of his cognitive horizons propels him to attempt to grasp and comprehend more about nature. The ultimate goal of intellectual activities is the discovery and construction of reality and the attainment not only of concepts of abstract relationships between properties of objects but also of the logical connections between concepts themselves. Piaget believes that man's concept of reality is obtained by successive approximations, beginning with the infant's early exercise of his innate reflexive behavior and continuing throughout the formative years of childhood. Every stage of cognitive functioning is thus more complex than the preceding one and less comprehensive than the one that follows. Changes are qualitative in that not only is the amount of experiential data greater, but these data are organized in a more complex manner. Generalizations and differentiations are of a higher order and closer to the actual properties of objects, and the knowledge of the interaction between the individual and reality is more accurate (Piaget, 1954).

The continuous, balanced coordination between the two processes of assimilation and accommodation is called "equilibration" by Piaget. In each stage of development, the cognitive system is in a state of equilibrium—that is to say, there is a hypothetical balance between the changes taking place within the subject and the qualities of the physical world assimilated by him. However, this equilibrium is an unstable one; further interaction between the child and his environment calls for the incorporation of newer data, more complex organization, and fresh accommodative efforts until such time as the child's concept corresponds with the knowable qualities of the objective world. For example, the infant at first behaves as if objects have ceased to exist when they are removed from his visual field. This level of comprehension represents a fragile state of equilibrium that is not sustained by further interchange with the environment. However, once the concept of object permanence is grasped, this understanding remains unshakable. From this point onward, the permanency of objects is a cornerstone of the cognitive edifice. The how and why of the equilibration process has not been fully explained by the Piagetian theory.

A distinguishing feature of Piaget's theory is his emphasis on action as the raw material out of which cognition is generated. One direct implication of this view is the belief that infants' sensorimotor activities are the beginning of attempts at actively seeking and organizing environmental stimuli and modifying and creating new cognitive structures (Flavell, 1963). The notion allows Piaget to conceptualize the innate motor and sensory reflexes as important early building blocks of cognitive development and to define the cognitive structure as "a class of similar action sequence" or schema. As the infant grows older, he is said to internalize his actions or sequences of activities, forming a mental image that, in combination with symbolic schemata, will give rise to conceptual thinking.

Another implication of the concept of intelligence as action concerns educational practices; according to Piaget, in order to teach a child general principles, he should first be encouraged to manipulate objects, discover the principles at work as the result of his own actions, and abstract and internalize his own activities. It must be noted that for Piaget learning about concepts and properties, whether by trial and error or through instruction, cannot account for cognitive development. Rather it is the stage of intellectual growth and the nature of available cognitive structures that determine what can be learned (Flavell, 1963). For example, the concept of volume is grasped only after concepts of length and width are acquired, even though the child's behavior may indicate that he treats volume as a distinct property of objects.

Affectivity and emotional states, although not a central part of Piaget's theory, are viewed as interdependent with cognition. Feelings are said to express the value and interest that are given to an act, while cognitive functioning provides the context and structure for it. Dreams, play, fantasies, and artistic endeavors are considered special forms of cognitive activities, although their contribution to both emotional and interpersonal lives is acknowledged.

Piaget conceives of cognitive growth as three successive periods that begin in infancy and continue into mid-adolescence. Within each period, one or more subperiods or stages can be identified. Although a rough estimate of time is provided for each developmental epoch, the only nonvariable characteristic of progression is the sequential order of stages, not their exact timing (Piaget, 1963). The three major periods are the period of sensorimotor intelligence (0–2 years); the period of preparation for and organization of concrete operations (2–11); and the period of formal operations (11–15).

Sensorimotor Intelligence. The neonate begins life with a group of motor and sensory reflexes that are his main tools for transactions with the environment. The adaptational task of the first two years of life are coordination and integration of sensory data and motor experiences; awareness of the external world as a permanent place with objects having properties that are independent of one's perception; and goal-directed, intentional activities. These tasks are achieved through the infant's use of his innate endowments in interaction with his environment. Maturational factors expand the number and the scope of infants' coping mechanisms; however, their influence cannot be separated from the impact of the experiential opportunities available to the child.

Piaget's minute observations and detailed interpretations of the activities of his own three children led him to postulate several propositions and assumptions regarding the evolution of infant behavior. He believed that certain early reflexes are mobile and flexible. That is, they have the potential to incorporate and assimilate some aspects of objects into their own patterns and are, in turn, gradually changed by them. Thus, through contact with the environment, these impulsive reflexes are transformed into basic psychological units called *schemata*. For example, the grasping reflex in the neonate is elicited by stimulation of the palm of the hand. As the infant grasps various objects, he comes in contact with different shapes, textures, temperatures, and weights. These qualities leave their imprint, or even impose themselves, on the reflex and ever so slightly change its pattern of activity. At first, the assimilative efforts of the baby—his attempt to make sense of the object, his accommodative activities, and the subtle adjustments caused by properties of different objects—are undifferentiated and confused. The external world and internal changes are one and the same.

Later on, the schema of prehension is coordinated with other schemata such as vision, hearing, and sucking. Information is now received through several channels simultaneously, or in close succession. Passive hearing and seeing give way to active listening and looking. The baby brings what he grasps to his mouth or tries to reach for what he sees. He interrupts his vocalizations and crying to look at a novel visual configuration or in the direction of a sound. However, these early impressions and sensations are at first intermingled. The infant remembers only sequences of motor activities, and his subjective world is not differentiated from external reality. Whoever holds the baby in a manner similar to that of his mother can expect the same kind of response from him.

As the sensorimotor period progresses, the child gradually begins to objectify his perceptions. He becomes aware of the properties of things and experiences his subjective sensations as emanating from his interaction with the external world. At this stage, the foundation of intelligent behavior has been laid. In Piaget's (1954) words:

> . . . intelligence thus begins neither with knowledge of the self, nor of things as such, but with knowledge of their interaction, and it is by orienting itself simultaneously toward the two poles of that interaction that intelligence organizes the world by organizing itself.

The coordination of various schemata, and the distinction between self and objects, makes it possible for the child to engage in goal-directed, intentional activities. Concurrently, through the ever-growing assimilation of and accommodation to more complex aspects of reality, the child's cognitive structures are expanded and a new level of organization is achieved. Although at this stage the child's adaptation is based on concrete and nonsymbolic behavior, nevertheless by the end of the sensorimotor period the child comes to a practical and orderly comprehension of such environmental invariances as object permanency, spatial relationships, time, and causality. The biopsychological evolution of the sensorimotor period paves the way for the appearance of the cognitive structures of the second developmental epoch: the period of preparation for and organization of concrete operations. This period is divided into two parts: the subperiod of preoperational representation (2–7 years of age) and the subperiod of concrete operations (7–11 years).

Preoperational Representation. The first and foremost task of this stage is that of internalizing the sensorimotor schemata that constitute the foundation of representational intelligence. The transformation of the intelligence of action into representational thinking, and the shift from the limited goals of concrete sequences of behavior to organization and contemplation of actions, requires the development of symbolic function. According to Piaget, the symbolic function includes language but is not limited to it.

The symbolic function is developed as the result of specialized forms of cognitive activities—namely, imitation and play. Imitation is viewed as predominantly accommodative, meaning that the child accepts and repeats a certain sequence of behavior that he has observed in a model. On the other hand, when a child is engaged in play, he does not show any regard or deference for the intrinsic properties of objects. He incorporates them into his own patterns of activities as he desires. Thus a stick can be a horse to ride on and a chair can serve as a boat. Imitation may be visible, deferred, or an invisible mental image. In his games the child pretends to imitate peoples' roles or activities, combining imitation and play or accommodative and assimilative activities. Mental images and pretend games provide the child with symbolic schemata: the child uses one thing to represent something else. When linguistic signs are first acquired, they are used with a variety of idiosyncratic and private meanings. A child may use the word *mama* to describe a number of vaguely similar acts, people, or objects. It is only as the child is socialized and environmental correction and modification take place that the conventional meanings of words are learned and language becomes a vehicle for communication. However, portions of the symbolic schemata remain nonverbal. These nonsocialized, idiosyncratic symbols are used in dream imageries, fantasy formations, and artistic activities.

Representational intelligence is characteristically concrete, bound by external appearances, and unconcerned with logical justification. The child's thinking is egocentric: he cannot consider points of views different from his own. He believes that his mother knows what he has done or how he feels, and therefore he expects to have his needs met without having to articulate them. The child is unable to avoid contradicting himself. If asked to describe his best friend, he may complain about this friend's aggression and abuse. During this period, the child's concepts are concrete and action-oriented. He may think that placing an object in a different context changes its identity. The child's attention is usually centered on one property of a thing to the exclusion of other characteristics. His reasoning jumps from a premise to a conclusion without logical links. His judgment is based on results and external appearances. For example, if two rows of coins are placed parallel to each other and spaced so that one row is longer than the other, the child will state that the longer row has more coins, even if his own counting reveals otherwise. The child is also more preoccupied with parts than with the whole. The idea of simultaneous membership in several classes is beyond his reach; he cannot understand that he belongs to a family, a city, and a country at the same time. His moral judgment is based on rigid notions of "good" and "bad." He cannot consider motives or circumstances when judging an act and feels that punishment or reproach is the natural consequence of a forbidden act. Words are, at first, taken very concretely and are most meaningful to the child when they refer to a real object or a demand for action. Later on, language becomes a tool in intuitive thinking, social intercourse, and interior conversation. The remnant of the child's belief in the literal meaning of the word is reflected in his conviction that if he is called stupid he might actually become stupid.

The world of dreams and fantasies may be considered an actual place, and at times, the distinction between dreams and reality is not firmly held. The child regards thinking as an internalized replica of actions and events. And, like concrete reality, cognitive organization is seen as irreversible. The child cannot change the initial premise in his mind and alter the sequence of his reasoning accordingly. While the child's behavior is orderly and organized, his thinking and perception of the external world are limited and flexible. Such environmental invariants as time, causality, measurement, and numbers are either not fully grasped or not uniformly applied.

Concrete Operations. From about the 7th to the 11th year of life, the child begins to structure and integrate his thoughts into a coherent system, to interpret and organize his present perceptions in the light of his past experiences, and to coordinate his concrete concepts into more complex totalities called *cognitive operations.* He can make numerous classifications of objects and their properties, is aware of transformational activities, and understands that changes of shapes do not necessarily imply changes of quantity or weight. Logical classes and relations are grasped and applied. Thinking becomes an absorbing activity since the principle of reversibility is discovered, so that a child can think about a particular solution from the beginning to the end and retrace his steps backward.

Concepts such as length, width, and volume are abstracted. Time is viewed as an independent dimension unrelated to perceptual data. Past, present, and future are appreciated as different points along the temporal continuum. Parts are now classified into larger wholes, either by the process of simple addition or by the organization of their interrelated links. Practical systems based on information, firsthand knowledge, and hearsay are constructed, although the logical implication of each system is not as yet grasped. Self-contradiction is avoided. Spatial and temporal proximity are no longer accepted as signifying causal relationship. Thinking is no longer predominantly egocentric, although increased objectivity in one area can coexist with egocentricity in other areas.

This new level of intellectual functioning is also reflected in the child's view of social behavior and interpersonal relationships. Having come to grips with the multiplicity of viewpoints, the child is now capable of true reciprocal interactions. Mutual respect replaces unawareness of the needs of others. The child tries to organize and master his own thoughts and feelings. The capacity for introspection and strivings for external and internal equilibrium are developed. Language remains an important tool for conceptualization and its communicative function is used to verify and comprehend reality. The syntactic structure of language gains significance and importance, although the ability to articulate lags behind the child's actual knowledge and comprehension. The concept of moral obligation enters the child's thinking, and concepts of right and wrong, rather than fear of detection and punishment, direct his activities.

Formal Operations. Piaget views formal operations as the most advanced form of cognitive activity, although he is quick to point out that this degree of intellectual sophistication may not be achieved by all people in some, or any, areas of cognitive endeavor. In an otherwise normal population, this failure may be due to a lack of environmental stimulation and cognitive nourishment; or it may be that after a certain level of intellectual development the individual's aptitude and area of interest will call for a different kind of cognitive ability (Piaget, 1972).

Formal operations are prerequisites for hypothetical–deductive reasoning and thus are necessary for understanding scientific experimentation and mathematical and logical propositions. This level of intellectual functioning is no longer bound by concrete objects and relationships but rather allows a person to concentrate on potential realities, the relationships between various propositions, and the implications of different assumptions. Each hypothetical premise can be viewed as a possibility, and solutions can be first worked out on theoretical grounds before they are put to action. Furthermore, the adolescent can generalize from one set of solutions to others, use the same cognitive strategies to solve problems of a vastly different nature, compute all the possible groupings of objects of various properties, and devise abstract systems (Inhelder and Piaget, 1958).

The implications of formal operations for adaptive behavior are also significant. Freed from the limitations of concrete reality, the adolescent can conceive of possible futures, plan for occupations of which he does not have any firsthand knowledge, and reject or adopt certain possibilities without becoming engaged in them. Piaget believes that this newfound freedom allows the adolescent to develop a strong belief in the efficacy of his own thought and the unlimited power of ideas for changing the world. At this stage, there is a new kind of egocentrism of thought, because the adolescent assumes that his own ideas and understanding are unique. However, this belief is gradually tempered by experiences with practical obstacles and the emotional maturity of adulthood. In interpersonal and social interactions, the individual is now aware of the subtleties of social contracts, views the spirit rather than the letter of the law as the more important in regulating society, and becomes interested in such questions as the purpose of the individual's life and the meaning of various endeavors.

Piaget's theory and investigative methods have been criticized on various levels. The data on infants' behavior are limited to Piaget's observations of his own three children, and while at times he recorded only what he observed, at other times he actively participated and elicited various responses. On the other hand, experiments regarding older children were designed for and applied to larger groups of schoolchildren, even though the results were not subjected to statistical analysis. It is further noted that Piaget's data did not always fit his particular theoretical assumptions or, at least, can be interpreted in accordance with a different set of hypotheses (Flavell, 1963). However, the importance of Piaget's contribution to the body of scientific thinking regarding child development is universally acknowledged. Furthermore, while Piaget's own experiments were limited to a relatively narrow population, his work generated a remarkable interest among psychologists and educators all over the world. His theoretical assumptions have been the basis of numerous investigations among dissimilar groups (Modgil, 1974). Piaget himself has used this new evidence to modify his own thinking. So that, at the present time, while reaffirming the basic tenets of his theory, he believes that only the order of succession of the stages of cognitive development remain fixed, while the rate of progression may be different in various groups and under different circumstances (Piaget, 1972).

LEARNING THEORY

All theories of child development include tacit or explicit assumptions regarding the cumulative effect of repeated experiences, even though the mechanisms involved in this learning process are not clearly described. Learning theorists, on the other hand, have attempted to discover the laws and principles governing the establishment of associative links between the environmental stimuli and the behavioral responses of the organism. Although differences in the genetic and constitutional makeups of individuals are acknowledged, these differences are viewed as independent variables that influence the rate of learning rather than the manner in which learning takes place.

The early, simple experiments of Pavlov and the more complicated hypothetical constructs of the social learning theorists are based on the common notion that the behavior of the organism is shaped and modified by a series of environmental variables that can be isolated and studied. The majority of behaviorists, therefore, purport to define behavior phenomenologically and to exclude or minimize the importance of such nonobservable concepts as memory, cognition, and other "mentalistic" notions. Every behavioral pattern, whether it is thought, feelings, or motor activity, is learned through repeated association with environmental stimuli. The more complex sequences can be analyzed into their simpler components, and the basic units can be shown experimentally to have developed as the result of stimulus–response association. According to these theorists, human learning is governed by the same principles as learning in nonhuman subjects in the laboratory. Child development can be viewed as the gradual modification of the newborn's behavior into the more socialized adult form (social learning).

The associative links between various environmental stimuli and the numerous behavioral patterns of the organism are established through two different, though complementary, forms of conditioning: classical and instrumental.

Classical Conditioning. Pavlov's experiments revealed that an innate physiologic response, such as salivation in the presence of food, can be made to appear following presentation of an unrelated stimulus, such as the ringing of a bell. In order to develop such a connection, Pavlov paired the ringing of the bell with the introduction of food. After a few trials, he noted that the animal began to salivate when it heard the sound of the bell, even though no food was delivered. In this experiment, the sound of the bell (auditory stimulus) was called a *conditioned stimulus* and the animal's response to it a *conditioned response* (Pavlov, 1927). Later on, Pavlov succeeded in establishing secondary links between the presentation of a light and the ringing of the bell, so that even though the light had never been paired with food, it came to elicit the salivating response from the animal. However, it was noted that repeated introduction of the bell ring or the light without the reinforcement of the delivery of the food led to the extinction of the response after several trials. Therefore the associative links can be weakened or strengthened by withholding or delivering the reinforcement.

Through conditioning, animals may learn to distinguish stimuli with minor differences (discrimination). Conversely, their responses may be broadened so that similar, but not identical, stimuli elicit the same behavior (generalization).

Language learning in children is particularly dependent upon discrimination and generalization. A child must learn to differentiate between various sounds with minute differences such as "b" and "p." At the same time, he must generalize his knowledge of language in order to make a variety of sentences with the same basic rules. Recently studies with chidlren have revealed that discriminative learning can be facilitated by giving verbal labels to learning tasks, while giving the same name to different stimuli assists in generalization (verbal mediating response). These principles have important implications for child development and human learning. In animal experimentations, learning may be facilitated when the subject has a high drive or motivation to carn a reward. For example, salivation is more likely when the dog has been kept without food for a few hours prior to the experiment than when it is satiated. Drive reduction is thus viewed as a type of reward or reinforcement for certain behavior.

The principle underlying classical conditioning is called the *contiguity principle,* meaning that when two stimuli appear in temporal proximity, one of them is able to evoke the response customarily elicited by the other one. This principle may be used to explain much of the nonintentional learning that takes place during childhood.

Instrumental Conditioning. Skinner's experiments have shown that the frequency of spontaneous and unsolicited behavior in an organism is dependent upon the environmental events following such behavior. This type of conditioning is called *operant* because the organism is not responding but acting upon the environment, and its activities are instrumental in bringing about subsequent occurrences. Behavior that is reinforced is repeated, while activities that are ignored do not recur. Extinction is brought about by withholding the reinforcement, while punishment inhibits a behavior in a particular setting. Totally new patterns of behavior can be produced by reinforcing gradual movements toward the designated goal and refining approximate endeavors. Behavior is thus modified and shaped by the experimenter's design (Skinner, 1969).

The concepts of reward and reinforcement have undergone several changes as the result of numerous experiments. Reinforcement is no longer viewed as an invariably enjoyable event or a biologically valued substance. At times, whatever seems to increase the frequency of recurrence of certain behavior in a predictable fashion is defined as a re-inforcement. Various objects and events may acquire a reinforcing quality by having been paired with other rewards. For example, it has been shown that tokens that can be exchanged for food may induce an animal to engage in designated activities. Furthermore, learning a par-ticular sequence of action may be occasioned by the animal's desire to avoid painful stimuli rather than its anticipation of rewards or rein-forcements. This is called *avoidance learning*. The important feature of avoidance learning is that it is self-reinforcing. That is, the animal who has learned that by pressing a lever it can avoid an electric shock will press the lever as soon as the signal comes on without waiting to discover whether the electric current has indeed been turned on. The principles underlying avoidance learning have been invoked to ex-plain certain phobic reactions in humans. Another significant finding about the reinforcement schedule is that a behavior that is partially or randomly reinforced is more resistant to extinction, although condi-tioning also takes longer to accomplish.

Social Learning and Child Development. Learning theorists have not as yet attempted to construct a systematic theory of personality. Some researchers, such as Eysenck (1960), have identified clusters of behav-ioral tendencies that are believed to reflect the outcome of the individ-ual's conditioning history and the differential reactivity of his central nervous system. The emphasis in Eysenck's conceptualization of per-sonality is on biological factors, which, in turn, influence the rate, ease, and quality of conditioning.

Another group of behavioral psychologists has attempted to map out a hypothetical course of child development based on extrapola-tions from laboratory studies and animals. Reasoning by analogy, these scientists held that the child's social milieu gradually shapes and modifies his behavior through the same mechanisms and based on the same principles as have been found to influence animal behavior. Al-though not all the relevant environmental variables have been iden-tified, the process of socialization is assumed to account for personal-ity development. However, these theorists have so far failed to construct a coherent theory of child development that explains the va-riety of changes that take place during the formative years. In addi-tion, even in the area of socialization, while stimulus–response link-ages are used as explanatory suppositions, the key concepts, such as dependency, imitation, and identification, are borrowed from other theories and do not fulfill the strict criteria set out by the proponents of the behaviorist school.

Dependency. Social learning theorists consider dependency the root of socialization and the long infancy of the human species as par-ticularly suitable to the establishment of dependency. Newborn in-

fants come to associate the presence of caretakers with feelings of sa-
tiation and drive reduction. Caretakers, on the other hand, willfully or
inadvertently reinforce those aspects of the infant's behavior that are
adaptive and socially desired. In such interactions, reinforcements are
bestowed at random; therefore the learned patterns are resistant to extinction. Simple sequences of responses are linked with each other to
create complex units of behavior called *habits*. Behavioral patterns or
habits determine the type of interactions that are customarily exhibited by each individual. Child-rearing techniques are the most influential factors in shaping such habits during the early years. For example, while in the first few months of life the infant's dependency is
reinforced and rewarded, later on parents attempt to inhibit or extinguish inappropriate expressions of dependency and reinforce independent behavior. Demands for attention and the exhibition of dependency needs may become associated with anxiety and anticipation
of disapproval. This anxiety may foster avoidance learning so that the
child learns more independent behavior in order to reduce the state of
tension. On the other hand, some children's behaviors seem to be instrumental in provoking negative attention from their caretakers. Such
children receive reinforcement for their dependency, and at the same
time parental disapproval or punishment causes a reduction of their
anxiety (Dollard and Miller, 1950).

Learning by imitation plays an important part in socialization in
that the child patterns his behavior after the available models in his
milieu and is rewarded for such behavior. Spontaneous repetitions
and imitations of parental activities and attitudes establish the nucleus
of the child's self-control and the internal regulatory mechanism that is
called *conscience*. Secondary drives, such as needs for approval and accomplishment, are developed through associations between reduction
of the level of biological drives on the part of the child and expression
of parental satisfaction and pleasure while administering to those
needs. Verbal approval comes to replace concrete physical rewards on
the same basis. In later years, marks, commendation cards, and pay-
checks become important incentives for accomplishments, while the
range of socially acceptable behavior widens and the number of secondary drives multiplies.

Aggression. The development of aggressive behavior has received
special attention from behavior theorists. Because excessive aggression
is socially undesirable and subject to severe disapproval, it cannot
simply be viewed as a response promoted by design and fostered by
the child-rearing methods. Behaviorists consider anger to be a primary
reaction to frustration and aggression to be goal-directed anger. In
early infancy, the angry outbursts of infants bring caretakers to their
sides, and even though the mother may express dissatisfaction and

annoyance, the frustrating agent is removed. The establishment of a link between annoyance and the expression of pain by others on one hand and the feeling of relief and satisfaction on the other is postulated as an explanation for the persistence of aggression in spite of social disapproval. Punishment inhibits the expression of aggression in the presence of the punishing agent. However, the behavior will continue to be exhibited in other situations. The inhibition of a response is thus different from its extinction. When the behavior is ignored—that is, reinforcement is withheld—the response is extinguished, while avoidance of punishment is the motivating factor in inhibiting the expression of a response. The particular forms of aggressive action may be learned through the imitation of various models (Bandura and Walters, 1963).

The failure or distortion of the socialization processes is viewed as a cause of various behavioral problems of childhood. Fortuitous associations between certain behavior and the reduction of anxiety are held to be responsible for the development of neurotic symptoms. Behavior modification techniques are devised in order to increase the frequency of occurrence of desired activities and the extinction of unacceptable habits. Neurotic symptoms are treated by weakening the associations between the anxiety state and the neurotic behavior. Attempts to shape and construct useful habits are directed at helping retarded or psychotic children to develop self-care and communicative skills.

While social learning theorists have succeeded in confirming some aspects of their hypotheses in experimental situations, their assumptions for the most part remain untested and unverified. Studies of child-rearing practices in different cultural settings have failed to lend credence to the notion that various personality types are produced by differences in child-rearing methods. Assumptions of multiple stimuli, multiple responses, and numerous associative links do not provide convincing explanations for such processes as cognition, language acquisition, or even various types of learning. However, while the elegant simplicity of the stimulus–response theories has failed to account for the complexity of child development, the methodology of the behaviorist school has exerted a significant influence in the field of behavioral studies. The emphasis on an objective, operational definition of behavior, the reproducibility of experimental designs, and the disconfirmation of certain possible correlations are aspects of behaviorist strategy that have contributed to the development of a science of behavior.

II
DISORDERED BEHAVIOR

4

Genesis and Etiology

In recent years, concepts such as mental health and mental illness, or normal and deviant behavior, have come under increasing scrutiny by behavioral scientists. Some psychiatrits claim they do not know what constitutes mental health (Pasamanick, 1968), while others consider mental illness to be a myth (Szasz, 1961).

Even when the broadest operational definitions of mental health and illness are considered, the relationship between deviant behavior during childhood and adolescence and the mental health or illness of adult years remains unclarified. However, it seems logical to assume that whether one accepts social effectiveness and a subjective sense of well-being as the sign of mental health or, conversely, considers the chronic inability to cope with life as the hallmark of mental illness, the personality of the individual and his habitual way of thinking, feeling, and relating to his environment play an important part in his behavior within any given context. An individual's behavior is in turn, a significant deciding factor in how he is judged and evaluated by others.

In studying a child's behavior, we observe the process of the making of his personality. Not only is any observable unit of behavior assessed as to its degree of deviation from the age-appropriate, culturally expected norm, but it is also evaluated as to its potential implications for the child's further development and his ability to cope with the social reality within which he will have to operate.

While the language of psychiatry has remained deeply rooted in a medical frame of reference, our concept of psychopathology or mental disorder is no longer a traditional medical concept. Rather, as Thorpe (1960) has pointed out, we conceptualize mental disorder as an hypothetical construct of dynamic interaction among biological, psychological, and social factors. In the field of child psychiatry, the parameter of developmental stage is a dimension added to this hypothetical construct. Developmental stage, while unquestionably age-dependent, cannot be equated with age. External and internal factors can and do hinder or facilitate a child's development.

In the following chapter, as well as throughout this book, disturbances and deviations of children's development are conceptualized as interdependent, interactional phenomena, with the child acting as a developing biopsychological organism within his social environment. As Glidewell (1968) has pointed out, the concept of mental health in children

> . . . transcends symptom formation but also provides a basis for a continuing inquiry into both the stability and the disturbance of the development of the motivational strength and direction, the emotional state and expression, the intellectual potential and utilization, and the personal enjoyment and skills of the school child.

No single external or internal factor can be said to have a direct bearing on the kind of personality that a child will develop (Murphy and Moriarty, 1976). However, the cumulative effects of a long-term undesirable environment and suboptimal biological endowment cannot fail to influence the child's emerging personality.

It is a well-known fact that all neglected children do not become socially deviant adults, nor does every premature infant become educationally handicapped. But we are also aware that the effective environment for the optimal growth of a mentally handicapped child is different from that needed for an intellectually gifted individual. Some biological or psychological factors limit the child's ability to cope with the most benign demands from the environment, while other children find ingenious ways to survive and develop in an intolerable situation. A well-socialized retardate is liked and protected by his peers; a hostile intelligent child is tormented and ostracized by his age group. The degree of self-respect and self-confidence of a child has far-reaching implications for his personality development, and one's attitude toward oneself is in part dependent upon how one is received and accepted by others.

In any discussion of childhood psychopathology, it should be kept in mind that the majority of children are fortunately well functioning and well adjusted. What concerns us is to identify and hopefully to correct those circumstances that hinder and distort the normal growth and the successful development of those children who are troubled.

Stress

In psychiatry, "stress" is frequently mentioned as a precipitating factor in the clinical appearance of a mental illness or is given implicit etiological significance in producing certain symptoms.

Selye (1950) defined *stress* as an event triggering certain physiological changes in the neurohormonal equilibrium of the body. He did not differentiate between desirable and pleasant happenings and unpleasant and unwanted accidents.

Psychological reactions following a natural disaster such as an earthquake or a flood are well known. World War I provided ample evidence of the emotional toll that the war may extract from individual soldiers. However, it was also clear that not all fighting men react with war neurosis. Therefore factors inherent in the premorbid personality of the individual had to play a part in that individual's reaction. This notion of stress could not be extrapolated to the ordinary peacetime lives of patients who developed psychiatric symptoms. The stressors therefore were conceptualized as undesirable changes, such as, for example, loss of job, physical ill health, divorce, and death in the family.

Dohrenwend (1973), following Selye's original idea, conceptualized all changes as stressful, while others considered the perception of the individual, regardless of the nature of the event, as being the decisive factor in how stressful a particular event might be. Meyers *et al.* (1972), in a two-year longitudinal study of stress and mental status in psychiatric patients, defined a set of "life events": "experiences involving a role transformation, changes in states or environment, and imposition of pain." The list of 62 life events was given to the subjects with the instruction that they could add any events that they found personally significant that had not been included in the list. The researchers found that patients who reported a greater number of life events within the preceding year were more likely to have a worsening mental status. Conversely, subjects with fewer life events showed a decrease in the number of symptoms over their previous mental status. The results indicated a relationship between the total number of life events and psychiatric symptomatology, even when the particular event did not depend on the psychological condition of the individuals. Meyers *et al.* concluded that "Apparently not only serious crisis, but almost any event requiring attention or some form of behavioral adaptation may be potentially detrimental to one's mental health."

The effect of life events on the mental health of children has not been systematically studied, although clinicians have found that events such as birth of a sibling, hospitalization of the child or a parent, divorce, change of school, and move to a new neighborhood have preceded manifestations of behavioral disorder. In studying the life stress of the psychiatrically ill mothers of young children, Cohler *et al.* (1975) reported a greater number of life stressors for the children of manic–depressive mothers as perceived by the mothers themselves.

Psychological reaction to life events in children may be loss of previous function, withdrawal, aggression, accentuation of previous symptoms, or the appearance of new sets of symptoms.

The age of the child or the stage of development may be an important factor in whether a particular event is perceived as stressful. For example, when children have just begun to develop friendships, the move to another neighborhood may be more stressful than when they are younger and are more interested in having playmates than special friends. Children who are more resistant to change and less adaptable to new situations may find such events taxing; when new situations occur frequently, they may be unable to cope with the demands placed upon them. Chronically anxious children or children who show signs of developmental lag or disturbances of the integrative functions of the central nervous system tend to be more vulnerable than others. The cumulative effects of life stressors and the constant need for coping with the new demands and new set of circumstances are more detrimental to the child's functioning than the aftermath of one hazardous event.

While the exact mechanism by which changes in life result in symptom formation is not clear, it seems that a certain amount of stability and predictability in the environment is necessary for the optimal functioning of any child (Robkin and Struening, 1976).

Constitutional and Genetic Factors

The familial occurrence of normal and abnormal behavior has always been known and commented upon. However, it is only recently that geneticists have begun to investigate the type of behavioral deviations that might be genetically transmitted and have attempted to form hypotheses regarding the mode of genetic transmission of such behaviors (McKusick, 1966).

Because controlled breeding experiments, which are scientifically the most satisfactory method of genetic investigation, are not possible in the field of human genetics, researchers have used such methods as analysis of family pedigree; studies of monozygotic and dizygotic twins reared apart and together; studies of cross-fostering (Wender et al., 1974); and investigations of biochemical aberrations and chromosomal anomalies of various patient populations (Rosenthal, 1970).

Cytologic studies of chromosomes have so far revealed that certain structural anomalies of autosomal chromosomes are associated with mental retardation. Aberrations of sex chromosomes, however, do not always lead to a lowering of intellectual functionings. These studies have so far failed to shed any light on the mechanism by which anomalies of chromosomes affect higher mental functionings. In some individuals, structural defects of the chromosomes are associated with somatic defects in various organs. One might assume that, similarly, structural defects of the central nervous system can account for the associated mental retardation (Daly, 1970). However, such defects have not been discovered, nor has it been possible to identify one group or a single chromosome as being invariably related to mental retardation and, by inference, as the agent responsible for the development of normal intelligence. Biochemical studies have identified mental retardation associated with such metabolic abnormalities as phenylketonuria and have discovered the genetic mode of transmission of the enzyme defect. Huntington's chorea is another neuropsychiatric disorder whose genetic basis is well established, although the pathogenesis is far from being understood.

In genetic studies of functional psychosis, neither chromosomal aberration nor consistent biochemical abnormalities have so far been identified. Therefore genetic inferences have been made on the basis of the occurrence of the same constellation of symptoms among various family members.

Schizophrenia. The methodological problems in these studies begin with the definition and diagnosis of schizophrenia. While there is high level of agreement regarding the diagnosis of the most severe forms of schizophrenia, the less severe forms, the borderline cases, and what has been referred to as the "schizophrenic spectrum" are not so easily identifiable. Furthermore there is no solid basis for the assumption that all forms of schizophrenia are etiologically related. Childhood schizophrenia is not a uniformly accepted category, and the relationship between childhood schizophrenia and adult forms of the disease is still unsettled. Phenocopies or environmentally induced forms of the illness, similar to what is said to be genetically determined, do occur. For example, toxic psychosis due to hallucinogenic drugs or amphetamine resembles schizophrenia.

Pedigree analysis of schizophrenia is usually based on the selection of an index case from the hospital records; therefore the results are based on a preselected group rather than on an epidemiologic study of a whole population. Furthermore, even in cases of monozygotic twins with identical genotype, 100% concordance for schizophrenia has not been found. This has led investigators to search for nongenetic congenital factors and experiential elements that play an important part in the phenotypic expression of the disorder.

From the overall results of various methods of investigation, the following conclusions can be drawn:

- The morbidity risk for developing schizophrenia among the blood relatives of schizophrenic patients is higher than the expectancy rate for the general population. For example, the risk for developing schizophrenia in children with one schizophrenic parent is about 8–10 times higher than the expected rate for the general population. Sibs of schizophrenics have a 6–7 times higher likelihood of developing schizophrenia.
- The concordance rate among monozygotic twins is higher when the illness is more severe, although it never approaches 100%.
- The concordance rate for monozygotic twins is always greater than for dizygotic pairs.
- Studies of children with schizophrenic parents who were raised by nonschizophrenic adoptive parents reveal the morbidity risk to be related to the biological parents' illness.
- Studies of normal children adopted by parents who were schizophrenics do not show any greater risk for schizophrenia than the general population.
- The full outcome of the longitudinal studies of children with high risk for schizophrenia, such as infants of schizophrenic mothers, is not yet known, although so far these studies have provided some indications that these children are indeed a high-risk group (Fish, 1957; Sobel, 1961; Mednick and Schulsinger, 1968).
- No particular genetic model can be found to account for the transmission of schizophrenia based on the results of these studies. A simple Mendelian single-gene theory does not explain the findings. Therefore either a modified Mendelian model or a quantitative, multiple-factor genetic theory must be postulated.

At this point, the possible genetic inferences based on family studies have been largely exhausted and new insights in this area may be expected to come from biochemical studies. The discovery of biochemical abnormalities may make it possible to define what is transmitted and what genetic mode of transmission is involved. A full theory explaining the genetic basis of schizophrenia would have to include a detailed analysis of the environmental factors that precipitate the clinical expressions of the illness; the mechanism operating in the natural remission; and the reasons for degrees of severity in symptomatology and the clinical subtypes (Rosenthal and Kety, 1968).

Manic–Depressive Psychosis. Genetic studies of manic–depressive illness have not been as extensive as those of schizophrenia, and the available investigations are not always comparable. Some researchers have included involutional melancholia and psychotic depressions along with classic forms of manic–depressive disorders, while others have limited their samples to manic–depressive patients.

Of the 100 pairs of monozygotic twins reported in the literature, the concordance rate for affective disorders has been as low as 50% (Harvald and Hauge, 1965) and as high as almost 100% in Kallman's sample (Kallman, 1953). Concordance rate for dizygotic twins have ranged from 2.6 to 38.5%. Most authors have refrained from any speculation regarding the genetic mode of inheritance of the affective disorders.

The field of behavior genetics in humans is in its early infancy, and the road ahead promises to be crowded with methodological obstacles. The role of heredity in normal and abnormal personality development can be conceptualized as facilitating or hindering the type and the range of responses that any individual can display under various environmental conditions.

Prenatal Risks

As the search for etiology or at least the antecedent events leading to behavioral deviations has become more sophisticated, it has become evident that development does not begin with birth. The intrauterine milieu in which the fetus grows, the length of pregnancy, the complications of pregnancy, the general health of the pregnant mother, and the process of delivery can all have a negative influence on the subsequent course of the child's development. As Pasamanick and Knobloch (1966) have pointed out, "There exists a continuum of reproductive casualty extending from death through varying degrees of neuropsychiatric disability." Sameroff (1975) has added the concept of a continuum of caretaking casualty to emphasize the interdependence and transaction between nature and nurture of the child.

Prenatal Factors. It is well established that at least some maternal infections during pregnancy are transmitted to the fetus and that the infant can be born with a variety of congenital defects ranging from gross mental retardation to more subtle indications of central nervous system impairment. Congenital rubella has resulted in a spectrum of neuropsychiatric deficiencies, such as hearing loss, blindness, mental retardation, autism, and motor deficit. Toxoplasmosis of the pregnant mother has produced infants with microcephaly, progressive hydrocephalus, and mental retardation. The list of known maternal infections with deleterious neurological consequences on infants is an expanding one, and new laboratory methods of isolating and identifying pathogenic viruses promise to make new additions to the list.

The effects of various drugs used by pregnant mothers on the fetal development can be studied only in laboratory animals or following tragic incidents such as the limb malformations in Thalidomide babies. Berlin (1969) reported chromosomal defects in infants whose mother had ingested LSD during pregnancy. Although the significance of such findings is not as yet understood, it does indicate that chemical agents ingested by the pregnant mother may, in fact, produce structural changes in the cells of the fetal body.

Narcotic addiction in mothers has resulted in the appearance of withdrawal symptoms in neonates ranging from irritability, restlessness, and sleeplessness to convulsions. Although these symptoms are not seen when the mother has undergone detoxification or has stopped using drugs for days prior to delivery, the effects of maternal narcotic use on the fetus's central nervous system during earlier months of pregnancy is not known.

Even drugs that do not necessarily affect the nervous system may increase the infant's susceptibility to other potentially hazardous occurrences. For example, large doses of aspirin prior to delivery have been shown to lower the albumin-binding capacity of the infant's blood and to increase the danger of hyperbilirubinemia, which, in turn, may cause brain damage.

Radiation during pregnancy can unfavorably influence the developing brain, although only exposure to extreme doses of radiation resulting in microcephaly and mental retardation have been documented (Yamazaki, 1966).

Metabolic disorders of the mother may create abnormal neurohormonal states in the fetus. This can cause direct impairment of the central nervous system or provide potentially hazardous conditions for birth leading to brain injury (as, for example, in the oversize babies of diabetic mothers).

Maternal toxemia with or without eclamptic fits can cause premature birth, fetal anoxia, or stillbirth. Bleeding, particularly during the first trimester, has been shown to be associated with neurological damage such as cerebral palsy, epilepsy, and mental retardation in children.

Perinatal Complications. Anoxia during the birth process, as assessed by the low Apgar score of the newborn infant, is associated with later neuropsychiatric disorders. Graham *et al.* (1962), in a follow-up study, found that a large percentage of full-term infants who had suffered anoxia during delivery scored lower in all tests of cognitive functioning on the Stanford–Binet as compared with a group with nonanoxic complications such as prematurity or erythroblastosis. Schacter and Apgar (1959) reported a significant correlation between prenatal complications, such as prolonged labor, difficult delivery, and neonatal problems, and low score on IQ tests of children at 8 years of age.

Pasamanick and Knobloch (1966), in a retrospective study of the birth histories of children with a variety of psychiatric disorders, found a significantly higher percentage of complications of pregnancy and labor in children with reading disability, mental retardation, cerebral palsy, epilepsy, and behavior disorders commonly associated with "minimal brain dysfunction." According to their studies, operative procedures during delivery such as Caesarean section and high or low forceps in and of themselves did not seem to be related with later complications. Only those complications that were anoxia-producing were related to possible central nervous system impairment.

The Small-for-Date Infant. Low birth weight in an infant may be due to premature delivery, retarded intrauterine growth, or a combination of the two. The mortality rate and the risk for various neonatal complications differ among children with low birth weight of various etiology. Maternal malnutrition is considered a major factor in the lower birth weight of children from poor families. However, the increase in birth weight because of better maternal nutrition or the decrease during acute food shortages is relatively small—only about 5–8%.

Recently the emphasis has been shifted away from studies of body growth to brain development during intrauterine life. Some authors have suggested that undernutrition during the period in which the brain undergoes its fastest growth rate may cause irreparable damage to the organism. In humans this period extends from the last few months of gestation through the first few months of postnatal life. The notion of a critical period for brain development has been experimentally proven in various animals. However, there is as yet no agreement among various researchers as to whether the time of maximum growth of the brain coincides with the critical period for rapid increase in the enzymes and structural changes of the cells in the central nervous system.

Studies of the brains of infants who have suffered severe intrauterine growth retardation have so far failed to show any signs of retarded maturation of the CNS. Minkowsky *et al.* (1966) concluded that cellular growth and maturation in the human brain during gestation are remarkably independent of unfavorable conditions that may affect the physical growth of the body.

Retrospective studies of children with low birth weight for gestational age have so far failed to show a significant relationship between birth weight and future intellectual functioning. In a prospective study of infants with low birth weight, Drillien (1970) found no difference in the IQ scores of 11 female monozygous twins with varying birth weight. However, the 8 male pairs in the study showed IQ scores correlating with lower birth weight. Postnatal feeding may also be a significant factor in the future neurological and intellectual status of these children. Children with low birth weight raised in poverty show the cumulative effects of pre- and postnatal malnutrition, while small-for-date infants raised in a more affluent environment can compensate for the effects—if any—of the intrauterine retardation and thus do not show any lowering of IQ in follow-up studies.

Another important factor in the later development of the small-for-date infant is the higher incidence of congenital anomalies in these children. In a study of a group of infants weighing 2000 grams or less, Drillien (1970) found that the number of both major and minor congenital anomalies increases as the weight for gestational age decreases and, that children with congenital anomalies, even when the anomaly is not handicapping in itself, are more likely to have mental retardation, neurological defects, or both. So far the most important etiological factor found in retarded intrauterine development is placental insufficiency, usually associated with toxemia.

Prematurity. The term *prematurity* refers to short gestational age and low birth weight in a newborn infant. The incidence of prematurity is several times higher among the low socioeconomic population. Etiology is varied. Infection, metabolic disorders, toxemia, and systemic diseases of the mother may all result in premature birth of the infant.

Studies of the neurological and psychological sequelae of prematurity have shown prematures to be a high-risk group for the development of various educational deficiencies and behavioral disorders regardless of the socioeconomic background.

To the possible effects of the etiological factors leading to premature birth, one must add the influences of the postnatal care of these infants, which until recently has consisted of isolating the infants in incubators and thus depriving them of the varied tactile, visual, and auditory stimuli experienced by full-term babies shortly after birth. It has been argued that had the premature infant remained *in utero,* he would not have been exposed to such stimuli. However, it is conceivable that the birth process changes the organization and the functionings of the sensory system, so that while the intrauterine existence shields the infant from such stimuli, it provides him with a series of appropriate stimulations that cannot be duplicated after birth. The premature infant is thus deprived of these stimulations as well as the postnatal experiences available to the full-term newborn.

Rubin *et al.* (1973) studied neurological abnormalities in four groups of children from various socioeconomic backgrounds. One group contained infants with birth weight under 2500 grams, and another contained infants with gestational age under 37 weeks (prematurity). The third group had birth weights over 2500 grams but gestational ages under 37 weeks, and the control group contained full-term, full-weight infants. The children came from an overwhelmingly white population. They were neurologically examined during the first week, at 4 months, at 12 months, and finally at 7 years of age. Psychological examination was done at 8 months, 4 years, 5 years, and 7 years of age. (The Bayley Scales of Mental and Motor Development, the Stanford–Binet, the Metropolitan Reading Readiness Test, the Illinois Test of Psycholinguistic Ability, and the Wide Range Achievement Test were used.) The group with low birth weight, with or without concomitant low gestational age, showed a higher proportion of children with neurological abnormalities. Some children who were neurologically abnormal during early infancy were considered normal at 4 years of age. Others showed persistent neurological signs at 7 years. Developmental quotients of infants with low birth weight and low gestational age were lower than those of children with normal birth weight or normal gestational age.

Between 4 and 7 years, the intellectual performance of children with low birth weight was inferior to that of children with full birth weight regardless of the gestational age. No difference was found between intellectual performance of boys and girls. On the other hand, a higher proportion of low-birth-weight boys than girls had academic, or behavior problems relating to school. The authors concluded that children with low birth weight are a high-risk group for neurological and educational problems. However, children whose low birth weight is accompanied with low gestational age seem to fare better than small-for-date infants. Their data suggest that two-thirds of male children with low birth weight and one-half of all small-for-date infants manifest problems of sufficient magnitude in school to warrant special class placement.

Epidemiological surveys show that low-birth-weight infants are usually born to young mothers with little or no prenatal care. The incidence of complications of pregnancy and delivery is high. Maternal toxemia, placenta praevia, premature rupture of the membranes, and maternal infections accompany these eventful pregnancies; respiratory distress, necessitating oxygen therapy, and elevated bilirubin plague the infants at birth. Postnatal malnutrition and infections are likely to occur, and the additive effects of all these unfavorable circumstances may indeed increase the risk of educational and neurological handicaps for the children of the poor in far greater proportion than can be caused by prematurity and low birth weight in higher socioeconomic families.

Postnatal Factors

Hyperbilirubinemia. When associated with hemolytic disease, such as erythroblastosis fetalis, hyperbilirubinemia has been shown to cause kernicterus and various neurological sequelae leading to neuropsychiatric disorders. The higher values of the unconjugated bilirubin are associated with higher risks of future neurological and intellectual deficits. The situation has been changed since exchange transfusion has become a routine procedure in cases of erythroblastosis.

Holmes *et al.* (1968) reported that hyperbilirubinemia without hemolytic disease does not seem to significantly affect the neurological status of children. Because hyperbilirubinemia is so often associated with prematurity, it is not possible to differentiate possible deleterious effects of hyperbilirubinemia from prematurity *per se.*

Infections of the Central Nervous System. Meningitis and meningoencephalitis during infancy may leave the child with residual damage to the central nervous system, resulting in specific or generalized deficits, lowering of intellectual ability, and various behavioral stigmata of brain damage.

Trauma. Birth trauma or head injuries during infancy and early childhood may cause chronic subdural hematoma, which, if unrecognized and untreated, can cause serious structural damage to the brain.

Malnutrition or Undernutrition. Hypoglycemia during the first 72 hours of life (blood value below 20 mg/100 ml) has been found to be associated with later neurologic and developmental sequelae. In fact, infants who show abnormal neurological status and hypoglycemia during the newborn period have a poor prognosis with regard to permanent neurological impairment.

Studies with experimental animals have provided ample evidence of the role of malnutrition in causing physical growth retardation, reduced brain maturation, and impaired learning ability. Dietary restrictions on rats and pigs shortly after birth have produced smaller brain size, decreased myelination, reduction in the number of brain cells, and abnormal EEG.

These experiments cannot, of course, be duplicated in human infants, and although studies of the intellectual functioning of mal-nourished children have demonstrated various deficits, the retardation cannot be solely attributed to low calorie intake or protein deficiency. Malnourished children come from poor families in which a variety of environmental factors, such as overcrowding, low-grade infections, and limited experiential opportunities, may be operative.

In most developing countries, children of the poor are breast-fed long past the time at which mother's milk can provide the necessary dietary requirements. When breast feeding is not supplemented, these children suffer generalized malnutrition. At times, the young child's diet may be insufficient only in protein. At other times, the caloric intake is inadequate. Kwashiorkor is a severe form of malnutrition in which the child is edematous, has abnormally pigmented and desquamating skin, and suffers from diarrhea and lack of appetite. He is un-interested in and apathetic toward his environment, or he may be ex-tremely irritable and restless. In children who are treated with a high-protein and high-caloric diet, kwashiorkor is reversible. How-ever, in one follow-up study of 20 children suffering from malnutrition in the first year of life, Stoch and Smythe (1963) found the head cir-cumference to be on the average 1 inch smaller than that of the control group of the same age and racial background. The smaller head cir-cumference was taken to indicate a diminished size of the brain. This assumption has been questioned on the grounds that since malnutri-tion causes retardation in bone growth, smaller head size in the chil-dren may not represent smaller brain size (Frisch, 1971).

According to Cravioto and Robles (1965), when kwashiorkor is seen in infants under 6 months of age, adaptive and motor behavior do not improve with treatment, while older children with the condi-tion tend to catch up after treatment. Scrimshaw (1969) reported re-tarded growth in height, weight, and head circumference in children from a number of poor countries in Africa and Latin America. These children, who suffered from chronic undernutrition, did not show the extreme degree of apathy seen in kwashiorkor.

In a study of preschool children in an Indian village in Guatemala, Cravioto et al. (1966) found almost all these children to show retarded physical growth. A series of tests assessing intersensory integration was administered to these children. The result showed that those in the lowest quartile for weight and height for their age invariably scored lower than those in the upper quartile for height and weight. Among the middle-class children of the Guatemala city, no such dif-ferences were found between those in the lowest and the highest quartile of height and weight. The authors concluded that while dif-ferences in height and weight in the middle-class children are due to genetic factors, in poor children such differences are the consequence of nutritional status and affect their intellectual functioning.

Klein *et al.* (1969) gave the same batteries of tests to children after first having demonstrated to them how to go about performing the task. The result showed no difference in the performance of the two groups. However, the authors found malnourished children to be more limited in their attention span and their concentration ability; they concluded that chronic undernutrition lowers children's energy level and their motivation for performance rather than their intellectual abilities.

Although acute and chronic undernutrition may not be as prevalent in the industrialized countries as it is in the developing countries of the world, it occurs among poor families regardless of geographic location. Furthermore children with growth retardation may suffer from undernutrition, not necessarily based on the general unavailability of food but because of other factors such as prolonged feeding problems or disturbed child–parent relationships.

Failure to Thrive. This is a syndrome of severe, chronic undernutrition in infancy and early childhood that is characterized by weight and height below the third percentile for age. The children have frequent feeding difficulties with occasional diarrhea and vomiting, are slow to gain weight, are irritable and easily fatigued, and have low energy levels. While there is no demonstrable etiology, there is retardation in bone age.

In some cases, maternal neglect and poverty result in children's undernutrition. In other cases, inadequate and immature mothers are unable to care for their infants, particularly when the babies are irregular and irritable. At times, this neglect is due to maternal emotional disorder or outright rejection of the infant.

Evans *et al.* (1972) did a follow-up study of 45 children who had been hospitalized with this syndrome. They found that when parental neglect was due to the mother's inability to care for the child, external help after the infant's discharge from the hospital improved the overall functioning of the mother and the child's subsequent growth was satisfactory. Where the mother–child relationship was pathological, retardation was chronic and the outcome poor to disastrous unless the child had been removed to a foster home.

What can be concluded from all the above studies is that chronic malnutrition, whether due to nutritional deprivation or secondary to chronic infections or systemic disease, can result in growth retardation, lowered energy level, difficulties in concentration, low motivation for achievement, and possible deficits in intellectual ability. Undernutrition may or may not lead to irreversible damage to the central nervous system, but there is little doubt that it interferes with the process of orderly interaction with the environment. Important aspects of experience are not registered, integrated, or used optimally. At best, learning becomes deficient and at worst fails to take place at all. Later academic difficulties, in turn, unfavorably influence the child's interpersonal relationships with peers and teachers, and this vicious cycle may result in a chronic state of dissatisfaction and unhappiness with self and environment.

Temperament

The formal study of temperament, as the concept now exists in the fields of child development and psychiatry, is of recent origin. However, the recognition that individuals differ behaviorally from birth onward dates back at least to Hippocrates' description of the four humors, and undoubtedly even before.

Temperament may be conceptualized as the behavioral style of an individual. It is the *how*, rather than the *what* (abilities and content) or the *why* (motivations) of behavior. When we refer to temperament, we are concerned with the *way* in which a child or an adult behaves. A group of children may all eat skillfully, throw a ball accurately, and have the same motivations for these activities. Yet, they may differ with respect to the intensity with which they act, the rate at which they move, the mood they express, and the readiness with which they shift to a new activity.

Temperament is a phenomenological term used to describe the characteristic tempo, rhythmicity, adaptability, energy expenditure, mood, and focus of attention of a child, independent of the content of any specific behavior. A formal analysis of behavior in terms of the *why*, *what*, and *how* has been used by workers such as Guilford (1959) and Cattell (1950). The latter identifies "the three modalities of behavior traits" as the "dynamic traits or interests . . . [including] basic drives plus acquired interests such as attitudes and sentiments"; "abilities, shown by how well the person makes this way to the accepted goals"; and temperament, "definable by exclusion as those traits which are unaffected by incentive or complexity . . . like highstrungness, speed, energy and emotional reactivity, which common observation suggests are largely constitutional."

A number of students of human personality have discussed the phenomenon of temperament, both in the past and in recent years. Thus in 1937 Freud asserted that "each individual ego is endowed from the beginning with its peculiar dispositions and tendencies" (1950). In the 1930s two pioneer workers in child development, Gesell

(Gesell and Ames, 1937) and Shirley (1931, 1933) reported significant individual differences in the behavioral characteristics of infants. Somewhat earlier, Pavlov (1927) and his followers postulated the existence of congenitally determined types of nervous systems as basic to the course of subsequent behavioral development. They classified different types of nervous systems according to the balance between excitation and inhibition, attempting to explain features of both normal and abnormal behavioral states on this basis.

In the 1940s and 1950s, a number of studies appeared that reported observations of individual differences in infants and young children in specific, discrete areas of functioning such as motility (Fries and Woolf, 1953), perceptual responses (Bergman and Escalona, 1949), sleeping and feeding patterns (Escalona, 1953), drive endowment (Alpert *et al.*, 1956), quality and intensity of emotional tone (Meili, 1959), social responsiveness (Gesell and Ames, 1937), autonomic response patterns (Bridger and Reiser, 1959; Grossman and Greenberg, 1957; Richmond and Lustman, 1955); biochemical individuality (Mirsky, 1953; Williams, 1956), and electroencephalographic patterns (Grey-Walter, 1953). These various reports emphasized that individual differences appeared to be present at birth and appeared not to be determined by postnatal experience. Abrams and Neubauer (1975) have more recently differentiated young infants on the basis of "person"- or "thing"-orientedness and have suggested that this characteristic influences the developmental process.

However, these researchers either did not formulate a systematic approach to temperament or failed to provide data on its functional significance, or both. For this reason, the discussion of temperament in this chapter deals with the concepts and data developed by Chess and Thomas and the findings of other studies derived from their longitudinal investigations. Dr. Herbert Birch joined Chess and Thomas as a senior research colleague a few years after their study began and participated actively in the work until his untimely death in 1973.

The New York Longitudinal Study of temperament, started in 1956 and still going on, began with the clinical observation that individual differences in child behavior are evident in the first few weeks of life. It was also noted that one-to-one correlations between a child's environmental influences and psychological development were impossible to make. And finally, there was concern about the psychological harm done by the then-fashionable assumption that mothers were responsible for all behavioral deviations and serious mental illnesses in their children.

The longitudinal study gathered data from parents on their child's behavior at regular intervals and verified these data with independent observations in the home and school, teacher interviews, and psychometric tests (Thomas *et al.*, 1963, 1968). Later samples included children born prematurely (Hertzig, 1974), children of working-class Puerto Rican background (Hertzig *et al.*, 1968), mildly retarded children (Chess and Korn, 1970), and children with congenital rubella (Chess *et al.*, 1971).

The identification of nine specific characteristics was achieved by an inductive analysis of the behavioral protocols. The nine categories of temperament are:

- *Activity Level.* The frequency and speed of movement of the child; whether wiggling in the bath or crib in early infancy or crawling, walking, or running in later developmental stages.
- *Rhythmicity.* Biological regularity or irregularity as seen in such functions as the sleep-wake cycle and the timing of hunger and defecation.
- *Approach/Withdrawal.* The immediate reaction of the child to a new experience—such as a new bed, place, person, or organization of schedule—in terms of his acceptance or rejection, without regard to the manner in which the acceptance or rejection is expressed.
- *Adaptability.* When a new experience has been withdrawn from or a new schedule imposed, does it require a short, moderate, or long time for adaptation to occur?
- *Threshold.* The minimum strength of stimulus required to engage the child's notice, without regard to the positive or negative direction or strength of his reaction.
- *Intensity.* The energy expenditure given to the expression of mood, without regard to the direction of the mood itself.
- *Mood.* The predominance, during waking hours, of positive mood as opposed to neutral or negative mood expression.
- *Distractibility.* The three scale points here are determined by the ease with which the child's attention is drawn from an ongoing activity by a peripheral stimulus, with cessation of the original activity and attention to the new one.
- *Attention Span and Persistence.* This is a double category, joined because operationally these two qualities could not be reliably differentiated for qualitative scoring despite having separate definitions. Attention span refers to the length of uninterrupted attention given to a single activity, such as gazing at a mobile,

playing with stacking toys, or working at a model or
homework. Persistence refers both to continuous, uninterrupted activity directed toward task completion and to spontaneous return to the task after its interruption.

It is of interest that frequency curves very similar to those identified in the original New York Longitudinal Study sample have been
found in different populations for those temperamental qualities. Such
populations include working-class Puerto Rican children (Thomas and
Chess, 1977), middle-class mentally retarded children (Chess and
Korn, 1970), children with congenital rubella (Chess et al., 1971),
children with neurologic damage associated with prematurity (Hertzig, 1974), and Norwegian twins (Torgersen, 1973).

Three major constellations of temperamental characteristics have
been found to be of importance during childhood in both normative
and problem development. These are the Difficult Child, the Easy
Child, and the Slow-to-Warm-Up Child. The Difficult Child is characterized by biological irregularity, predominance of negative mood,
high intensity of expressiveness, withdrawing reactions to new stimuli, and slow adaptability. These behaviors make for stormy withdrawals from new experiences and a need for repeated exposures to
encourage adaptation. Once adaptation occurs, such children are
usually delightfully expressive in their positive appreciation of the
events in which they participate. During infancy, when nurturing
centers around sleep, eating, diaper changing, and toilet training, biological irregularity makes for stressful days and nights for the parents
and a possible feedback of their negative attitudes to the infant.

The Easy Child, in contrast, is usually described by parents as a
"good" baby. He is biologically highly regular and predictable, has a
predominantly positive mood, expresses moods with mild or moderate energy level, approaches new situations, and adapts quickly. Thus
early child-rearing practices tend to go smoothly and the parents feel
properly rewarded for having been loving and nurturing, with behavioral evidence that can easily be appreciated by the onlooker. The
parents of the Difficult Child, in contrast, often believe themselves
responsible for their child's style of behavior. They all too frequently
believe the conventional wisdom that negative reactions of babies are
ipso facto proof of parental rejection. The stormy responses of the child
to new situations and demands then undermine their confidence that
they did indeed want and love the baby. Even without such guilt reactions, they may feel robbed of the expected pleasures of parenthood
and begin to anticipate contacts with the child with dread or dislike.

The Slow-to-Warm-Up Child has the characteristics of the Difficult Child with the exception that negative reactions are mildly expressed. These children are shy: they withdraw from new situations by hiding behind mother and quietly moving apart from the group. They are often called "anxious" when in fact they are participant observers who, given an opportunity for repeated exposures to the new stimuli, gradually and spontaneously draw closer. Adaptation is slow, but unless such a child is rushed more quickly than is consonant with his style, his tendency is to move into the new situation with growing outward evidence of quiet enjoyment. Should a new element enter the situation, however, there may be another period of withdrawal, with a gradual return to active participation as before.

In the course of these various longitudinal studies, it has been possible to identify several interactive considerations that have pertinence to the theoretical and practical concepts of developmental dynamics, with particular relevance to normal and pathological behavioral outcomes. These involve such issues as the influence of the child's temperament on parental child-rearing practices; the selective impact of different events and attitudes on individual children, vulnerability to the formation of behavior disorders; the role of anxiety in the genesis and maintenance of behavior disorders; symptom selection; and the continuity and discontinuity of temperament over time.

Influence of Child-Rearing Practices. There is a tendency to regard children's reactions to parental attitudes and events, such as the birth of a sibling or separation, as if they evoke similar responses from all or most children. Child care practices had largely been predicated on the suppositions of the universality of reactions: stranger "anxiety" around 8 months, need for a single female caretaker throughout early infancy, one set of rules for weaning and toilet training. However, with the variety of temperamental patterns that children show from early infancy on, it has long been clear to mothers, baby nurses, and indeed most pediatricians that child care practices, to be successful, must differ for different children. As a simplified example, given an intense, highly active, biologically irregular baby, the old style of toilet training, which involved placing the baby who was motorically capable of sitting in comfort—at, say, 10–12 months of age—on a small potty seat up to one-half hour after each meal, was doomed to failure for several reasons. The timing of the bowel movements was unpredictable, the child's ability to sit for more than a few moments in comfort was nil, his protests were guaranteed to be loud and clear. If this baby was also persistent, the scene of the protest would go on for a long time. On the other hand, the more current opinion that toilet training should be deferred until 18 months, 2 years, or later is unnecessary for those babies who are biologically regular, have low or moderate activity level, and are moderate or low in intensity of mood expressiveness. Such babies may very well be able to deposit their bowel movements in a potty at the predictable time daily, with pleasure in the accomplishment and no stress whatever from the procedure. Thus the same child care practice in bowel training may produce widely different experiences. For one child it may be highly stressful, while for another it may be a happy experience leading to quick mastery. In similar fashion, the temperamental constellation of the child influences the sequence and the impact of the parental handling in the areas of socialization, nurturing, discipline, and the like.

Selective Impact. The above example also illustrates the issue of the selective impact of events and attitudes on children's reactions to their experiences. As a further illustration, a child's temperamental qualities largely determine whether he feels alarm, little concern, or great pleasure when, at 3 or 4 years old, he becomes separated from his mother in a large store. An approaching youngster, with positive mood, for whom all new experiences and new people are welcome, usually ends up having a friendly adventure from which he draws the confirmation that people take care of him. The lesson to him may be that getting lost is great fun. The withdrawing child, on the other hand, reacts negatively to the friendly overtures of the strangers who suddenly surround him. If, in addition, he is intense in mood expressiveness, the experience may be one of great stress with long-lasting fear of parental separation.

Vulnerability to Behavior Disorders. Within all of the groups studied, it has been found that the temperamental constellation of the Difficult Child creates a greater risk for stressful interaction with the environment and hence for the development of behavior disorder (Thomas and Chess, 1977). These children made up 7–10% of the New York Longitudinal Study sample but provided about half of those who developed behavior disorders by age 5 years. Children with intellectual or physical defects plus even mild manifestations of the difficult child constellation were especially vulnerable to the development of a behavior disorder. The vulnerability of a handicapped child can be expressed quantitatively. This is done by categorizing an individual child in terms of how many of the five signs of the difficult child he shows: biologic irregularity, predominance of negative mood, high intensity of mood expressiveness, high withdrawal from new situations, and slow adaptation. With this method of comparison, it was found that one less sign of the difficult child was required in the mentally retarded sample to evoke the same probability of behavior disorder development as in the New York Longitudinal Study sample (Chess and Korn, 1970). A similar comparison showed that the congenital rubella children with behavior disorders showed a high incidence of four or five signs of the difficult child (Chess et al., 1971).

It is essential to emphasize, however, that a child with *any* temperamental pattern may, under specific circumstances of environmental expectations and demands, prove vulnerable to behavior disorder development. This may occur most frequently in children with the difficult child constellation, but even a child with diametrically opposite temperament traits—that is, the easy child—may not be able to master certain types of situational stresses and conflicts.

In analyzing the nature of the temperament–environment interactive process, Chess and Thomas have found the evolutionary concept of "goodness of fit" as elaborated by Henderson (1913) and the related ideas of consonance and dissonance to be very useful. Goodness of fit results when the properties, expectations, and demands of the environment are in accord with the organism's own capacities, characteristics, and style of behavior. When *consonance* between organism and environment is present, optimal development in a progressive direction is possible. Conversely, poorness of fit involves discrepancies and *dissonances* between environmental opportunities and demands and the capacities and characteristics of the organism, so that distorted development and maladaptive functioning occur. Goodness of fit is not an abstract concept but is based on the values and demands of a given culture or socioeconomic group.

It should be stated that goodness of fit does not imply an absence of stress and conflict. Quite the contrary. Stress and conflict are the inevitable concomitants of the developmental process, in which new expectations, demands for change, and progressively higher levels of functioning occur continuously as the child grows older. Demands, stresses, and conflicts, when consonant with the child's developmental potentials and capacities for mastery, may be constructive in their consequences and should not be considered inevitable causes of behavior disturbance. The issue involved in disturbed behavioral functioning is rather one of *excessive* stress resulting from a poorness of fit and dissonance between environmental expectations and demands and capacities of the child at a particular level of development.

Thus each temperamental trait or cluster is capable of entering into an excessively stressful and pathogenic interaction with specific environmental expectations or demands. The highly active child is vulnerable to the demand that he sit quietly for long periods; the easily distractible youngster finds it difficult or impossible to concentrate for long periods when peripheral stimuli are abundant; the highly persistent child becomes very frustrated when forced to terminate an ongoing activity in which he is absorbed. The easy child can develop a behavior disorder if there is conflict between the behavior patterns he learns at home to conform to parental goals and the contradictory expectations of teachers or peer groups. The slow-to-warm-up child is vulnerable to any new situation that demands rapid adaptation.

"Goodness of fit" may depend on more than the temperament–environment interaction. A physical handicap, a perceptual or cognitive defect, or multiple or continuous environmental traumata may make it difficult or impossible for a child to cope with the environmental demands that other children usually master smoothly.

Even though the difficult child is most vulnerable to the development of behavior disorder, this does not imply a negative prognosis for preventive or therapeutic intervention. In each instance, the crucial question is whether the parents or teachers are capable of understanding the excessively stressful character of their demands on the specific temperament of the child and are willing and able to make the changes required to enable the child to cope successfully and constructively with these demands.

Anxiety. When the group of children under five years of age who had behavior disorders were examined, there was no evidence that anxiety consistently preceded the onset of symptoms. The dynamic progression appeared to be from, first, clear behavioral expression of the child's temperamental individuality to, second, parental handling that was dissonant with the youngster's temperament to, third, the emergence of a behavior disorder whose symptoms reflected the child's temperament and the parental style. Thus a withdrawing child who in infancy had rejected each new food initially but accepted it after repeated contact showed this withdrawal response at his first exposure to nursery school. Pushed into abrupt exposure to this totally new situation, with new children, new teacher, and the first experience with an authority and nurturing figure outside of the family, this child withdrew more and more from the group's activities. With no opportunity for a gradual adaptation to these many new social expectations, a behavior problem characterized by nonparticipation in play with other children developed. Anxiety then became a secondary, but increasingly important, feature that acted to exacerbate the behavior problem.

At later ages, it was found that the child began to use more sophisticated defenses and symbolization began to appear. As the behavior disorder continued, poor self-image also became prominent.

Symptom Selection. Why one symptom as opposed to another appears in an individual has been long an issue of interest. It would appear that a knowledge of a child's temperament sheds some light on symptom choice, although it still leaves many unanswered questions.

Under stress, a child reacts with a more extreme expression of his individual behavioral style. Thus a quiet child becomes withdrawn, while a highly active youngster may show hyperactivity when events and/or attitudes are stressful. The slow-to-warm-up youngster may be at particular risk for school phobia. The distractible youngster with short attention span is more likely to exhibit school learning difficulties than is a nondistractible youngster of the same age and intellectual level.

Social class and ethnic membership may influence the degree of consonance or dissonance between a child's temperament and environment and the nature and severity of symptom development. Child-rearing practices may differ, and the resources available to the family may give greater or lesser flexibility in relation to the individual child's temperamental attributes. For example, a financially comfortable middle-class family with a high-activity child may be able to move to a suburban house with grounds or play areas that give this child's activity expression. In contrast, a poor urban family, just as concerned with the welfare of its children but without this option of moving to the suburbs, may have to keep a highly active child confined to a small apartment for his own safety. This may easily create excessive stress for the child, with the risk of a metamorphosis of high normal activity into pathological hyperactivity.

The effect of group differences in child-rearing practices on symptom development can be illustrated by a comparison of the New York Longitudinal Study (NYLS) sample and a similarly studied sample of New York City children from Puerto Rican working-class families (PRWC) (Thomas *et al.*, 1974). Complaints about sleep problems in the NYLS sample were most numerous in the preschool years. As a group, these parents were not tolerant of deviant behavior in this area and demanded that their children establish regular sleeping habits early. By contrast, the PRWC parents tolerated late bedtimes and night awakening in their preschool children, and few sleep problems developed. When these children approached school age, however, the situation changed dramatically. As they began school at age 6 years, they had to go to sleep and get up promptly at regular hours, eat without dawdling, dress quickly, and arrive at school on time—all functions that they had not previously been required to perform. This sequence correlated with the finding that almost half of the PRWC sample that came to notice between the ages of 5 and 9 presented sleep problems, whereas only one child under 5 had a sleep difficulty.

Discipline problems were significantly more frequent in the PRWC children, whose parents were concerned about the risk of delinquency in the East Harlem community. Learning problems, on the other hand, were more common in the middle-class children, whose parents frequently had overriding concern with scholastic success and exerted considerable pressure on their children for superior cognitive performance.

These findings emphasize the need for understanding the social and cultural background when evaluating what constitutes excessive stress for any individual child. The incidence at any age period and the types of presenting symptoms may reflect parental expectations as much as they do problems of functioning intrinsic to the child.

Temperamental Stability. The identification of temperament becomes more complex as the child grows older. Behavioral characteristics become increasingly affected by the continuously evolving interaction of the temperament with motivations, capabilities, and special life events. Nevertheless, temperamental qualities continue to be a significant element of the individual's behavior and influence his style of reaction to the increasingly complex demands of the environment. It becomes important, therefore, to know whether the temperamental assessment in infancy and early childhood is consistent over time and can be assumed to remain the same during middle childhood, adolescence, and/or adult life periods. One of the most difficult issues with regard to making this determination is that of definitional identity. Thus phenomenologically identical behaviors at widely spaced ages may not have the same meaning, whether it be temper tantrums or such temperamental qualities as attention span or speed of adaptation. Within the New York Longitudinal Study, this question has been examined through an analysis of development in middle childhood (Thomas and Chess, 1972), a study of the relationship between temperament, school functioning, and learning (Chess *et al.*, 1976), and on examination of the evolution of behavior disorders into the years of adolescence (Thomas and Chess, 1976). Five patterns have been defined: clear-cut consistency in temperament; consistency in some aspects of temperament at one period and in other aspects at other times; distortion of the expression of temperament by other factors, such as psychodynamic patterns; consistency in temperament but qualitative change in temperament–environment interaction; and finally, change in a conspicuous temperamental trait. It was found that individual children might show a combination of several of these five possibilities.

Thus no linear, predictable sequence in temperament from infancy onward can be assumed. This is hardly surprising, considering that all other psychological phenomena, such as intellectual competence, coping mechanisms, adaptive patterns, and value systems can and do change over time. What is predictable is the process of organism–environment interaction. Consistency in development comes from continuity over time in both the organism and the significant features of the environment. Discontinuity results from changes in one or the other or both that make for modification and change in development.

Further Studies of Temperament. Categories of temperament delineated by the New York Longitudinal Study have generated significant interest in the fields of child development and psychopathology of childhood. Modified strategies have been used in accordance with the research question addressed. For example, Katcher (Thomas and Chess, 1977) has determined that temperamental individuality could be identified and rated during the neonatal period. By using two periods of observation on the second and fourth days of life in 16 normal neonates and a semistructured interview with the nurse, he found that seven of the nine categories could be scored.

Kringlen and Torgersen have studied the possible origins of temperamental qualities in their twin study of a group of Norwegian children (Torgersen, 1973). The persistence of temperamental individuality in a uniform child-rearing milieu was confirmed by Marcus *et al.* (1969). The relationship of temperamental characteristics to such pediatric issues as night awakening and colic has also attracted attention (Carey, 1974).

The identification of temperamental categories and their significance for psychological development requires detailed and lengthy data gathering and analytic methods. For practical clinical usage, more economical procedures are necessary. Consequently questionnaires have been developed that can be given to parents and teachers. These require 20–30 minutes for completion and approximately 10 minutes for scoring. With such questionnaires, the determination of temperament can be parsimoniously achieved by psychiatrist, pediatrician, educator, or other child care professional (Thomas and Chess, 1977). A pediatrician, William Carey, (1972) has already constructed a questionnaire for birth to 18 months, while Chess and Thomas have developed one for the 3–7 year periods. Work is in progress on similar questionnaires for the other age periods of childhood.

Sex

Epidemiologic surveys and clinical studies have shown that behavior deviations during childhood occur with different frequency among boys and girls. Furthermore, stressful life events may exert differential influence on the two sexes.

Sex differences in behavior and personality have been widely reported, although cross-cultural studies have tended to show these differences to be more the results of cultural sex typing than intrinsic to different sexes (Whiting and Edwards, 1973). Whether the higher aggressiveness of the male is a biological or sociocultural issue remains undecided.

Of the psychiatric disorders with male preponderance, developmental disorders such as speech problems, enuresis, and early infantile autism are invariably noted. The cause of such preponderance is a matter of conjecture.

The higher frequency of antisocial behaviors in boys has been explained partly on the basis of presumed aggressiveness in males, although girls are by no means exempt from manifesting such problems. Furthermore, changing social circumstances seem to produce changes in the available statistics of delinquency, with reports of an increased rate of delinquency for girls. Feeding problems, sibling rivalry, phobias, and hysteria all have been reported to occur more in girls. Differential sex ratios for various psychiatric disorders (suicide and homicide, for example) are also reported in adults. So far no overall hypothesis that accounts for these differences has been presented.

Intrafamilial Factors

A most important environmental and experiental base for a child's personality development is the quality and the nature of his early human environment—that network of interdependent group relationships that is called the family. The child may be born into a nuclear family and be the first of many to come, or he may remain the only child. He may have only one parent as caretaker, or he may be a member of an extended family with several generations living together. His care may be the responsibility of one or more people in a household, or he may be cared for in an institution by a series of caretakers, with or without any opportunity for a continuous stable relationship.

The complexities and subtleties of the infant's interaction within various caretaking arrangements defy any simple categorization. While the global concept of maternal deprivation has been frequently used to explain the genesis of psychopathology in children, it is now quite clear that loss or absence of the biological mother or variations in caretaking practices are only one among the multitude of factors influencing the child's future development (Rosenthal *et al.*, 1975).

From the standpoint of personality development, an effective environment should meet the child's physiological needs; provide him with appropriate cognitive, motor, and perceptual stimulation; and prepare him for emotional give-and-take with other human beings. We consider the concept of emotional relationships to be broader than socialization, since we believe that capacity for affective experience—that is, to feel sympathy and empathy and have a sense of belonging to the human race—is more than conformity with social expectations and competence in performing various social roles.

The infant's early environment may be deficient in one or more areas. Neglected children may be under- or overstimulated. Abused children may be well fed and cognitively and perceptually well developed; they may be well behaved and socially skillful, even though they are overwhelmed by chronic parental hostility and possibly by physical violence. A child reared in an institution may receive all the necessary care except for an opportunity to form an emotional bond with an adult, or he may indeed be more fortunate in this respect than a child raised by a seriously disturbed mother.

Maternal Deprivation. The concept of maternal deprivation as ctiologically significant in a variety of psychiatric disorders of childhood and later life has undergone numerous refinements and has lost much of its explanatory appeal since first espoused by Bowlby in 1951.

Cross-cultural studies have discounted the view that multiple mothering may be detrimental to the child's emotional growth (Mead, 1962). The presence of the mother does not guarantee bond formation, and the infant's characteristics exert a powerful influence on the shaping of parental attitudes. A placid and quiet infant may invite a frenzy of activities from an overconcerned mother, making the infant irritable and frightened and leaving the mother with a sense of dissatisfaction with the child and insecurity regarding her own inadequacy as a mother. Conversely, a very alert and vigorous infant may not be well appreciated by a mother who prefers quiet babies. The father's expectations and preferences may be quite the opposite of those of the mother, and the infant may thus become more intensely involved with and attached to the father. Since there is no way by which one can assess the likelihood of temperamental compatibility between an unborn infant and his biological mother, the chance for smooth bond formation is greater when more than one or two caretakers are available to the infant for developing attachment.

Schaffer and Emerson (1964) reported that among a group of 18-month-old children, principal bond attachment was not always to the mother; also, children showed multiple attachments even when their strongest bond was with the mother or the father. In reviewing the caretaking arrangement of kibbutzim children, Bowlby (1969) concluded that the intensity of interaction seems to be a more important factor in bond formation than the length of time that a child spends in parental company. Feeding and bodily caretaking is not a necessary condition for bond formation (Schaffer, 1971), although it is assumed that any pleasurable interaction that gratifies needs increases the likelihood of attachments.

The notion of a sensitive and critical period for bond formation has been held by most workers in the field, although the evidence is mainly based on studies of children's reactions to separation from their mothers and a familiar environment. Children under 6 months of age do not seem to react with distress when they are removed from their homes or are in the company of strangers, while most children between 1 and 2 years of age react unfavorably to the separation. However, even for these children, prior acquaintance with the new caretakers or the presence of a younger sib may lessen the amount of observable distress. Only a minority of children show the reaction of protest, despair, and detachment that Bowlby has reported. Furthermore, the occurrence of such reactions depends upon the degree of stress inherent in the circumstances leading to the child's separation from the family, as well as the age of the child and the amount of preparation and information that he has received prior to the actual separation.

Studies of the effects of the length tend to suggest that long-term separations may be more stressful than short-term ones. Children who have had previous unhappy experiences with separation are more likely to react with distress upon the repetition of the experience.

The long-term consequences of early separation cannot be differentiated from the circumstances preceding or following the actual bond disruption. Although maternal deprivation has been said to lead to mental and physical growth retardation and delinquency, it now appears that the children studied had suffered other adverse conditions, such as lack of stimulation, failure to thrive because of malnutrition, and long-standing parental conflicts, before they were actually separated from their mothers.

Distortion of bond formation may be a more detrimental factor than disruption of the affective bond in children's future emotional health and sense of self-confidence and self-worth. In fact, children of rejecting parents show more distress upon separating from them than children who have enjoyed parental acceptance.

It is probably a safe assumption that a continuous, loving relationship with a limited number of individuals is necesary for an infant's emotional development; discontinuous early experiences with people hinder development either by depriving the infant of a necessary experience or by taxing his capacities for reciprocal interactions and adjustments.

After a lengthy review of the literature on maternal deprivation, Michael Rutter (1972) concluded that "The most parsimonious explanation of the research findings suggests that a child needs to have the presence of a person to whom he is attached, but it is irrelevant whether or not this person is his mother."

However, the idea that a young child cannot relate to others in the absence of the person to whom he has been attached and is therefore bound to suffer certain deficiencies cannot be accepted uncritically. While it is true that young children's memory and language are not fully developed, it may be that once the experience of bonding has been felt, what is important is the unarticulated ability to relate to others rather than the continuation of an emotional tie with a single person.

Fatherless homes. The permanent absence of the father, whether because of desertion, divorce, or death, usually leaves the mother as breadwinner as well as the sole adult caretaker of the children; this tends to lower the family's socioeconomic status. The adverse effects of the permanent absence of the father on the children, therefore, can be related not only to the lack of an important individual in the child's life but to the impact of conditions associated with the broken home. Furthermore, it must be remembered that every two-parent family does not provide the child with ideal relationships with both parents. In fact, in some families the fathers are "psychologically absent" to their children and their wives; in other families chronic conflict between the two parents creates an emotionally unhealthy environment that is more stressful than a home that is actually broken.

Studies of fatherless children have emphasized the role of the father in sexual identification, particularly in boys. On a number of personality inventories and projective tests, these boys are found to have lower masculine identification than boys living with their fathers. However, the significance of such findings for the future development and the mental health of the child is not clear. There are some claims in literature that fatherless male children are disproportionately represented among adults with disturbed sexual orientation. The consequence of the father's absence on sexual identification of girls is even more unclear, although sex typing and reinforcement for sexual role acceptance seems to be dependent on both parents' behavior for girls as well as boys.

Since a higher proportion of delinquents come from broken homes, there has been some speculation regarding the role of the father in socializing the children. However, studies of this type consider only one aspect of the multitude of adverse conditions surrounding such children. In a thoughtful review of research regarding fatherless homes, Herzog and Sudia (1968) concluded that: "existing data do not permit a decisive answer to questions about the effects on children of fatherlessness." In a comparison of 105 children from fatherless homes and 53 children living in intact families who were all attending the University of Florida Mental Health Clinic, Kogelschatz *et al.* (1972) found that the fatherless children were more withdrawn and showed poorer peer relationships than the children with fathers. In studying the mental status of the two groups, the authors stated, "It appeared in most cases that father absence was no more singular than economic class membership in its influence upon the nature and severity of a fatherless child's problems."

So far we have seen that father absence cannot be studied as an independent variable in the adjustment or maladjustment of children. The impact of the absence of the father depends on such factors as the previous relationship of the child with the father and the mother's subsequent reaction to the child. When the father is absent through death or socially acceptable causes, the effect on the household and the emotional climate of the home is quite different than when the father has deserted the family or is in a mental or correctional institution. The absent father may in fact remain a positive or even idealized person when the mother presents a positive image of him to the children. On the other hand, the mother may come to project the undesirable traits of the father on a particular child, or she may turn to a child for the kind of support that the father was expected to give. Some mothers may sexualize their relationship with their sons or become extremely concerned about the sexual interests of their daughters, fearing that lack of father may actually give the daughter a license to engage in unacceptable sexual activities. Other mothers turn for support to their own family, and children's discipline and care are thus shifted to the grandparents, with continuous disagreement among the grandparents and the mother as to the goal or the mechanism of child-rearing practices.

The age of the child is also an important factor in his subsequent adjustment to the father's absence. Younger children may be more capable of accepting the continuation of the mother's authority than adolescents, who are in the process of seeking their own independence.

Another male member of the family or an outsider may come to be a substitute father for the fatherless child, with or without the mother's agreement and encouragement. In such situations, the child's conflict stems from his own wishes and his mother's preference and is not related to the father's absence *per se*, since the same situation might have occurred with the father in residence.

What can be irrefutably assumed is that the presence of an adequate and affectionate father is desirable for the normal personality development of a child, but his absence may be compensated for by the remaining adults in the family with little permanent psychological sequela.

Divorce. Divorce is an unpleasant, distressing experience for all children and for the majority of their parents. Since divorce is usually the consequence of long-term conflicts and disharmony between the parents, the psychological reactions of the children cannot be solely related to the final breakup of the home. These children have usually lived through the painful dissolution of the parental relationship, have found themselves involved in the conflicts, and, at times, have been forced to take sides.

The children's immediate reaction to the divorce may be grief over the loss of their intact family, concern and guilt regarding their own role in the breakup of the marriage, shame and uneasiness with their peer group, and anxiety regarding their own future and continuing relations with both parents (Wallerstein and Kelly, 1975). In most cases, this stage is of transient nature and children soon make the necessary adjustment to their new status. Some children remain enmeshed in the postdivorce conflicts between the parents. Some parents exploit the presence of the children to continue their conflictual relationship. They expect their children to take sides regarding the money, visitation rights, and other matters related to the divorced parents' personal lives. Furthermore, these children receive contradictory messages regarding the parents' desire to continue their relationship even though the final steps to end the marriage have been taken. In more than one-third of divorce cases, the turbulent relationship between parents continues after the divorce, and studies show that these are the cases in which children exhibit the greatest incidences of maladjustment following the divorce.

Of 153 consecutive children referred to the University of Wisconsin Child Psychiatry Clinic, Westman *et al.* (1970) found that 23, or 15%, were children of divorced parents. Although in the majority of cases the divorces had taken place two years prior to the referral, in 8 cases the postdivorce interaction between the parents had remained conflictual. The remaining 15 had lost complete contact with one parent, usually the father, and had thus been abandoned. None of the children came from a background in which divorce had been satisfactorily handled.

In reviewing the clinical status of these children, the authors found that their subjects continued to wish for parental reunion even though in some cases the parents had actually married new partners.

The children had an exaggerated view of their own responsibility for the divorce and considered the expenses of their own upkeep or their bad behavior to have been the cause of parental disagreement.

When there are postdivorce legal procedures related to custody and visitation rights, the contesting parent usually casts doubts on the moral character or adequacy of the other parent in relation to children. This places the child in a dilemma as to which parent to believe and how to interpret his own perception of the situation when the two important adults in his life have such differing views.

The divorce *per se* need not be more than a transient stress to the child when the parents can achieve a satisfactory arrangement for dissolving their marriage and continuing their shared responsibilities as parents. However, when children are used as pawns in postdivorce struggles, the divorce becomes pathogenic in that it will present a continuous source of stress to the child and seriously distort the parent–child relationship.

Adopted Children. A review of literature regarding the adjustment of adopted children shows that most studies tend to reveal a higher rate of emotional problems among the adoptee than in the general population. However, most studies are open to methodological criticism. In the absence of a well-planned epidemiologic study, Lawton *et al.* (1964) concluded after reviewing the literature that the data from clinical impressions and studies of clinic populations cannot be uncritically accepted.

Bohman (1972) chose a sample of 168 adopted children (98 boys and 75 girls) from the registry of the Stockholm Adoption Agency and was able to conduct interviews with 122 parents living in Stockholm and the teachers of all except 5 of the children attending schools. Information regarding the biological parents was collected from various official records. The children had all been placed before 1 year of age, with the majority adopted before 6 months of age. Of adoptive parents, 71% were from the professional and managerial class. The reason for childlessness in the majority of cases was infertility of one or both parents, although the cause of infertility had not been ascertained in 26% of the parents, and 5% reported childlessness to be due to voluntary contraceptive practices.

Dissolution of the marriage due to the death of one parent or to divorce had resulted in one in every six adoptees being raised in a one-parent family. This is roughly the same ratio as that for the general children population of Stockholm.

The studies of school records and teacher interviews showed the same percentage of academic difficulties for adopted as for nonadopted children; however, of the adopted boys, 22% were considered maladjusted by teachers as compared to 12% of their nonadopted classmates. Another 35% were reported to have moderate difficulties, while only 18% of the nonadopted children fell into this category. These differences were statistically significant.

Adopted girls showed the same trend for higher level of maladjustment in comparison with their same-sex classmates, although the difference was not statistically significant. Of the adopted children, 80% had been informed of their adopted status before age 7.

The author concluded that adoptive status, particularly in boys, seems to be associated with a higher percentage of maladjustment. None of the biological or environmental factors studied showed a significant correlation with emotional maladjustment in this group.

Speculations regarding the reasons for the higher rate of maladjustment have been based on the nature of the parent–child relationship; the possible contribution of parental disharmony and dissatisfaction regarding the parent's own or the spouse's infertility; the out-of-wedlock status of the child implied in the adoption; and societal views and reaction to adoptive families and adopted children.

Children may be preoccupied with their own fantasies of two sets of parents, with their desire to know their biological parents, and with their opinions of themselves as being unwanted and abandoned. Among the 118 children studied by Schechter *et al.* (1964), only a small percentage reacted positively when informed about their adoptive status, while 12% reacted negatively, and the majority did not show any immediate reaction.

Some adopted children are involved in a continuous interaction of a testing nature with their adoptive parents in order to reaffirm their own status and to be reassured that they are wanted. Others use their adopted status as an excuse for defiance of their adoptive parents' values and standards. During adolescence, some children decide to pattern themselves after their fantasies of their absent biological parents and are thus involved in a conflictual relationship with the adoptive parents.

Some adoptive parents may in turn relate the child's undesirable characteristics to his supposedly biological and hereditary background, thus reinforcing the child's desire for identification with the absent parents.

When parents do not inform the child of his adoptive status, the discovery may be extremely painful to the child because he feels both betrayed by the adoptive parents and abandoned by the biological ones.

There is complete agreement in the literature regarding the following aspects of adoption: (1) children should be placed with adoptive parents during the first two years of life; and (2) the fact of adoption should be revealed to the child as soon as it is within his ability to comprehend the concept of adoption.

The Child's Role in the Family. The family is a culturally defined unit that links the individual to the larger community around him. As a unit, the family strives for self-preservation as well as the preservation of its individual members, with their various ages, sexes, personalities, needs, and aspirations. In a healthy family, members share compatible values and realistic goals and are aware of their own and others' needs. They provide each other with support and gratification, facilitate each other's growth, and are able to search for appropriate solutions for the inevitable conflicts that arise within a network of interdependent individuals. In such a family, the child's birth is planned or desired, his sex and physical characteristics are acceptable, his growth is encouraged, his needs are fulfilled, and, in turn, he is expected to learn to share the value system of the family, to adjust to the appropriate demands placed upon him, and to accept the collective aspirations of the family group. When there is a conflict between the parents' expectation and the child's abilities, it is the parents who have the obligation to reevaluate their demands and to readjust their expectations in order to provide a continuous source of support and encouragement for the child.

In such a family, the child gains a sense of self-confidence and self-esteem. He receives his first and most reliable training in sensitivity to and respect for others. He participates in finding appropriate solutions for intrafamilial conflicts. He is able to tolerate the limits placed on his desires and impulses by the necessity of living and interacting with other people. He perceives interpersonal relationships as mutually gratifying and comes to consider his family as a source of support in dealing with the uncertainties and stresses of life. He is not subject to excessive, chronic guilt nor a victim of self-doubt and anxiety. He grows within the family and with the family.

Unfortunately families are not always healthy, and indeed they may be the breeding grounds for various defects in personality and for behavior deviations. The parents may have married on account of an unwanted pregnancy. They may have fled their own emotionally destructive home atmosphere through hasty marriage, or they may find the close relationship with a spouse confining, destructive, or unsatisfactory. Some children are born unwanted. Their appearance on the scene is at best an undesirable inconvenience and at worst a source of family misfortune. Other children are conceived with the idea that their birth will save the parents' shaky marriage, by providing either a goal for the aimless, unsatisfactory life of the mother or possibly a stabilizing influence on the half-hearted commitment of the father to the marriage. At times, it is only to satisfy the grandparents' desire that a child is conceived, and one or both parents may consider the child as an imposition on their lives.

However, because the family is in a constant state of dynamic interaction, an undesirable child may indeed become desirable; a shaky marriage may become more stable for reasons related or unrelated to the child; or a child who is welcomed at first may become a source of conflict later on.

In a healthy family, the role assigned to the child is compatible with his level of personality development and appropriate for his age. The role is therefore flexible and realistic. On the other hand, the child may be assigned an inappropriate role in a family in conflict. These roles are usually inflexible and unrealistic and serve the family's pathological interaction more than they serve the child. The complexities of role assignment and role fulfillment in the circular system of feedbacks within the family defy any simple categorization. The parents' attitudes, particularly the mother's perception, may be crucial. However, the father and sibs reinforce the assigned role and the child fulfills the expectations placed upon him to varying degrees. The determinants of role assignment and role acceptance or rejection are not always clear, but they are of crucial significance in the child's personality development and the nature of the psychopathology that will be exhibited.

Rollins and Blackwell (1973) described a variety of roles that children may play in their families and the consequences of the role assignment on the child's personality. Children who are referred to as "pet" in the family are showered with love and attention and are praised without having deserved the reward. These children are manipulative and ingratiating and learn to induce guilt in order to gain their purpose. Other children are designated as "baby." They are considered in need of excessive protection. Their misbehavior is tolerated and not disciplined. These children in turn come to view themselves as helpless and in need of protection. They remain emotionally immature and overly dependent on their families. They withdraw from interaction with their peers and find the safety of their home to be the only true place for themselves. The child who is the "peacemaker" is given the role of diverting the family's attention from the underlying conflicts that threaten to break to the surface. Such a child is pressured to deny the realities of the situation, to avoid harsh feelings, and to make light of every unpleasant encounter. He is in a constant state of vigilance and considers any unpleasant clash in the family a sign of his own inadequacy. Children who are scapegoated may come to view themselves as the source of all troubles; since their efforts at change are unsuccessful, they may be chronically dissatisfied and depressed.

Deviant behavior in children may be a direct reflection of an assigned role, such as the anxiety and feeling of inadequacy in an overprotected child, or it may be an effort to escape a particular role designation. Some behavioral symptoms develop as a bargaining position within the family; others are generalized to extrafamilial milieus. In some children, symptom formation serves the function of bringing the drifting parents together; other symptoms reflect the child's desire to escape or to bring outsiders to intervene.

Child-rearing practices are not directly related to role assignment, although the former may be modified in order to reinforce what is expected of the child. For example, parents who are strict disciplinarians may show high tolerance for the misbehavior of the child who is the "pet" or the "baby," while children who are scapegoated may receive unduly harsh punishment for minor infractions of parental rules. Some children are seen as the "reincarnation" of their grandparents or other members of the parents' original families and may be the recipients of favorable or unfavorable treatment by parents because of this fancied resemblance. Mother or father may project the undesirable qualities of the respective spouse on a child, who thus becomes involved in constant bickering that in reality is directed at the other parent.

Inadequate and insecure parents may expect children to provide them with attention and understanding that are beyond the child's capacity and may become resentful and criticize the child for his inability to fulfill such expectations. In families with a high level of disharmony between the parents, the children are exploited. Either their welfare is sacrificed or they are made to feel responsible for maintaining the family equilibrium. Some families are highly intolerant of individual differences among their children and create emotional distance or jealousy among brothers and sisters by constantly comparing the nonconformist child with his or her sib.

In some families, the child's desire for autonomy and independence runs counter to parental wishes, and a variety of subtle or overt pressures are used to keep the child in a dependent state. Children's reality testing may be seriously impaired when one or both parents are psychotic. They may incorporate deviant forms of thinking and communication or may learn to use defenses that are characteristic of the family. The depressed mood of the parents may be contagious for the child, who may reflect the home atmosphere without knowing the cause of it.

The evaluation of a child's deviant behavior must include an assessment of his family. The child's desire and drive for individual growth cannot be separated from his need to be accepted by his family. Family dynamics and expectations are powerful forces that impinge upon the child and may in fact be the source of the problem. The child's perception of his parents, his anxieties regarding the well-being of the family unit, and his ideas about the role assigned to him within the family unit are important factors in diagnosis and treatment.

Child Abuse. The battered-child syndrome was originally identified by pediatricians, who found that the multiple skeletal injuries of some children brought to the hospital could not be satisfactorily explained by the accidental mishaps reported by the parents. In a follow-up study of 50 children who had been hospitalized in Children's Hospital of Pittsburgh from 1949 to 1962 with multiple skeletal injuries, Elmer and Gregg (1967) were able to locate 33 children. Of these, only 20 cases had been unanimously judged abused. Of these 20 children, 8 were diagnosed as seriously disturbed by other physicians; 10 children had IQs below 80. Only 2 children out of the 20 had remained normal in all areas, while one-third of the sample had physical defects clearly related to abuse. Of the 20 children, 10 had been healthy babies at birth, 6 were of low birth weight, 3 had serious illnesses from early life, and 2 were premature. Of the 10 children who had remained with their parents, 6 had remained or fallen below the third percentile for physical growth, while the 10 who lived away from home showed normal physical growth. Of the original 50 children, 5 had been institutionalized with mental retardation; 2 were known to have died at the hands of their own mothers; 3 had died as the result of intracranial trauma; and 1 had died of malnutrition.

Studies of the families of abused children have revealed that while child abuse is not rare among middle-class families, poor, unemployed, and underprivileged families are more likely to inflict excessive physical punishment on their children (Garbino, 1976). Mothers are more frequently the abusive parents, reflecting the fact that caretaking is often the responsibility solely of the mother. Abused children are usually unwanted, although they may have become undesirable only after birth because they were sick, retarded, or difficult to care for. In this respect, premature children, or children who have spent a long time away from their mothers, are at particular risk. The age of the child is an important factor. Children under 3 years of age are more likely to be abused since they are more dependent, less able to defend themselves, and more likely to sustain physical injuries with excessive physical force.

In some families, inadequate mothers feel overwhelmed by life pressures and may actually lose control when angry and inadvertently inflict injuries on a difficult child. Other children develop a pattern of aggression and counteraggression with the parents and, being younger, are less able to withstand the parents' reaction. The stressful life circumstances plaguing some families may result in child abuse. When the parents find themselves unable to cope with the harsh realities of their own lives, the children's demands are a source of irritation and additional stress for them.

Child murder may be an accidental result of child abuse or it may in fact be an intended killing of the child. The first six months of life are particularly risky for children of mothers who are themselves suicidal and who consider murdering the child an altruistic act performed to spare the infant from future disappointments and misery.

In a study of filicide (killing after the first 24 hours of life), Resnick (1969) reported the presence of psychiatric disorder in three-quarters of parents who had murdered their children. The combination of suicidal intention on the part of the parent and an overvalued child was particularly ominous because most parents decided to kill the child as an act of mercy.

Psychological abuse of children is more difficult to define although by no means of less consequence. A child may be exposed to verbal attacks, may be repeatedly punished by starvation, or may be the subject of abusive sexual practices. Apart from the physical defects resulting from repeated injuries, the child's psychological well-being may be in serious danger in an abusive home. Abused children are hostile, tense, and insecure. They may experience a chronic state of rage, which at times is easily expressed. Their view of themselves and of other people is colored by their early painful experiences. Some children protect themselves by inattention to pain and become insensitive to others' sufferings. The failure to trust the parents and the inability to empathize with others are the most lasting sequelae in the child's personality makeup.

Sociocultural Issues

The most consistent finding reported in the psychiatric literature relating to social class is that among the children of poor families there is a higher rate of educational deficiency, low intelligence-test scores, and delinquency than among families from higher social classes. Because some ethnic minorities, such as Afro-Americans, are over-represented among the low socioeconomic strata, the etiology of these behavioral deviations is a subject of controversy between the social pathologists on the one hand and the behavioral geneticists on the other. Both groups consider the research findings basically valid. Their differences are related to the meaning and the significance of the data. Behavior geneticists treat the results of IQ score as meaningful genetic traits indicating genotypic differences among the races, while social pathologists espouse the notion that environmental factors are responsible for the phenotypic heterogeneity of the genotypically homogeneous groups (Deutsch, 1969; Zigler, 1970).

Recently the validity and reliability of the data themselves have come under question on a variety of methodological grounds. It has become evident that the diagnostic processes and assessment procedures are not free from the cultural biases and expectations of the evaluators (Cole and Bruner, 1971). McDermott *et al.* (1965) reviewed the psychiatric evaluations of 263 children of skilled and unskilled blue-collar workers attending the University of Michigan's Children's Psychiatric Hospital. They found that although there were slightly more broken homes, desertions, and divorces in the family background of the skilled workers as compared to the unskilled group, twice as many families among the unskilled group had been rated as unstable and conflict-ridden. Furthermore, children of unskilled laborers had been frequently diagnosed as showing personality disorders and borderline psychosis. These differences among the two subgroups of the lower socieconomic class were not explainable on the basis of data on the record and could be accounted for only by the expectations of the evaluators.

In another study by McDermott *et al.* (1967), the psychiatric records of 853 children from different social classes were searched for the incidence of prenatal and postnatal difficulties associated with diagnoses of mental retardation and chronic brain syndrome. No significant differences in the incidence of reproductive casualties were noted among the members of various occupational groups; however, diagnoses of mental retardation and organic brain syndrome were less frequent in the lowest and the highest social class than in the middle-class children. The authors argued that because it is a well-established fact that the rate of severe mental retardation due to organic damage is not related to socioeconomic backgrounds, the findings of this study again point to the factor of examiners' expectations and biases in interpreting the data. The examiners did not expect to find severe intellectual impairments among the children of the uppermost occupational group and consequently failed to make the appropriate diagnosis. On the other hand, their low expectation regarding the intellectual and educational performance of the children of the poor made it impossible for them to identify their organically caused retardation.

Most behavioral scientists make the implicit assumption that the social class of an individual is totally dependent on his personal characteristics and attributes. The single most important factor in low-social-class status is habitual unemployment—or unskilled and semi-skilled labor—which, in turn, is considered an indicator of little education and, by extension, of a low IQ score. The basic flaw in this assumption is that it ignores the economic system and the capacity of various sectors in the labor market. As long as the size of the labor force is used as a regulatory mechanism in the management of the economic system, the unemployable and the unemployed are an integral part of the system, and the availability of jobs in different occupational classes does not necessarily reflect the individuals' abilities and disabilities. For example, it is by no means certain that a substantial increase in the number of high school graduates would increase the number of jobs available in the clerical and lower white-collar categories. The surpluses of the labor force tend to discourage the entrance of the newly qualified members. This occurs in professions also; a decrease in the demand for engineers is followed by a drop in the number of applicants to schools of engineering and a shrinkage of funds for scholarships and loans to engineering students. Although in the case of lower occupational classes the process of feedback and the regulatory mechanism are not as obvious and as well articulated as the drying up of funds for attracting new recruits to the school of engineering, the same socioeconomic forces are operative. Just as one would not assume that fewer applicants for engineering means that there are fewer people who have the intellectual ability to become engineers, one cannot conclude that all members of the low socioeconomic group are intellectually inferior even though they may not have finished high school or learned a trade, for which the incentive and encouragement must come from job opportunities.

The validity of explanatory hypotheses such as "cultural deprivation" as a cause in educational deficiencies or "cultural conflict" as leading to juvenile delinquency is questionable on the grounds that even if their existence were accepted, the mechanism by which these factors affect human behavior and personality development is not clear. Furthermore, the concepts of cultural conflict and cultural deprivation are vague and untestable (Schultz and Aurbach, 1971; Katz, 1969; Clark, 1970). While it may be postulated that socioeconomic and cultural factors play a decisive role in personality development, the nature and the extent of the influence of each single factor or combination of factors must be clearly delineated, and the mechanisms by which these environmental variables hinder or facilitate healthy adaptation and adjustment must be conceptualized. For example, poverty in an urban area is likely to be associated with substandard housing in crime-ridden inner-city ghettos, while in rural poverty, residence in old, dilapidated buildings does not necessarily expose children to the same degree of violence and insecurity. On the other hand, the rural poor have less and lower-quality medical care than that available to disadvantaged families in large cities.

Some poverty-related disadvantages can be easily observed and effectively remedied. Deficient and nonexistent pre- and postnatal care is associated with a higher incidence of prematurity, low birth weight, and other reproductive casualties that show a significant relationship to neuropsychiatric problems. Poor physical health and insufficient diet produce low energy level and deficient responsiveness to the environment, including academic learning. Furthermore, schools in poor neighborhoods are substandard in the quantity of educational mate rials; instead of compensating for the children's lack of familiarity with educational requirements, they fail to provide the optimal atmo sphere for learning. Living in overcrowded and dilapidated housing not only creates a sense of hopelessness and despair in parents but may indeed result in chronic lead poisoning leading to brain damage. The high crime rate of the inner-city ghetto makes the streets and parks unsafe for children, depriving them of opportunities for play and recreation and exposing them to the stressful trauma of observing death and destruction and being victims of violence themselves. For adolescents, the dangers of identification with criminals and involvement in various delinquent activities are always present. When parents cannot successfully counteract such influences, occasional, if not habitual, delinquent behavior follows.

Joblessness of parents in the family creates feelings of dissatisfaction and powerlessness that may seriously affect their parenting function. Children may become easy targets for the parents' discontent and anger. Childish behavior and demands for attention are experienced as impositions. The irritable parents may actually inflict harsh corporal punishment on the child or withdraw from any interaction with him and thus neglect him. Deficient medical and psychiatric care of the parents indirectly affects the lives of their children by failing to improve their ability to care for the child.

Quantitative statements regarding the incidence or prevalence of particular behaviors within defined populations are the grist of epidemiologic surveys. But as psychiatrists it is our task to also understand the qualitative nature of mental health and normal development in particular situations. It is with such understanding that we must view behavior as reflecting life circumstances. For example, the cautiousness of a ghetto child may be a normal and highly adaptive trait borne out of life experiences rather than an irrational mistrust or paranoia. The relucance of parents to allow their children to play in unsafe streets may be a wise decision rather than a sign of overprotection and a symbiotic relationship with the child. The extended family and reliance on friends in the caretaking of children is not always an indication of parents' overdependence on their own family to be used as a "pseudoexplanation" for certain behavioral deviations in their children. It may be a beneficial system of mutual cooperation in child fostering in unpredictable situations. Irritability, short attention span, and aimless wandering in a child from a lower-class family may well be due to chronic lead poisoning rather than a sign of maternal neglect or "stimulus overloading" in a chaotic home environment, although one might decide that neglect or lack of supervision has played a part in the child's ingestion of lead-containing paint. The immediate course of treatment for such a child obviously depends on whether or not the correct diagnosis has been made.

The above discussion should in no way be construed to mean that all or even the majority of children from poor families manifest deficiencies in personal growth and adjustment. Certain factors within such life circumstances may indeed facilitate personality development. Some of these children show a high degree of mastery in their encounters with stressful situations. Others have learned to be caring and sensitive in their interactions with their peers. They are willing to take responsibilities, are motivated to survive and succeed, are capable of sympathizing with the plight of others, and are remarkably able to solve those concrete problems of life of which their more fortunate peers can hardly dream. Their firsthand experience with hardship has provided them with a sense of self-assurance and a keen awareness of their environment that cannot be measured by their scores on intelligence tests. Their limited vocabulary is compensated for by their creative use of simple language, which serves them well in formulating their unique experiences and conveying them to each other.

The "culture of poverty" is not created by a series of distinct values and standards. Rather, to the extent that such a culture can be said to exist, it is a valid set of perceptions and conceptualizations of the reality of being poor in an affluent, industrialized society.

Minority Group Affiliation. The influence of ethnic group membership on the child's emerging personality can be related to two major factors: first, differences in language, cultural values, and standards from those of the dominant culture; and, second, the undesirable sterotype image of a particular minority group held by the majority culture.

When the language spoken at home is different from the language of school, the child's task upon entering school is made difficult because he must learn the new language in its spoken and written form at the same time. Children with language disorders or problems with auditory and visual perception find the scholastic demands particularly stressful. Other children may manage to learn the oral language to only a limited degree and shy away from active particpation in those academic activities that depend on oral presentation. Or they may receive more instruction and stimulation in the majority language and not develop their native tongue beyond the limited extent necessary for understanding simplified forms of intrafamilial communication. However, children of educated parents, and those with high verbal ability, learn to be fluently bilingual and are in an advantageous position.

In any evaluation of a bilingual child, the assessment must be made in the language in which the higher level of proficiency has been achieved. In tests of verbal performance, the factor of bilingualism must be taken into consideration. For psychiatrists, it is particularly important to remember that difficulties in communication may account for much of the child's bewilderment and deviant behavior. He may become restless and bored when the discussion in the classroom is incomprehensible to him, or he may become highly distressed when he cannot make his feelings or thoughts understood by others. Backwardness in learning may result in the child's reluctance to attend school and in his lonely wandering in the neighborhood. When school attendance is stressful, truancy is a self-protective maneuver rather than an indication of the child's antisocial attitude or his lack of regard for established rules.

Value systems and cultural attitudes do not in themselves lead to deviant personality formation, although they play a part in the manner in which any individual perceives and responds to reality. Belief in the supernatural or in faith healing may explain the meaning and significance attached to a particular phenomenon, but it does not cause the phenomenon. Parents of a hysterical child may believe that he is possessed, but there is as yet very little evidence to prove that such cultural beliefs are the sole etiology of symptom formation.

Child care practices of various ethnic groups have been linked to the prevalence or absence of certain deviations among their children. For example, the relative rarity of juvenile delinquency in the Chinese-American community is said to reflect early suppression of aggression (Sollenberger, 1968). However, assertions like these are based on clinical impressions; no research project has been reported that evaluates all the factors operative in a particular community at a particular time, in comparison with a control group. Furthermore, it has been shown that child-rearing practices do not remain fixed even over the life span of one generation. Mussen and Maldonado (1969) showed, for example, that a shift in the father's occupation changed child-rearing practices among a group of Puerto Rican industrial workers coming from a rural area.

The undesirable stereotype image of the minority held by the majority may or may not have far-reaching social and economic implications for particular minority groups. By far the most devastating impact of the undesirable stereotype image on personality development and eventual adjustment is felt by children of minority groups who are considered intellectually inferior, morally deviant, and consequently subject to discrimination by persons and institutions of the majority culture. The views, prejudices, and expectations of the majority are pathogenic factors in the personality formation of these children. The child is born into a poor family, is surrounded by dissatisfied and outraged or powerless and resigned parents, and resides in a community with little service, high unemployment, and rampant crime. Parents transmit their own impressions and experiences of futility and hopelessness to their children. The early encounters of children with the majority culture and institutions reinforce these impressions and crystallize their vague ideas about how they are viewed and what is expected of them. When there are no means at the child's disposal with which to counteract stereotyped designations, the child may come to accept them with little resistance. Or in order to escape these images of inferiority, he may totally reject the majority culture and consequently fail to learn the adaptive skills necessary for entering the mainstream culture. Minorities without effective heroes, glorious history, and living examples of achievement and power have children who are deprived of a source of inspiration and focus of imagination. While it is not easy to measure the influence of these internal motivating factors on the achievement needs and success orientation of children, one can cite numerous examples from the biographical accounts of great men in which the lives of historical characters or the examples of successful adults around them provided the driving force and orienting focus for their future activities.

Any claim regarding generalized traits, personality types, propensities for certain behavioral deviations, or inferior performances of a minority ethnic group, whether couched in sophisticated statistical terms or handed down by tradition, is invalid because the roles of historical, social, and economic factors and the complexities of human behavior under various conditions cannot be simplified and neatly categorized.

When parents are satisfied with their lives, they impart a sense of pride and satisfaction to their children and they create family legends that are congruent with their own pride. They reinterpret the majority culture in harmony with their life experiences. They find heroes and retell their history in a manner that nurtures hope and optimism in their children. By the same token, parents' hopelessness, their inability to change what they do not accept, and their shame about their own past and present status within the culture adversely affect their children's outlook on life and create the conditions for their future failure.

5

Presenting Symptoms

Children and adolescents are referred to a psychiatrist for a variety of deviant behaviors. These deviancies are the direct or indirect consequences of developmental disorders with, or without, complex emotional reactions. More often, the deviant behavior is the outcome of distorted, faulty interactions with other people. The child's unpleasant experiences determine his intrapsychic world and color his perception of external reality. Happy, carefree children have a better chance of learning through their experiences and achieving a level of social adjustment that is satisfactory for both the individual and society. By contrast, society pays a high price for the sufferings of an angry, unhappy child who may grow into a dependent or hostile and maladjusted adult.

Depression, anxiety, and aggression are not well-differentiated and separate entities within the spectrum of mental anguish; rather there is always a mixture of these emotions in which only the relative proportion may change. An anxious child is depressed by his awareness of his inability to cope with his environment and angered by his plight. An aggressive adolescent fears the ever-present possibility of retribution by society and his victims and is helpless in controlling his destiny. Fire setting, for example, is an aggressive and destructive act, but it may be the last desperate attempt of a deprived, abused child to bring attention to himself even though he risks being destroyed in the process.

In the following discussions, aggression, depression, and anxiety have been separated only for the purpose of clarification.

AGGRESSION AND HOSTILITY

Whether aggression in man is a biological instinct, as some ethologists and psychoanalysts believe, or a response to frustrations, as some behaviorists postulate, it is clear that aggressive behaviors in all their variety are of special concern to society. Ethologists like Lorenz who consider aggression as a biologically necessary instinct believe that the higher intellectual abilities in man and the collective values and rituals inherent in every culture provide avenues for the sublimation and utilization of aggression. In this view, rational child-rearing practices channel the child's aggression into socially acceptable behavior.

Psychoanalysts who accept Freud's theory of the death instinct and those who are more at ease with his earlier formulation of aggressive drive emphasize the taming power of libido and believe that successful fusion of the libido with the aggressive drive will save society from the more destructive manifestations of the individual's aggressive tendencies.

For behaviorists, the development of aggressive behavior in a child is an indication of a high degree of frustrating circumstances in his early life and the differential reinforcement that he has received for aggressive responses.

Lauretta Bender (1953) expands the concept of frustrating situations to include the child's failure to master various developmental tasks. Furthermore, according to her, a child's aggressive reaction in a depriving environment is essentially a counteraggression, since the child views the failure of the environment to provide for his needs as the equivalent of hostile and aggressive acts directed against him.

It must be noted that none of the above hypotheses has been able to account for the fact that boys are overrepresented in all varieties of aggressive behaviors from childhood through their adult lives. Bender's view cannot explain the reported findings that children coming from disharmonious households and receiving inconsistent discipline are more likely to be aggressive than children raised by consistently harsh or indifferent parents.

The young child's desire to assert his own wishes and preferences has to be modified because he is a member of a group and his need to explore the world around him must be supervised. Training and discipline are methods of transmitting these facts to the child and of teaching him about potential dangers. The family is the first agent of socialization but it is not the only one. School, religious organizations, peer groups, and a variety of other social institutions have important functions in socializing the child, teaching him the limits of his rights and a concern for the rights of others. The role of television in promoting violence has become a source of serious concern for parents and educators in recent years (Siegel, 1972). Mental health professionals and correctional organizations are called upon when the conventional agents have failed in this task. The deviant behavior of an un-socialized child is not merely a reflection of his failure to incorporate the norms of society but also a series of maladaptive mechanisms by which he is trying to gain entrance to group membership and to ward off isolation. Lacking a workable guideline, he continues to use his own wishes as the yardstick for his actions; to the extent that these are inappropriate and unacceptable, they further alienate him from his group. Such a child feels himself victimized and attacked. Since the frustration and hostility thus evoked call for revenge, the aimless, diffuse aggression of earlier years can become vicious and goal-directed. The child may now find companionship alongside other children of the same bent. He may be hardened in his attitude toward the suffering of others and not feel any guilt over his transgressions. However, the sense of loneliness and futility never leaves him. Self-destructiveness in a direct or indirect manner is always present in such a picture (Szurek and Berlin, 1969; Redl and Wineman, 1952).

Manifestations of failure in socialization depend on the child's stage of development and the environmental circumstances. Attempts at habilitation and correction of deviant behaviors have to be directed at the milieu as well as the individual. The prognosis for each child can be conceptualized as the degree of flexibility in environmental circumstances and the individual's responsiveness to these changes.

Preschool Children

Aggressive behavior is a common presenting complaint among children under 6 who are referred for psychiatric evaluation. Parental concern centers on the child's negativistic behavior, destruction of objects, lack of concern for other children's possessions, physical aggression against younger sibs, cruelty to animals, and, even, running away from home or separating from parents in potentially dangerous situations. Temper tantrums, general unhappiness, and physical or verbal aggression against parents or other adults may also be a part of the picture. The general impression is of a child who is unmanageable and wild. Parents usually state that the child is agile, well coordinated, and intelligent and consider his behavior calculated and purposeful.

On clinical examination, in cases where the child is not clearly retarded or psychotic, one may notice defiance and negativism in the manner in which he responds to the examiner. The child may refuse to play or talk, or, conversely, he may show a lack of inhibition, quickly feel at home, and exhibit aggressive and destructive behavior in the office. When the child is observed in interaction with his parents, it becomes obvious that they are locked in a conflictual relationship in which parental response occurs only when the child's activities have approached a point of no return (e.g., the child has already begun to throw an object). At times, a parent seems to give the child suggestions in disguise—like a mother who upon entering the playroom with her 4-year-old child turned to the psychiatrist and said, "If you don't take that ashtray away, he is going to break it." The child's response was almost immediate. He disregarded everything else in the playroom and picked up the ashtray.

Aggressive behavior on the part of these children can be best understood in the context of their intrafamilial relationships. McRae and Lowe (1968) found that of the 33 preschool children referred for aggressive behavior, in "the largest group (33%), the parent–child relationship was of a hostile, rejecting type." In this group, parents, particularly mothers, had rejected the child either because of dissatisfaction with their marriage or the responsibilities of mothering, or disappointment regarding the child's sex, appearance, or some aspects of his personal style. A few of the mothers blamed their untimely pregnancy for keeping them from finishing school, obliging them to get married, or causing rejection by their own families. In these cases the child seems to have been rejected at conception and the series of events following the child's birth were a self-fulfilling prophecy. When one or both parents are disturbed, the distorted relationship with the child may be caused by the parents' global disturbance in interpersonal relationships, without any particular resentment against the child.

Case History

A 4-year-old boy was brought to the hospital by the police with the presenting complaint that he had broken all the furniture in the apartment, had chased his mother with a knife, and had thrown flowerpots out of their 12th-floor window. The mother, unable to stop him, called the police and requested protection. When seen in the emergency room, the child was exhausted and sleepy, but the mother's first sentence to the psychiatrist was "I will not take him home." She then gave a long list of the child's misbehavior, saying, "I never wanted a child. My husband insisted that he wanted to be a father and then walked out on me as soon as the baby was born." This child proved to be a frightened, unhappy boy who was eager to please other adults and seemed surprised and pleased by the amount of positive attention paid to him in the hospital, where he did not exhibit any aggressive behavior.

Inexperienced parents may create a conflict in their relationship with a child by misinterpreting normal development. There are parents who consider a toddler's lack of empathy and sympathy with other children as an alarming indication of "emotional disturbance." They try to understand the causes of the child's behavior by asking him for an explanation or by consulting popular books on emotional disorders of children. These parents may inadvertently encourage and reinforce what was initially age-appropriate behavior beyond the appropriate age by giving inordinate amounts of attention and asserting their love and devotion to the child whenever he is engaged in aggressive behavior. Other parents assume the presence of unvented anger toward parents as the cause of a toddler's assertive, aggressive behavior and encourage the child to verbalize his anger. The child dutifully obeys, only to be rejected by other adults or even his own parents when such verbalization occurs.

CASE HISTORY

Three-year-old Lee was brought for a psychiatric evaluation because both parents were disturbed by her lack of consideration for other children, destructive fantasies, and chronic anger. The mother was a guidance counselor and the father a stockbroker. They had married in their 30s and eagerly planned to have two children. Lee was the first born, loved and cherished by both parents. They had avidly read child psychology books and were pleased with their daughter's normal development until she was 2 years old and the mother became pregnant. Now both parents began to think about ways to prepare Lee for the birth of the sibling, which they were convinced would be a serious psychological trauma, since "she would feel dethroned." When the mother was in her sixth month of pregnancy, the parents decided that it was time for Lee to be toilet-trained in preparation for attending nursery school. Lee did not accept the mild suggestions to use the toilet and once threw a temper tantrum when the mother became insistent. Both parents were alarmed by this show of temper and decided to suspend further effort. However, Lee began to have temper tantrums whenever she did not get her way. With the birth of the second child, another girl, the parents began to consider the tantrums Lee's expression of discontent with her loss of status. They explained to her their understanding of her feelings and tried to reassure her by heaping attention on her. The tantrums did not cease; the parents began to think that Lee was angry with them and told her to feel free to "get it off your chest." Lee obliged and the parents were alarmed at the intensity of her anger.

Lee was a normal, highly intelligent, and verbal child. She explained that she had been brought to a doctor because "I am always angry." When pressed for the meaning of her statement, she said, "Because I scream." She proudly reported that her parents let her do everything and she was very happy with them. However, she thought if she could change her parents, she would choose parents who "did not talk so much." She said that when she was "bad" her parents gave her a "long talk with big words."

In children in whom aggressive behavior emerges after a period of satisfactory family relationships, the cause of the aggression may lie in

the child's feeling of abandonment when the parents become preoccupied with the problems of a sibling or with other stresses. These
children quickly learn that aggressive behavior is the quickest and
surest way to reengage their parents. Aggressive behavior is the most
common strategy of young children for combating the effects of the
psychological absence of the parents. This absence at times is due to
parents' depression and withdrawal.

When a child suffers early physical illness or fragile health, some
parents are inhibited from making any demands on the child. Setting
limits becomes more and more difficult. As the child senses parental
uncertainty, he exploits his physical status to avoid conforming to any
external demand. These children may engage in aggressive behavior
when the parents finally become insistent. Parental reaction to this
aggression may be counteraggression followed by guilt and a lessening of demands, which leaves the child confused and frustrated, and
thus a guilty, resentful interaction begins on both sides (Finch, 1962;
Makkay, 1962).

Treatment. Since there are many possible causes of aggressive behavior in preschool children, the specific therapeutic intervention
must be appropriate for each case. It is important first to identify those
elements in the parent–child interaction that create frustration and encourage aggression. For some parents, a series of counseling sessions
discussing normal development, combined with specific suggestions
for parental handling, may be sufficient. It is neither useful nor psychologically sound to advise parents to be "firm" or "permissive."
Rather, segments of the child's behavior and the parents' customary
reaction should be discussed and analyzed. The psychiatrist should
point out how the child may be interpreting the parents' behavior.

In other cases, rejective, hostile parents are not likely to accept the
therapist's view of the child's behavior since they have an emotional
investment in proving that the child deserves to be rejected. These
parents may dutifully appear for appointments and agree to give the
child another chance, but they are likely to distort the meaning of the
therapist's suggestion for firm discipline and become even more punitive and rigid; or they may agree to try leniency, only to prove that the
child's behavior will not immediately improve. For these parents,
treatment should be directed at the roots of their own unhappiness.
Simultaneously, it would be helpful to provide other sources of socialization for the child, such as a well-structured nursery program.
Parents who are depressed and withdrawn need psychiatric help
themselves before they can be expected to engage in altered interactions with their children. Any available source within the family, such
as an older sib, should be recruited as a partial substitute for the

parent, and outside support for the child in the form of a preschool program should be sought.

When parental preoccupation with a sick sibling is the cause of neglect and abandonment of the aggressive child, assisting the parents with the burden of caring for the sick child may be sufficient to reestablish equilibrium within the family. Individual psychotherapy with these children is not necessary. If one believes that undivided attention from an adult may be helpful to the child, any interested adult could serve such a purpose.

Successful treatment of aggressive behavior in preschool children prevents the myriad of distorted and harmful interactions between the child and his surroundings and supports normal development.

School-Age Children

Children who are referred for evaluation of aggressiveness during the school years usually have a long history of such behavior dating back to their early childhood. Parental neglect or high tolerance for disruptive activities in large chaotic families may have permitted the child's behavior to go unchecked or unnoticed. Some young children in these families spend most of their waking hours on the street; it is only when they have to remain within the confines of a classroom that their aggressive interactions come to the attention of their teachers and are communicated to their families.

Another group of aggressive children come from families in which harsh punishment by the parents has succeeded in inhibiting any expression of aggression at home; these hostile, angry children give free rein to their aggression at school. Furthermore, these parents tend either to discount reports of the child's misbehavior at school or to encourage the child to "stand his own ground and fight back." If the child's aggression is considered a justifiable defense of his own rights, his attitude may soon be generalized to include disobedience and defiance toward the teacher. Parents may then blame the teachers for lack of understanding or a prejudice against the child.

Aggressive children soon alienate their peers and teachers, find school an unfriendly or even hostile place, and lose motivation for learning academic subjects. They consider every criticism and correction by adults another expression of personal hostility and respond with further hostility and defiance. They may be assaultive and destructive and sooner or later find themselves unpopular and behind the academic level of their peers. Some children hold the school responsible for their parents' angry reaction when they are informed of failing marks or poor behavior. Cut off from any rewarding experience within their family or school, these children seek the company of those who "understand" them or do not condemn them; these are usually other children with the same kind of behavior. The child thus becomes involved in a variety of unacceptable actions either by himself or with a group of companions. He may steal, stay out late, avoid school, and search for excitement in such dangerous activities as setting fires, trespassing, and vandalizing.

In a clinical interview, the child may be negativistic and uncooperative, complain about his teachers and schoolmates, deny any responsibility for his actions, but admit to feeling unhappy and lonesome. He considers himself "bad," a source of trouble for his family, unloved, and unwanted. Lack of warm emotional relations has left the child with an underlying emotional immaturity that at times gives a picture of a child who vacillates between being a tough bully and a whimpering, whiny baby. He is defensive about his failure in school, saying either that he does not find any value in learning or that he finds the work beneath him, even though he may not be able to read. He justifies his behavior as not wanting to be "pushed around" or "bossed." He cannot project ahead to his future as an adult nor think of what he wants to do or be.

In some of these children, a chronic state of anxiety and depression is easily apparent. They have nightmares, are unduly concerned about physical injury, and have various somatic complaints. Their depression may be frankly expressed in suicidal ideation or through their recklessness in engaging in dangerous activities.

While fantasies and games involving aggressive, violent themes are abundant in younger children, older ones may be reluctant to reveal their fantasies or may phrase them as the desire to be a policeman or go to war.

These children are usually of average intelligence, though they may have reading retardation of various degrees. Some authors (Bender, 1972) have noted the presence of reading disability, perceptual motor problems, and other developmental pathology as possible contributing factors in the creation of chronic frustration and hostility in these children. Others have remarked on the apparent lack of anxiety associated with the unsocialized aggression. However, Robins (1966), in a follow-up study of such children into adulthood, found anxiety to be among the lasting characteristics of the group.

Aggressive reaction in a previously socialized or inhibited child is always an indication that the level of intrapsychic and/or environmental stress has surpassed the child's capacity for adaptation. Prompt investigation and intervention is necessary to help the child regain his previous state of functioning.

Fire Setting

In a preschooler, fire setting may simply be an act of exploration by a poorly supervised child even though it can lead to tragic consequences. The extent of damage or loss of life cannot be equated with the degree of disturbance in the child. For some children, playing with matches is as tempting as other prohibited acts, such as ringing other people's doorbells, flooding the bathroom, or pulling the cat's tail.

Among school-age children, fire setting may be one distinctive aggressive act among a myriad of unacceptable behaviors, such as stealing and using obscene language. For these children, fire does not have any symbolic meaning, nor is there a preoccupation or fascination with it. However, once these children discover the destructive force of fire without personally suffering from it, they may deliberately choose fire setting as a means of revenge on people who have deeply angered them.

Some children, on the other hand, are obsessively preoccupied with fire and draw pleasure from its awesome destructiveness. These children may use fire and their ability to set a fire to compensate for their feelings of impotent rage against their environment. Inadequate in every area of functioning, they feel isolated and unable to relate to others; their unrelieved rage and chronic depression find spectacular expression in starting a fire. They want to watch the fire, but they run away to safety, more out of fear of retaliation than a desire to save themselves (Vandersall and Wiener, 1970).

CASE HISTORY

John, an 8-year-old boy of superior intelligence, had set his first big fire at the age of 6. He had started the fire under the bed, lingered to watch the flames, and then left the apartment, taking his favorite toy with him. He had remained in the lobby until the firemen arrived, then walked across the street to watch the fire from a hidden corner. The apartment was totally burned, though his parents managed to escape unharmed. John's second substantial fire was set when he was 8. He had awakened one Sunday morning before his parents, made himself breakfast, and got dressed. While in the kitchen, he had seen a book of matches and had gone to his parents' bedroom with them. The parents were asleep. John tried to light the match, failing several times. Finally he managed to set fire to the fringe of the bed quilt covering his parents. He said, "When the blue flames started going up, I thought I should leave before my parents catch me." This boy did not deny that his parents could have died in the fire. He said he would have felt bad but he would not cry: "My father says I am grown up and should not cry."

During the interview John tried, but failed, to avert his gaze from the lit matches in the examiner's hands. When invited to examine a lighter, he said, "Aren't you afraid that accidentally I may set fire to your office?"

In adolescence, fires may be set deliberately to cover a crime, to show the violent intention of a group against authority, or to provide a thrilling spectacle for diversion. While the terror and excitement associated with fire setting may lead to an erection in the adolescent, the sexual arousal is not necessarily the motivating force behind the fire setting. Once the association is established, however, sexual excitement may become the primary purpose, especially for an inhibited and inadequate adolescent.

As we have seen, fire setting cannot be assessed solely on the basis of its obvious danger. It is the study of the particular child or adolescent who has set the fire that can unravel the significance of the act and the possibility of its future repetition. When the fire setter is a timid, withdrawn child, he must be helped to feel less isolated and to participate in gratifying relationships with his peers. Aggressive, hostile children are in need of close supervision and structure in their activities in order to find more constructive avenues for expression of their feelings. Depressed, inadequate adolescents are most responsive to efforts that provide them with means of bolstering their self-esteem. Children who are fascinated with fire can be helped to find more appropriate ways of being associated with fire without endangering their community.

In psychoanalytic literature much emphasis has been placed on an association between fire setting and enuresis as the symbolic manner in which the repressed sexual drive is expressed. Studies of children who have set fires fail to substantiate such consistent association. Some authors have regarded the triad of enuresis, fire setting, and cruelty to animals as having predictive value for occurrence of violent behavior in adulthood. Follow-up studies have not proved the validity of these claims.

Homicide

Young children's actions may lead to the death of another person under a series of unusual circumstances. The victim is usually a younger child—a sib or a playmate. In describing a group of 33 children and adolescents who had killed, Bender (1959) reported that in all cases involving children under 11 years of age, social and familial disturbances abounded in the background history. Homes were chaotic and inadequate; parents were rejecting or ineffectual; some children were clearly brutalized and neglected; and in several cases, prior psychiatric evaluation had noted the child's unsocialized, potentially dangerous behavior, although recommendations for intervention had never been carried out.

Younger children do not have the concept of death as being final. Their wishes for the death of others are only a desire for the offending person's removal from their immediate environment. When such a child causes the death of another child, he is shocked and disturbed. His reaction is in many ways similar to a psychotic depressive state lasting from a few months to years. Some such children manage to make a successful adjustment after long-term psychiatric care. Others become involved in repeated aggressive crimes as adults.

Older children and adolescents may also cause accidental death. However, the majority are intent on harming their victim, even though their intention may have been a response to an impulse of the moment. Such adolescents may kill because their impulse goes unchecked and they find a weapon or an object that can be used as a weapon. They understand the nature of their action, although they may deny any guilt and anxiety following their act. In the group reported by Bender, a few of the adolescents who had been involved in murdering another person later on developed epilepsy, and some were diagnosed as schizophrenics in their adult life. Bender considers the following combination of circumstances possible antecedents of homicidal aggression:

- Organic brain damage associated with lack of impulse control.
- Chaotic home and personal experience with violence and death.
- Inadequacies in other areas of functioning, such as poor school performance.
- Preoccupation with death and violence in a schizophrenic child.
- Compulsive fire setting.

In a poorly supervised setting, the presence of an irritating victim may lead to a homicidal act by an aggressive, depressed child or adolescent, even though the intent to commit murder has not been previously entertained.

CASE HISTORY

Clarence, a 5-year-old boy, was admitted to the hospital following the killing of his 2-month-old sister. Clarence lived with his 20-year-old mother, who had spent eight years of her life in a mental institution and had become pregnant with Clarence shortly after her release. She did not know the boy's father and was supported by welfare. She could not find her way around the neighborhood and was totally illiterate, and though chronically hallucinating, she refused to go to the follow-up clinic for fear they would give her medication. She claimed that she had become "dumb" as the result of the heavy doses of medication given to her in the hospital. Clarence had been a healthy baby who had begun to take care of himself at around 3 years of age. The mother relied on him to make sandwiches for both of them, to remember to put out the garbage, and at times to nurse his mother when she would remain in bed for days staring at the ceiling. She had become pregnant with her second child by another chance meeting with a man. Clarence had not shown any undue reaction when the baby was born, but the mother had felt more tired and unable to take care of the baby. On the day of the accident, the mother had not got out of bed and the baby had not been fed. The baby's cry had disturbed Clarence, who had tried to calm her down. He had tried to arouse his mother to no avail. Finally, he had decided to carry the baby to his mother. However, the baby had begun crying louder and louder. Clarence had begun to hit the baby with a pot. The hitting continued until the baby stopped crying.

On admission to the hospital, Clarence was confused, incoherent, and extremely frightened. He repeated over and over that the baby cried too much. He asked to go home to see the baby and wanted his mother to bring the baby to the hospital. He had nightmares and at times refused to go to bed because he did not want to fall asleep. He withdrew whenever approached and did not play with other children. His activities consisted of aimless wandering around the ward or staring out of the window. At times he did not even pay attention to his mother. His situation remained essentially unchanged for two months, until another 5-year-old boy arrived on the ward. Clarence began to follow this new boy around and slowly accepted his invitation to play. He then began to respond to adults' overtures, and although he remained detached and sad looking, he was able to attend school and after two years was placed in a residential treatment center, where he has continued to make slow progress for the past four years.

Case History

Terry was first seen at the age of 8 at the request of the guidance counselor of his school because following a minor fight with another child, Terry had threatened to kill himself by leaping out of the window. Terry was the only child of his parents. His father was serving a life sentence for a murder that he had committed shortly after Terry's birth. The mother was working in a supermarket and was not home when Terry returned from school. She became angry and abusive whenever called by teachers because of Terry's behavior. Although she stated that she could not control Terry, she blamed the teachers for picking on him and thought other children were responsible for his numerous fights. On this occasion, she reluctantly agreed to take Terry to the hospital, and although she agreed to have him admitted, she decided to sign him out after a week. Terry was a depressed, irritable, and anxious child who felt threatened and reacted with aggression every time another child made an approach toward him. He complained bitterly about how everybody was against him. He said he would end up in jail like his father and repeatedly wished that he were dead, though he denied any suicidal intention. He cried when his mother came to visit him because he wanted to go home. He said that he worried about his mother's safety.

Terry was next heard from at the age of 12. He had been remanded by the juvenile court, where he had appeared following a mugging incident during which he and a 14-year-old boy had stabbed an elderly woman, causing her death. Terry was extremely hostile upon arrival at the hospital and demanded his immediate release because "I am not crazy." He threatened to kill someone in the hospital in order to get discharged. He related that on numerous occasions he had managed to snatch women's purses or take money from children by threatening them with a knife. He blamed his partner's ineptitude for their having been caught by the police. He did not think that he had done anything wrong: "The woman was almost dead of old age." Terry was placed in a correctional institution, from which he had to be referred to a more closed setting because of his aggressive and assaultive behavior.

JUVENILE DELINQUENCY

Juvenile delinquency is a legal term defined by the laws of each community and applicable to persons of a certain age who are found guilty of engaging in behavior that would be considered a crime if committed by an adult. Some behavior that is not considered against the law for adults is considered delinquency for children and adolescents, such as running away from home, truancy from school, and the use of alcohol. On the other hand, such acts as homicide or fire setting by a child under 7 are not considered criminal or delinquent. In practice, repeating offenders and those engaging in more serious crimes have a higher chance of being officially adjudged delinquents. Therefore studies of officially designated delinquents cannot provide a valid basis for generalizing about all juveniles who break the law. It has also been noted that children of lower-class families, particularly those in which the father is absent from the home, are more frequently arrested, more frequently appear in court, and are more likely to be adjudged delinquents. This fact casts serious doubts on whether the statistics for the prevalence and incidence of delinquency in various communities and neighborhoods truly reflect the amount of crime committed or are a result of other sociocultural factors.

Juvenile delinquency is reported in every country and culture. In nations with an accelerated rate of sociopolitical change, delinquency is on the rise. In Western Europe and the United States, the statistics of delinquency fluctuate in various years and locations. The urban areas of industrialized societies have shown a higher rate of reported delinquency than rural communities. However, these and other statistical facts may always prove to be, at least in part, the artifact of identifying and reporting the delinquent person. As in all other varieties of aggressive behavior, boys outnumber girls in juvenile delinquency, and for this reason most of the reported studies have been done on boys.

Theories of Etiology

Juvenile delinquency has been studied by various disciplines and from various perspectives. Psychiatrists are interested in the psychodynamics of the individual delinquent, although they then try to generalize their findings to explain the possible intrapsychic and interpersonal forces leading to delinquency. Sociologists, on the other hand, study delinquency as a social phenomenon and try to identify the sociological factors associated with the development of delinquency in various communities.

The role of genetic and biological endowment in the causation of delinquency has attracted sporadic attention. However, at the present time, the available data are extremely meager and the mechanism by which a particular biological deviation or constitutional type could result in a pattern of deviant behavior has not been postulated.

Plans for remediation and treatment of delinquency primarily reflect the philosophy of the legislators who allocate tax resources to finance these programs and are more likely either to be based on a combination of all available theories or to swing from one pole to the other as the expected results fail to materialize.

Psychological Theories. Psychological theories set themselves the task of explaining the reasons that juvenile delinquents have failed to abide by cultural norms and have learned a particular pattern of unacceptable behavior. Since parents are the earliest agents of cultural transmission to their child, it is logical to assume that antisocial parents produce antisocial delinquent children (Van Amerongen, 1963). While there is some evidence for this hypothesis, all delinquent children do not come from antisocial families, nor do all antisocial parents have delinquent children.

Some psychiatrists have postulated that in those families in which the child's delinquency develops in a socialized milieu, the parents have failed to enforce some cultural taboos or have unconsciously encouraged specific acts of delinquency. Szurek and Johnson (1969) have called this phenomenon "superego lacunae," which in children mirrors the lacunae in parental superego. Learning theorists have postulated that as a pattern of behavior, delinquency is learned from parents or peers. Others have considered delinquency a pattern of aggression first directed toward the family and later against society. For these theorists, delinquency is an individual's reaction to unmet and unfulfilled dependency needs. For some psychoanalysts, delinquency is a substitute for neurosis, and the psychodynamics of the delinquent can be understood on the same basis as those of the neurotic.

Other authors have pointed out that delinquent behavior can be caused by a child's failure to identify with the parents. Bowlby's (1944) term "affectless personality" describes a group of juveniles who, because of numerous separations, had failed to develop the capacity for rapport and identification with parents or parental surrogates and substitutes; therefore they could not be expected to develop an intrapsychic mechanism by which the standards and norms of society could regulate their behavior.

The psychological characteristics of delinquents have been the focus of numerous studies. Following the development of IQ tests, some studies reported lower intelligence for delinquents, and for a while it seemed that low intelligence could explain the delinquent's failure to conform with the societal norms. These findings were later proved to be either unsubstantiated or of minor dimension. Other investigators have studied such areas as time orientation, impulsivity, and responsiveness to social rewards in different groups of delinquents. The results of all these studies may provide a composite picture of the delinquent child, but they have so far failed to account for the phenomenon of delinquency.

Sociological Theories. As was noted earlier, delinquency is more prevalent in the slum areas of industrialized cities, and the lower socioeconomic class contributes the largest percentage of delinquent youths. These facts have attracted the attention of anthropologists and sociologists, who are interested in development of sociocultural phenomena within the larger context of any given society (Quay, 1965).

Durkheim, in 1897, described the conditions under which cultural norms no longer have an inhibiting influence on the behavior of individuals or groups of individuals. Cloward and Ohlin (1960), following the same orientation, pointed out discrepancies between the goals and standards of society and the meager opportunities available to children of the lower social class to achieve these goals. For these authors, delinquency is the logical, though unwanted, by-product of the social organization in which delinquency becomes a means of achievement.

Miller (1959) considered delinquency from an anthropological perspective. He described a distinct lower-class subculture with a set of values and standards according to which some delinquent acts are not considered deviant. This subculture values toughness, smartness, momentary excitement, and the ability to remain out of trouble, that is, out of reach of the established authorities. These values are quite different from—in fact, the opposite of—the values of the middle class, which stresses academic achievement, concern with the rightness and wrongness of an act, and delayed gratification. Given this clash of values, lower-class families cannot be expected to transmit majority values to their children, and schools and religious organizations are also unable to promote conformity among the youth of this subculture.

In describing juvenile gangs, A. K. Cohen (1955) stated that group delinquency is a collective reaction of the disadvantaged group to a set of standards and values that they cannot achieve and therefore must try to devalue. This collective reaction formation allows gang members to escape feelings of helplessness and entrapment in their socioeconomic situation. Some sociologists have considered the phenomenon of gang formation the result of long financial dependency of youth, their delayed entrance into the world of adulthood, and the lack of any clear demarcation between the end of childhood and the beginning of adult life. For these authors, delinquent acts by gang members are incidental to their primary function, which is a collective expression of masculinity and a declaration of independence of and equality with adults.

Sociological theories of delinquency are essentially theories of group formation that draw their basic data from gang membership and gang activities. They do not explain delinquency among middle-class children, cannot account for delinquency in girls, and, most importantly, fail to explain the fact that all children living in slum areas and all people belonging to the lower socioeconomic group are not delinquent and antisocial. Like psychological theories of delinquency, sociological theories do not offer any explanation for the observation that a good percentage of juvenile delinquents become stable, functioning members of society in their adulthood.

Predelinquent Children

The predelinquent child is usually a 7- to 8-year-old child who is referred by the school or other agencies with the presenting complaints of aggressive behavior toward peers, defiance of teachers and other authorities, little regard for the rights of others, and lack of concern for rules and regulations even when they are for his own safety. He lies even when lying does not seem to serve any purpose. He has stolen money from other children and merchandise from stores, at times objects for which he does not have any use. He may have engaged in sexual activities and may have spent most of his time on the street on the periphery of older delinquent children. Although he has average intelligence, he is uninterested in schoolwork and may be behind in reading. He is ill informed despite being "street-wise." His family lives in a slum area of the city; his home is overcrowded and dirty. His father has deserted the family, has served time in jail, or is unemployed. The father may be drinking excessively and having continuous conflict with the mother. The child's mother is neglectful or unavailable. She may have been delinquent herself and may have spent time away from her own home sometime during her own childhood or adolescence. Discipline is more dependent on the parents' mood than on the child's activities. He may be punished for any infraction of the parental commands, although no effort is made to censure his misbehavior outside. He may be shielded or lied for when neighbors and police are concerned, only to be brutally punished for having caused trouble for the parents. He is punished if he takes money from his parents' pockets, but nobody seems to notice that he has brought a new toy home.

Delinquent Adolescents

This is an older child, 13–15 years-of-age. He has been repeatedly involved in delinquent acts and has been arrested several times. He may have appeared in court on one or more occasions, charged with robbery, assault, or possession of stolen goods. He may have used narcotics and alcohol. He may have engaged in a variety of sexual misbehavior, such as rape and sodomy. He now uses his home only as an occasional place to sleep, either not seeing or totally disregarding his father. He may show more concern for his mother, although she can no longer count on his obedience. His attendance in school is irregular and only for the purpose of meeting with his companions. He shows contempt for those who spend their time in pursuit of academic studies. His social relations are limited to association with others like himself.

In a psychiatric interview, he may present a facade of cooperation in order to "con" the psychiatrist into helping him avoid the consequences of his behavior. He may express regret about what he has done or make promises for the future; however, his plans, when fully described, do not seem to be quite realistic. He has very little tolerance of frustration and becomes irritable when he fails to achieve his purpose. He may lie unnecessarily, so that one questions his ability to appreciate the reality and the limitations of individual liberty.

A delinquent girl is more likely to have been engaged in sexual misbehavior. Pregnancy, prostitution, use of drugs and alcohol, and shoplifting may be the presenting complaints. She may have run away from home on numerous occasions. Her relationship with her parents is usually unsatisfactory. She may complain of depressed mood and nervousness or various somatic symptoms.

Psychological Testing. On psychological tests of IQ, delinquents show a wide range of intelligence. They may have superior ability or be on the borderline of mental retardation. While some authors have tried to construct a psychological test profile of delinquency, others have failed to duplicate their results. Recently more attention has been focused on the possible qualitative differences in the intellectual functionings of delinquents, but the differences found so far are not sufficient to account for the development or maintenance of delinquent patterns of beahvior.

Objective tests of personality development have been used to map out the area of deviancy within the personality makeup of delinquents. So far, what has been learned from these tests does not give a more penetrating insight into the problem of delinquency than that gained through simple observation or clinical interview.

The Course of Delinquent Behavior. In a follow-up study of the adult status of 524 white children who were referred to the St. Louis Child Guidance Clinic for antisocial behavior, Robins (1966) has provided significant information in regard to the course of socially deviant behavior. According to her analysis, "Antisocial behavior predicts no specific kind of deviance but rather a generalized inability to conform and perform in many areas." There is no clear connection between the form of deviancy in childhood and the deviant behavior exhibited in adult life. Of all the children referred for antisocial behavior, 28% were diagnosed as sociopathic in adulthood with chronic inability to function as parent, spouse, worker, or member of the armed forces. They were isolated from their relatives, did not have any friends, and did not belong to any organization. Their death rate was twice that of the general population in the same area. They had divorced more often and their children had been frequently involved in antisocial behavior. Another significant percentage of the original group had been diagnosed as chronically alcoholic or schizophrenic during their adult life.

On the other hand, about 50% of the children with antisocial behavior had grown up to be functioning members of society. It appears that while the absence of antisocial tendencies during childhood can almost guarantee their absence in adult life, the same cannot be said about the predictive value of deviant behavior in childhood. Children who had engaged in more varieties of antisocial activities and over a longer period of time were more likely to become antisocial adults. When mothers and fathers were antisocial, the antisocial behavior of their children had a higher likelihood of continuing into adult life. Poor neighborhood, membership in gangs, and low socioeconomic status of families did not seem to be the deciding factors in the outcome of delinquent behavior in later life.

In this sample, boys outnumbered girls (5 to 1). However, girls who had engaged in repeated delinquent behaviors fared less well as adults than did boys. Disharmonious homes, sociopathic parents, and inconsistent discipline are factors associated with the continuation of childhood antisocial behavior into adult life, but we know very little about the factors that prevent other children from becoming sociopathic adults.

Prediction. Glueck and Glueck (1950) designed a scale for predicting future delinquency based on information and observations collected at 6 years of age. The three areas studied were family background, character traits, and personality traits. Character traits were isolated from responses on Rorschach tests and personality traits observed in clinic interviews. The children with a higher risk of future delinquency had hostile, overstrict fathers and indifferent or hostile, rejective mothers; they showed suspiciousness, destructiveness, and aggressiveness on their Rorschach responses; and they were adventurous, stubborn, and emotionally labile. The scale was reported to be 87% predictive of delinquency. The Gluecks' predictive scale has been criticized on methodological grounds, and its validity and usefulness have been seriously questioned (New York City Youth Board, 1961). Glueck and Glueck (1968), conceding the necessity for some revision in their scale, reported that this device had been shown to be "reasonably effective in distinguishing boys with a high delinquency potential from those with a relatively low risk." Kvaraceus (1961) devised a checklist for rating delinquency-proneness, but studies have not been carried out to validate the predictive value of the checklist. To date, the prediction of delinquency in individual children is at best an educated guess based on family background, psychiatric status of the parents, and some psychological factors in the child's personality (Ferracutti and Dinitz, 1972).

Treatment. For the predelinquent child, treatment must be directed at integration within the school system and provision of role models, preferably within his community, to aid identification. When the family is willing or able to cooperate, they can be helped to provide close supervision and a more predictable and supportive environment for the child. Foster home placement may be indicated when the family is clearly unable to deal with the child's needs. Psychotherapy may be useful when the child has internalized a poor self-image and his delinquent behavior can be traced to his feelings of hopelessness and futility. In older delinquents, external control may be best provided in a structured setting in which the delinquent is protected from further risks of involvement in antisocial activities while every attempt is made to help him with his deficiencies. When the adolescent's delinquency is traceable to intrapsychic and neurotic conflicts, individual psychotherapy and parental supervision will help him to control his acting-out behavior.

Social programs aimed at removing poverty, creating jobs, cleaning slums, etc., are commendable goals and may in the long run be effective in combating juvenile delinquency. However, the psychiatrist's expertise can be best used in studying the individual's difficulties in his relationship with his society and providing suggestions and programs to help him.

DEPRESSION

Mood, in psychiatry, refers to a chronic psychobiological state that is to be differentiated from the immediate or short-term affective responses evoked by external or internal stimuli. While sadness, disappointment, joy, and excitement are appropriate stimulus-bound responses, depression and mania are considered pathological states, even though there may be precipitating events appropriately evoking sadness or elation.

In disorders of mood, deviations in psychological and biological parameters are concurrent. Although our knowledge of the biological or, more accurately, neurohormonal changes is at present extremely meager, clinically the biological disturbances associated with disorders of mood are manifested in changes in appetite, digestive functioning, level of motor activity, and sleep. However, the biological deviations related to mania and depression are not necessarily of an opposite nature. The agitated, depressed patient does not show slow motor activity, and the manic patient may not eat and sleep very much. One major consequence of this irregularity is that, for the most part, the diagnosis of disorders of mood must be heavily dependent on the psychological parameter.

In depression, the triad of symptoms is depressed mood, psychomotor retardation, and difficulty in thinking. Depressed mood is subjectively felt, verbally reported, and behaviorally expressed in sad faces, indifference to personal grooming, weepiness, and so on. Difficulty in thinking is manifested in slowness of verbal response, scantiness of speech production, and the patient's assertion that his thinking process has slowed down. Psychomotor retardation is an objective assessment on the part of the observer to which the patient may also allude. A variety of other symptoms are associated with depression, such as feeling of fatigue, lack of enthusiasm and energy, and vague, unsubstantiated somatic complaints. An important consideration in the symptomatology of depression is the patient's own subjective feelings and ideas. Other symptoms are essentially of a corroborative nature. This dependence on the patient's account of his own illness is a serious disadvantage because unless the patient is able or willing to identify and report his own state of mind, the presence or absence of depression cannot be reliably established.

The existence of depression in childhood has been a matter of controversy. Some authors have claimed that depression as it is known in adult psychiatry cannot or does not appear in childhood. Others, lacking any neurohormonal evidence and acknowledging children's inability to identify and report their subjective feelings, have attempted to delineate the behavioral equivalents of depression in childhood.

Psychological theories of depression in adults have drawn attention to some similarities between grief reaction and depressive states. The concept of loss of a valued object in one form or other has provided the basic framework for various theories of depression. The first designation of depression in childhood is based on similar conceptualization. Spitz and Wolf (1946) reported apathy, weepiness, withdrawal, insomnia, and failure to thrive in several infants who had been separated from their mothers for a period of up to three months. This picture, which resembled adult depression, was called *anaclitic depression* (loss of support), and the authors reported that reunion with mothers was followed by a disappearance of the symptoms.

The immediate impact of separation from the mothering figure caused various degrees of disruption in the behavior of young infants observed by Yarrow and Goodwin (1973). In some infants between 6 and 9 months of age, the reaction to a change in mothering figure was manifested in disturbances in feeding, sleeping, social interactions, emotional state, and development. Studies of primate behaviors following the separation of infant monkeys from their mothers have revealed a similar disruption in the activities of these infants.

The reaction of 2- to 3-year-old children after separation from their mothers was described by Bowlby (1944) as three phases of behavior: protest, despair, and detachment. In his initial discussion, Bowlby equated this picture with the mourning reaction of adults. Later he moved toward agreement with those clinicians who pointed to discrepancies between the above picture and normal grief reaction and stated that separation reaction in these children resembled pathological grief in adults. Observations of children's responses to the death of a parent have shown that in younger children death is totally denied; they fail to show any prolonged reaction to the event. In older children, affective changes are not very obvious; instead there are behavioral changes such as hyperactivity, restlessness, aggressive behavior, temper tantrums, and delinquency. These behaviors have thus been designated as possible equivalents of the depressive mood in children. Glaser (1967) considers a variety of behavioral disorders masked depression. He includes school phobia, failure to achieve academically, and vague somatic complaints, such as headache, dizziness, and abdominal pain, among the possible manifestations of depression in childhood.

Malmquist (1971) described children with irritability, high sensitivity, willingness to condemn themselves, and general unhappiness as suffering from depression, even though they may try to deny their unhappiness by clowning, engaging in provocative behavior, or episodic aggressive acting out.

In reporting 14 cases of overt depression in children, Poznanski and Zrull (1970; Poznanski *et al.*, 1976) set the following criteria for their diagnosis: sad and unhappy look with periods of crying; withdrawal and apathy; sleep disturbance; and feelings of being rejected and unloved, with concomitant feelings of low self-esteem or negative self-image. In 12 out of these 14 children, there were episodes of other-directed aggressive behavior, though self-destructive ideation could also be elicited. The authors described these children as having been the overtly rejected children of families with a high incidence of depression. The children's symptomatology developed slowly and insidiously over one or more years.

Three levels of disturbance in childhood depression are described by Cytryn and McKnew (1974):

- Depressive themes in fantasy, dreams, and responses to projective tests such as the Rorschach and the Thematic Apperception Test. These themes include such fears or preoccupations as worries about death, personal injury, abandonment, and rejection.
- Verbal expressions of unhappiness, unattractiveness, worthlessness, and helplessness.
- Behavioral manifestations, such as disturbed sleep, loss of appetite, and psychomotor retardation, or, conversely, hyperactivity, aggressiveness, and delinquent behavior.

The authors stated that the presence of depressive themes in fantasy is the earliest indication of depression in childhood and the last to disappear with improvement in the child's mood.

CASE HISTORY

Blinda, a 7-year-old Puerto Rican child, was referred to the hospital for hyperactivity, aggressive behavior directed at children and adults, and frequent temper outbursts. Although she had been a difficult child from the first day at school, the teacher reported a definite worsening of her behavior over the previous four weeks. Blinda's mother gave a similar account of the child's behavior, stating that she had become a management problem in the year since her father had been shot. It was reported that the father had been shot during a drinking brawl and that the bullet that had lodged in his brain could not be removed. He had been discharged from the hospital with no provision for follow-up, and the mother reported that "he acts crazy since his accident." A month prior to the youngster's hospitalization, a playmate of hers had been murdered by her own father and Blinda had attended the funeral. The mother stated that she had taken Blinda to the funeral because the two children had been close friends, but she did not think that her daughter had been disturbed by that experience, although she noticed that Blinda had remained next to the child's open coffin longer than anyone else.

In the hospital, Blinda began to kick and spit as soon as the psychiatrist approached her. She refused to talk or play and threw the toys wildly. She quieted down when told that she would have to remain in the hospital, although she still refused to talk. On the following day, it was noted that Blinda would usually sit alone with downcast eyes and sad appearance and at times cried softly to herself. She did not seem hyperactive; in fact, she would not engage in any activities. She ate very little and refused candies offered in the classroom. Her teacher's report in the hospital indicated that Blinda was below grade level academically and did not like to do any schoolwork. During one of her crying episodes, Blinda agreed to talk to the psychiatrist and told the story of her dead friend. She said she could not sleep at night because she was afraid that her own father would do the same thing to her or to her mother. She thought that her father was "crazy" and that like her friend's father, he could not be trusted. She had a vivid memory of the dead child, talked about her and the games they had played together, and added, "I dream about her every night. I don't want to die. When I think about her, I go mad in my head." Blinda remained depressed and weepy for two months. Then her mood began to change slowly and she increasingly interacted with other children, despite continuing concern about death. She worried that her mother would die, stating, "Then I will be all alone; nobody will take care of me; I will just have to die."

In adolescents, depression may take the form of refusal to leave the house, aimless wandering, truancy from school, and delinquent acts, such as stealing, driving at high speed, and reckless behavior. In older adolescents, the symptoms of depression begin to resemble adult depression, with complaints of loneliness, boredom, depression, and suicidal ideations.

Suicidal Behavior

Successful suicide, suicidal attempts, and suicidal threats are rare occurrences in children under 12 years, but the incidence of these behaviors increases with age. Toolan (1962) found 102 admissions for suicidal attempts and threats among the 900 admissions to the Bellevue Hospital child and adolescent psychiatric units. Of these, only 18 children were under 12 years of age.

Children may express the wish that they were dead, but they do not have the concept of death as a finality and their death wishes are usually an expression of dissatisfaction with and a desire for a change in their immediate situation. Of the 100 children under 12 years of age referred to the child psychiatry unit of Bellevue Hospital in New York during a 15-month period, 9 were said to have threatened to kill themselves. The threat usually was communicated to the teacher or the mother; in each situation, the child seemed to have hit upon the idea as a manipulative and coercive measure to deal with the demands placed upon him. All these children either denied having suicidal ideas or said they would not have carried out the threat. When pressed, they all thought that others would have stopped them or, if they had managed to injure themselves, that the injury would not have been of a serious nature. One 11-year-old boy said, "I wouldn't let myself die, even if I jumped, only my leg would be broken and it could get fixed in the hospital." This boy was a very defiant child who had threatened to jump out of the window when his teacher would not allow him to leave the classroom. When a child's suicide attempt results in serious consequences, it is usually caused by a combination of unfortunate factors in the environment rather than the seriousness of the child's own self-destructive desires.

In adolescents, suicide attempts and threats are more frequent among girls. But the relatively rare successful suicides in younger adolescents are usually carried out by boys. The incidence of suicidal threats or attempts in children and adolescents is unknown. During a two-year period (July 1963–July 1965) in the metropolitan area of Cleveland with a population of 1.5 million, 75 cases of attempted or threatened suicide were referred to the 24-hour emergency clinic of the child psychiatry department of the University Hospital of Cleveland. The ratio of girls to boys was 3 to 1. Boys had made more threats and girls had made more suicidal attempts. During the same period, 7 cases of successful suicide had been reported for the Cleveland area in adolescents, all of whom were boys (Mattsson *et al.*, 1969).

Suicidal attempts and threats, while possibly not life-threatening, are always an indication of great disturbance in the immediate environment and a sign of the child's or adolescent's inability to cope with the situation in a less dramatic and more constructive manner (Ackerly, 1964).

Mattsson *et al.* (1969) described the following causes for the suicidal threats or attempts in their sample:

- Acute or prolonged grief following a loss, desertion by a parent, death of a parent, or the breakup of a highly valued relationship with a peer, usually of the opposite sex.

- Long-standing difficulties at home and in school leading to a sense of worthlessness with little hope for a better future. This group may show other signs of depression.
- Serious, unbearable tension within the family, in which the adolescent may feel entrapped and resorts to a suicidal attempt in the hope of attracting outside attention to his or her plight.
- Anger expressed by suicidal or homicidal threats with the idea that those left behind will suffer the consequences of the act and "pay for their insensitivity" and "learn a lesson."
- Psychosis, usually schizophrenia, with rather insidious onset and feelings of internal disintegration.
- A reckless, potentially dangerous act engaged in as a desperate maneuver to impress peers and provide a sense of invulnerability for a shaky and insecure adolescent.

The majority of suicidal attempts are done in the presence of others or are reported to parents, peers, and teachers shortly after the attempt (Shaffer, 1974). Ingestion of various chemicals is the most frequently used method, though superficial slashing of wrists or lacerations with knives are not uncommon.

Indications of mounting tension are usually present a few weeks before the act of suicide. In retrospect, teachers and parents remember the adolescent's falling grades, irritability, lack of interest in work, and depressed mood (Toolan, 1971; Connell, 1965).

Of particular importance is the possibility of suicide in adolescents who have a chronic physical illness or deformity that is expected to continue into the future. These adolescents, after months of apparent adjustment to their disability, may begin to realize the irreversibility of their condition and be overwhelmed with feelings of despondency and helplessness. Suicidal attempts or threats on the part of these patients may indicate a serious desire to end their own lives and to put an end to the hardship inflicted upon their family. Failure to keep appointments with the physician and refusal to take medication or continue with the therapeutic regimen may be the early warning signals of future suicidal intention in these adolescents.

Treatment. Treatment for suicidal behavior in children and adolescents begins with a carefully considered diagnosis of all the contributory factors. Hospitalization is not always necessary, provided that one can be reasonably certain of the parents' cooperation and the child's lack of strong motivation for further attempts.

Family therapy may be extremely helpful when the source of tension lies within the network of intrafamilial relationships. Even in those cases in which the basic problem is the child's difficulty in coping with intrapsychic and/or extrafamilial stress, the family is the logical source of continuous support for the child, and their cooperation is necessary as an adjunct to other forms of treatment.

Placement in a residential treatment center or foster home may be indicated when the severity of the child's psychopathology or a rejecting or chaotic home warrants such a measure.

Antidepressant drugs have not as yet been approved for the use in children under 12 years of age by the regulatory agencies in the United States. Available studies from European and American sources have reported some beneficial effects, although these studies are open to criticism on methodological grounds. In older children, chemotherapy for depression should always be undertaken under close supervision and only as an adjunct to psychotherapy (Annell, 1972).

ANXIETY

The concept of anxiety as a specific emotional response is a central issue in theories of personality development and maladjustment. Fear and withdrawal, as normal reactions to intensely unpleasant and painful stimuli, are experienced by both animals and human infants. But anxiety appears to be a peculiarly human response that develops as the result of the prolonged physical dependency of the human infant on his parents and the continuing psychological interdependence.

Negative reaction to strangers or the "8-month anxiety" can be observed in most children, although not necessarily at 8 months of age. After months of indiscriminately interacting with a variety of people, infants of around 6–9 months of age withdraw from advances made by strangers and show their displeasure by crying and clinging to their mothers. The intensity of this reaction and the circumstances of its appearance are dependent upon several factors. Many infants seem to show a transitory period during which they are reluctant to interact with those whom they have seen only sporadically. Some authors have postulated that the appearance of such reactions coincides with the time that the child has begun to relate to his mother as a distinctly separate identity and feels a rudimentary sense of well-being in her close proximity. Others consider this phenomenon as an expression of affectional tie and infant–mother attachment. It has been noted also that the presence of the mother can potentiate the toddler's willingness to explore a new environment. When the human environment is kept constant, children are able to ignore most disruptive occurrences in their surroundings. Conversely, when the mother is not present, even a nonthreatening but novel situation may be disturbing to some children; thus nursery school, as well as hospitalization, may evoke separation anxiety.

An intense dependence on familiar figures (mother, father, and other family members) is a prerequisite for socializing the child. The feeling of anxiety and insecurity that is associated with physical separation is gradually replaced by a fear of affectional distance, so that the presence of the parents is no longer needed to assure the child of his security but is replaced by an abstract, internalized concept of being approved of and belonging to the family.

The process by which this change from the concrete presence to the abstract approval of the parents is achieved is among the most complex issues in child rearing and child development. The effort to maintain and regain parental approval is later generalized to other significant adults and peers. Fear of disapproval and loss of parental affection is a prototype for all anxiety reactions in children. When parental norms and, by extension, the norms of the culture are internalized, anxiety is experienced as having an internal source. Now the threat of loss of parental approval recedes into the background and the growing child is concerned about the threat to his own self-esteem and self-image.

Avoidance of anxiety is a potent force in the development of conformity to cultural and societal demands and standards. Failure or inability to conform to the expectation of parents, peers, and culture creates anxiety. When the resultant anxiety is not so overwhelming as to inhibit the child, it is constructive in that it leads to a state of high arousal and strong motivation to learn the expected behavior. On the other hand, crippling anxiety is detrimental to the child and his future development.

Parental rejection of the child, particularly after he has developed dependence on their approval, can cause extreme insecurity and disorientation. On the other hand, overprotective parents can create anxiety for the child by tacitly implying or explicitly stating that the child cannot hope to receive approval from people other than his parents. In symbiotic relationships between mother and child, the most damaging result is the child's insecurity in relating to his peers and other adults. Overdemanding parents who fail to respect the limitations of a child's ability and make their approval contingent upon impossible achievement may produce perfectionistic and insecure children. Capricious parents who fail to provide their children with predictable demands set the stage for the child's chronic state of uncertainty. Anxiety is experienced in cases of developmental lag when the child is aware that he is unable to achieve what is normative for his age and doubts his own competence and acceptability as a person.

Clinically we may expect anxiety to be a part of most behavioral deviations for which parents refer their children. During psychiatric examination, anxiety may be manifested as restlessness, timidity, and refusal to speak or even to enter the office. Children may avoid eye contact, demand to have their mothers present, or complain of being nervous. They report difficulty in sleeping and may have nightmares. Speech may be under pressure, ideas disjointed, and associations difficult to follow. Phobias, concerns about physical safety, and preoccupation with death are commonly reported. Fantasies are sometimes populated by destructive, malevolent, supernatural forces. The child may show his insecurity by repeatedly asking for direction and approval. When asked to perform simple tasks, such as drawing a picture or writing a few words, he may refuse, or he may preface his attempts by stating that he is not good at this particular subject. Anxiety may diminish the effectiveness of his performance on psychological tests and thus lower the obtained IQ. Some children manifest their high tension by biting their nails, pulling their hair, or masturbating.

An anxious adolescent may be negativistic and defiant, although his worried look and clammy hands speak of his basic tension. Vague somatic complaints may be blamed for feelings of fatigue and irritability. Other adolescents complain of incomprehensible changes in themselves (depersonalization) or in their environment (derealization).

Panic reaction associated with the emergence of overpowering sexual impulses or in reaction to what is viewed by an adolescent as sexual advances by others should be differentiated from the extreme anxiety due to the experience of psychic disintegration in acute schizophrenia.

Situational anxiety can be best understood by reviewing the nature of the patient's interpersonal relationships and uncovering potential threats to his self-esteem.

Unrelieved chronic anxiety of intense quality may be an early signal of a psychotic process. In some cases, diseases of the brain (tumor, epilepsy) may be first manifested by unexplainable anxiety. A careful physical examination in adolescents presenting what clinically appears as anxiety reaction is always necessary if one is to rule out such metabolic disorders as hypoglycemia or hyperthyroidism, in which the subjective state may be similar.

For further discussion of anxiety, see Chapter 11, "Childhood Neuroses."

6

Assessment

CLINICAL EVALUATION

The purpose of psychiatric evaluation in children, as in adults, is to obtain information both about the nature and severity of the functional impairment and about the more normal aspects of the personality. The majority of adult patients, even when not self-referred, can give an account of their own problems. However, children are usually judged to be in need of a psychiatric assessment by adults such as parents, teachers, or law enforcement agencies. The fact of the referral does not provide convincing evidence that the child is psychiatrically ill, since factors such as ignorance of age-appropriate behavior or exaggeration and misinterpretation of the child's activities may color the views of those in close association with him. Also, the attitudes and practices of the caretakers may play a significant role in causing the maladaptive behavior for which the psychiatric evaluation is requested. Furthermore, because children's behavioral repertoires are limited, presenting symptoms are unreliable guides to the nature and severity of the underlying problems. Psychiatric examination of children, therefore, requires both careful collection of information from all the available sources and also direct observation and evaluation of the child. An interview with the caretakers usually precedes observation of the child, although at times this order may be reversed because of various contingencies.

An interview with the parents requires patience, discretion, and understanding from the child psychiatrist in order to assure that all the factual data regarding the child are obtained. A nonjudgmental, sympathetic atmosphere allows the parents to reveal their own concerns and thoughts about their parenting function. It is usually desirable to see both parents together, even though each parent may request, or can be invited for, an individual session. When parents are in disagreement as to the nature of the problem or even the necessity for an evaluation, it is up to the child psychiatrist to convey to the dissenting member his own impartiality and respect for the differences of opinion between the couple.

Interview with the Parents

When parents have been pressured by outsiders such as teachers to bring a child for psychiatric assessment, they may view the child psychiatrist as a part of the system that is trying to label their child and exclude him from social institutions. They may therefore be hostile, uncooperative, and mistrustful and either minimize the child's difficulties or blame others for them. Other parents may have developed an oversensitivity to any indication of problematic behavior and give an exaggerated picture of the child's symptoms. Some parents' objectivity is marred by their conviction that the child's troubles are created by parental mishandling or neglect, and their guilt and fear of the psychiatric findings render them unreliable informants.

The emotional tone of the parents while giving information about the child is a significant part of the interview and must be carefully noted. However, the fact that parents are anxious, aloof, on the brink of tears, or angry may show their reaction to the situation rather than their prevalent mood or style of interaction. The knowledge that one or both parents have histories of psychiatric problems in and of itself does not indicate that the child's behavior is caused by parental handling or that his impaired functioning is genetically determined. Children of alcoholic parents or those with major psychiatric disorders, although admittedly under stress, may not fare worse than youngsters whose parents suffer from other chronic medical illnesses. All information and observations must be recorded, though their relevance and importance may become clear only after direct examination of the child or when treatment strategies are contemplated.

The following outline is suggested as a guide for obtaining pertinent data from the parents. Modifications and elaborations will be needed according to specific circumstances surrounding each case, and information may be gathered in a different sequence.

Identifying Data. These should include the age and sex of the child; his grade placement in school and the number of years that he has attended the particular school; the number of sibs, their ages, and ordinal position; the parents' occupation and their educational background; and the child's address and living accommodations. When parents are divorced or separated, it is important to ascertain whether legal guardianship has been contested or is under consideration by the court. The frequency of the child's visits with the nonguardian parent gives an indication of the value that can be attached to her or his description of the child's behavior. For example, when the nonguardian parent visits regularly and frequently, he or she may be expected to observe the child's customary behavior, while when visits are limited to vacation times each year, the child's activities may be vastly different from what the other parent describes. Such differences do not necessarily reflect the interactional patterns with each parent but may be due to lack of pressure from academic obligations or peer relationships.

When the child is adopted, the circumstances leading to adoption, the child's age at the time of adoption, and whatever is known about the biological parents must be recorded. Most children know about their adoptive status; however, the question must be specifically asked of the parents, and the child's reported reaction to the fact of adoption must be explored. Some guilt-ridden adoptive parents may reconstruct their memories of the child's early years to fit a possible picture of genetic and constitutional peculiarities. However, the same parents become accepting of the child once their fears and guilt are put to rest.

Foster parents may be defensive and resentful when they believe that their adequacy and qualification for child rearing is being questioned. They may exaggerate the severity of the child's disturbed behavior in order to vindicate themselves, or to expedite a child's removal from their home without being viewed as unqualified for fostering other children.

Source and Reason for Referral. Preschoolers are frequently referred by their pediatricians, while school-age children may have been sent at the advice of the school personnel. In either case, parents have been aware of the child's problem or the difficulties have been brought to their attention before a consultation is sought. Details regarding the presenting complaints, the duration of each symptom, and its evolution over time must be carefully explored. Parents must be asked to describe in an objective manner the behavior, the precipitating factors, and their own attempts to correct and handle the behavior. Some parents tend to give interpretations of what they believe to be the child's motivation in engaging in a certain behavior; others use psychological jargon, assuming that technical terms have higher communicative values. Such interpretive statements can lead to misunderstanding by the psychiatrist and lock the parents' perception of the child into a particular mold that may not be applicable to the situation. It is therefore necessary to insist that parents give concrete examples. When previous consultations have been sought, one must inquire about the conclusions that have been conveyed to the parents, the kind of intervention proposed, the child's response to any treatment that was undertaken, or the parents' reasons for ignoring or not accepting the previous recommendations. In addition to clarifying the course and nature of the presenting symptoms, such information allows the practitioner to avoid the pitfall of presenting the parents with the same unacceptable plan or repeating the unsuccessful treatment.

Developmental History. Circumstances in the family, including the length of marriage, the number of previous pregnancies and live births, the parents' age, and the planned or accidental nature of conception, are significant aspects of the environment in which a baby is born. Some children, conceived after years of childless marriage, are at the risk of being overprotected and overindulged. Other youngsters are born at a time when one or both parents feel overburdened and unwilling or unable to care for them. The parents' age, particularly the mother's at the time of conception, may be a contributing factor in such disorders as Down's syndrome. Conversely, a mother's young age may account for her real or imaginary feelings of inadequacy and hesitancy in mothering.

A history of previous miscarriages and post- or premature delivery may give a clue to possible intrauterine risk factors. Length of pregnancy and maternal health during the period are important aspects of prenatal life, while the duration and nature of delivery may indicate the presence or absence of fetal distress. The birth weight, as well as immediate postnatal events such as resuscitation, exchange transfusion, and incubation, gives valuable information regarding the normality or physical ill health of the baby.

Following the immediate neonatal period, parental attention is focused on caring for the infant and attempting to discover the tempo and the style of his activities and to accommodate to and regulate the schedule of his biological needs. Problems with feeding, elimination, and sleep are usually remembered when they have been of protracted nature and have necessitated frequent changes of formula, although at times parents may forget these early inconveniences only to be reminded of them when questioned. Conversely, some parental memories are slowly and inadvertently changed in order to place the child's early behavior in a continuum with his present status.

Developmental landmarks such as the age of walking and talking are usually remembered when parents considered them too slow or precocious. Rate of language acquisition is developmentally significant, not only because it is so closely associated with the child's intellectual ability but also because communicative skills play an important role in the child's socialization. Toilet training is a major parental effort to impose socially prescribed regulations on the child's physiological activities. The ease or difficulty with which toilet training is accomplished reflects the child-rearing practices of the parents and the infant's adaptation or maladjustment to them.

Separation from the mother and participation in such outside institutions as nursery school or kindergarten are indicative of the child's level of social and emotional readiness at certain points in his life. Even though some children are not sent to nursery school for other reasons, some are considered too fragile and sickly by their parents, and still another group are not accepted because they do not function at an age-appropriate level. The history of interactions with peers may be explored by asking parents about any comments made by nursery school teachers in this regard or the availability of playmates at home or in the neighborhood.

A significant medical history, particularly of those incidents that have necessitated the child's hospitalization or exclusion from normal activities, is important. Such incidents may be contributary factors to the physical status of the child, or they may be a significant reason for the kind of parental handling that he has received. Inquiries into the types of stressful situations to which the child has been exposed give information about the physical and psychological illnesses and marital or financial problems besetting the household. The birth of sibs, a death in the family, or the departure or arrival of new members is at times given as the beginning of the child's problematic behavior. Careful investigation may reveal a drastic change in the child's status as the result of such occurrences, or it may show that in their search for etiology parents have come to attach undue significance to such inevitable happenings.

The child's school history provides information about his social, intellectual, and adaptive functioning. It is most helpful to request that such reports be specifically obtained for the purpose of the psychiatric evaluation. However, some parents are reluctant to inform the school that they have sought psychiatric help for their children, particularly when the child's problems are said to be limited to his home environment. In such situations, the child's report card may be searched for descriptions of the child's behavior and his academic standing.

Present Functioning. To ascertain the present functioning of the child, the psychiatrist asks the parents to describe his daily routine, peer group activities and affiliations, areas of nonproblematic functioning, use of leisure time, hobbies and interests, and what the parents consider to be the child's special strength.

The child's interactions with various family members and relationships with both parents are questioned in detail. Some child-rearing techniques, such as the parents' tolerance of aggression or their prevalent method of disciplining may come to light or be inquired about when each parent describes his role and relationship with the child.

The degree of responsibility for self-care and help with household chores that are assigned to the child and his compliance or rebelliousness with set routines are explored. Furthermore, parents are asked to describe the child's predominant mood, the ease with which he adjusts to new situations, the predictability of his responsiveness and reactions, and their view of his overall functioning. Such inquiries may encourage the parents to take a fresh look at their child and may set the stage for their active participation in the treatment plan that will be presented to them.

The history of major neurological or psychiatric disorders in the family may have a direct bearing on the child's problem. While some disorders are genetically determined, others may be significant only to the extent that their occurrence in the family background has sensitized the parents to any behavioral deviations exhibited by the child.

The internal consistency of the account of the child's behavior given by the parents is the most important index of its reliability. Parents may forget significant data and be vague about certain facts regarding themselves or their child. They may disagree with each other's account of the child's behavior or appear to have no interest in what the psychiatric evaluation may reveal. The child psychiatrist must attempt to learn as much as possible about the child without alienating the parents. Although he may note certain obvious signs of psychiatric disorders in the parents, his task is to assess the manner in which such psychiatric symptoms may inhibit the child's normal growth or contribute to the creation of his deviant behavior.

Preparing the Child for an Interview. Finally, it is important to ask the parents how they intend to prepare the child for the visit to the psychiatrist. Some parents believe that children must be kept in the dark as to the purpose and the nature of the examination. It is necessary to advise the parents that the child must be told the reason for the consultation. Children are usually aware that some aspects of their behavior are subjects of parental concern and do not find it strange that their parents have sought professional help. Some youngsters are eager to find ways to modify their behavior; others can be told that no advice can be given until their side of the story is known.

The hesitation and anxiety of some parents can be removed when they are assured that the psychiatric interview will not expose their progeny to undue pressure and that the youngster may in fact play or talk about whatever concerns or interests him.

The issue of confidentiality in child psychiatry is not easily solved and no firm guidelines have been set by the professional bodies. Parents must be told about any information that has clear implications for the child's safety and protection. On the other hand, both parents and the young patient need reassurances that they can express their feelings and ideas without fear of exposure. Such balance can be achieved by informing the youngster that while the child psychiatrist cannot withhold certain vital materials from the parents, the patient will be told in advance of any such exposure, and the issues and the necessity for such action will be discussed with him. This is of particular value for adolescents, who must be convinced from the outset that the psychiatrist will not betray their trust but must not be given a sense of false security.

It is necessary for the child to know that his parents have reported all the pertinent data about themselves and their child's background so that the patient can feel free to discuss whatever concerns him without feeling that he is giving out a family secret or letting down his parents.

Interview with the Child

The ultimate goal of the psychiatric interview with a child is to collect the data necessary to formulate some conclusions about the patient's mental status. Such interviews cannot be rigidly structured, but it is also not helpful to leave a child without any direction. While more than one interview session may be necessary to formulate an accurate diagnosis, an experienced child psychiatrist is expected to use the allotted time in such a way that a statement can be made about the child's normality or the need for further psychiatric investigation after the first encounter. In very young children, when developmental lag or deviation is suspected, reassessments at six-month intervals are necessary to clarify the picture.

Ideally the child should be seen alone, although some children become extremely anxious when separated from their parents and the intensity of their fears inhibits their functioning. In these situations, a parent is allowed to remain with the child for the beginning of the interview, or for the whole session if separation is too distressful. Preschoolers can be tempted with toys and the invitation to play with them. With the school-age group, it is sufficient to inform the child that he may choose to play while talking. The invitation may be repeated to those children who initially choose to sit and talk and become restless as the discussion progresses.

Following the greeting and introduction, questions about the child's age, school, likes, and dislikes are asked to put the child at ease and establish the child psychiatrist as a person who is interested in getting to know the youngster. Some patients are poorly prepared for the visit by their parents. Others choose to profess ignorance about the purpose of the visit for reasons of their own. If the child insists that he does not know why he has been brought to the psychiatrist or has only a vague and distorted notion about it, a simple explanation is needed about the nature of the alleged problem, the concern of the parents, and the psychiatrist's role in trying to understand and help both the child and his family.

When the patient is seen in the hospital at the request of his primary physician, the concern of the child's doctor must be conveyed as the reason for the consultation, and the child must be assured that he will still remain under the care of his own physician. Children who are hospitalized for psychiatric reasons may be frightened, hostile, and defiant and may view the hospitalization as evidence of abandonment or punishment by the parents. They need reassurance, clarification, and explanation as to their safety and their parents' continuing responsibility and interest before they can be expected to trust the psychiatrist.

Most children find general questions difficult to answer, so inquiries must be simple and concrete. At times, a sequence of actions can be questioned step by step so that the psychiatrist may gain an understanding of the child's mental processes. Inquiries about emotional reactions to various events are frequently answered by vague statements such as "It made me feel bad" or "I was upset." To clarify such responses, the child may be given a choice among a few words that may more precisely indicate his feelings. For example, *sad, angry, hurt, sorry,* or *guilty* are alternatives that may replace the word *bad* or *upset* in the above statements. Further refinement of concepts may be achieved, particularly with inarticulate patients, by asking the child to describe the activity that accompanied the feeling, such as crying, hitting, or desiring to do so.

A record of observations and conversation with the child include the following items.

Appearance. The child's size, his state of nutrition, and any obvious defects and scars must be noted. Tics, mannerisms, facial expressions, and the way they change during the interview may provide clues about the child's mood or state of tension. Unconventional attire or hairdo and other striking features may reflect parental preferences at young ages or the youngster's desire for self-expression during adolescence.

Level of Motor Activity. Gross movements around the room, fidgeting in the seat, or hypoactivity and rigid posture must be recorded. In some patients the driven quality of motor activity is noticeable only when the child appears to lose control while engaged in an activity. For example, a child may begin to paint or draw carefully and painstakingly; gradually he uses less-coordinated brushstrokes or produces shakier lines; this builds up to the point where he splashes paint indiscriminately over the paper or scribbles to fill the page. If the psychiatrist identifies such a process at an early stage and manages to distract the child, it may save him more strenuous efforts at limit setting for these patients.

Mood and Affect. These include the predominant mood during the session, the depth and range of affective expression, and their relation to the child's verbal or nonverbal activities. Additional information about the emotional state may be gathered from the child's response to questioning. Children are usually able to identify their moods of sadness, happiness, anger, and fear and to give elaboration such as wishing to be dead, contemplating suicide, wanting to hurt a particular person, or being very worried.

Thought and Verbalization. The child's verbal ability is reflected in the vocabulary and sentence structure he uses. Some children with articulation defects are nevertheless capable of conveying their ideas through sophisticated vocabulary and grammatically correct sentences. But attentive listening may reveal subtle deficiencies of language such as word approximation, anomia, or other indications of central language disorder. Immediate echolalia is easy to identify, while delayed echolalia may appear as an irrelevant statement within the context of the child's activities. In adolescents, neologism is clearly distinguishable since language acquisition is complete, while very young children may delight in playing with words or may distort the pronunciation of a word to the point of nonrecognition. In preschoolers, a clinical estimate of verbal age can be achieved by comparing the child's vocabulary and sentence structure with the age-expected range.

The child's thinking processes are judged by his ability to organize his perceptions, impressions, and activities. This may be reflected in his speech or his use of toys. Irrelevant answers to questions may be due to the child's lack of comprehension, while incoherent statements require attention, patience, ingenuity, or educated guesses to unravel. School-age children are expected to use language as a means of social communication; therefore irrelevancy and incoherency of speech are less likely to occur in their conversation. Loose association or frequent changes of subject may be due to short attention span and distractibility and are not necessarily indicative of psychotic thinking in young children. Concreteness is a normal quality of pre-adolescent thinking, and abstract concepts such as the cause-and-effect relationship are not mastered beyond the child's daily experiences. The child's logic is a reflection of his personal view of his environment and is not comparable with the formal logic of adults and adolescents.

Objective criteria for the assessment of thinking disorder in children are nonexistent. In fact, some theories of disordered thinking in adult schizophrenics are based on the premise that schizophrenic thinking in adults resembles normal children's thinking. The judgement that there is a disordered quality to the child's thinking is made on the basis of highly fragmented, disorganized, and bizarre verbal and nonverbal activities and the child's inability to keep his age-appropriate concepts from merging into each other. For example, while a normal preschooler may indeed become so involved in his fantasies that his affective responses and expectations become colored by his daydreams, a school-age child is expected to remain aware of the distinction among reality, fantasy, and pretend games. An 8-year-old child waking from a nightmare is anxious and frightened. However, the same child is able to fantasize about his encounter with powerful men from outer space without overwhelming anxiety.

Bizarre content must be differentiated from the child's idiosyncratic view of the environment. Questioning the child about his statements usually provides the psychiatrist with clues about how a youngster has drawn conclusions from what he has seen or heard from others and how he has combined or organized his ideas. A psychotic child cannot explain the process by which he has come to a specific conclusion, and his attempts at justification reveal his inability to organize his perceptions. Nancy, a 9-year-old psychotic girl, in response to the question "What would you like to be when you grow up?" says, "An ice cream." ("Why?") "Becuase I am sweet." ("What is good about being an ice cream?") "People eat ice cream. I like people to eat me." Bruce, a 6-year-old boy, says, "A part of my brain is loose inside my head." ("How do you know") "I got shot in the head." ("When?") "In my sleep. This boy didn't like me. I got shot." ("You dreamed that you got shot?") "Yes." ("How come you don't have a bullet wound?") "Because the bullet just went inside, a part of my brain is loose. I hear it going around, making a boom-boom sound."

Cognitive errors, such as attaching a literal meaning to figurative words, associating concepts based on their spatial or temporal contiguity, and misinterpreting information, are factors that may result in the formulation of idiosyncratic views. An example of an uncommon personal view in a normal child is Mark's response to the question ("How many brothers and sisters do you have?"): "I have one sister." ("How old?") "I don't know, she is not born yet." ("You mean your mother is going to have a baby?") "Yes." ("How do you know it is a baby sister?") "My father told me." ("How does he know?") "The doctor told him." ("How did the doctor find out?") "Because he has X-ray eyes. He looks at something and can tell right away." The child's parents had indeed told him that he would have a baby sister following the result of an amniocentesis done to rule out fetal abnormalities.

Senses and Perceptions. Reports of unusual sensitivity to various sensory stimuli such as sound, smell, or texture may be related by parents. In nonverbal children, the reactions of the child to noise, touch, and attempts at physical contact must be observed and recorded. Older children can be directly asked about the reasons for their avoidance of certain foods, reaction to sounds, and hallucinatory experiences. Some children report having heard their names being called or being told such things as "Don't be bad" or "Everything will be fine." Others report seeing monsters and ghosts in a semidarkened room. In preadolescents, such phenomena are usually benign unless the content of the auditory hallucinations are bizarre and morbid or the visual experiences happen in well-lit rooms when the child is fully awake. Furthermore, the child's reactions to frightening experiences give a clue as to whether such events can be dismissed as the by-products of the child's vivid imagination and efforts to amuse himself. Imaginary companions in young, lonely children may be described as carrying on a conversation or sitting and playing with toys. Older children may engage in such fantasies, but they are either reluctant to divulge such information or express the view that it is a make-believe game. In adolescents, hallucinations are rarely innocuous, even though they may be transient.

Self-Image. The child's view of himself includes such areas as his gender identity, his description of himself as "good" or "bad," his feelings about his standing with his peers, and his competence or deficiencies in school. Most children can project themselves into the future by answering questions about what they would like to do when they grow up and whether they would like to marry and have children or would prefer to remain alone. Exploring the child's reasons for his choices gives the psychiatrist additional information about the child's present state of mind and his impressions of life within the family. For adolescents, such choices are more realistic and the patient's responses more revealing of some aspect of the reality with which he is struggling.

Feelings about Family Members. The child's opinion about his parents and siblings must be carefully explored. Some children are reluctant to give their views about their parents but may be willing to accept the psychiatrist's invitation to describe what they would like to change about their parents' behavior. A certain amount of aggressive feeling toward siblings is usually expressed very freely. However, at times the child gives such a negative picture of his relationships with sibs that one must try to solicit positive aspects of the interactions in order to obtain a balanced view. The same children may reveal that they fight with others in support of their sibs or insist that their parents buy something for the brother or sister who has been excluded from a shopping trip. When the child describes his altercations with his sibs, it is important to inquire about the parental handling of such situations, since some children's resentment against their sibs originates from or is compounded by what, in their opinion, is parental unfairness. Taken to its logical conclusion, these youngsters will express their belief that their parents do not like them as much as their brothers and sisters.

Children coming from broken homes usually wish for parental reunion, even though they may report that life before the separation was full of bickering and disharmony. When a stepmother or stepfather is a member of the patient's daily environment, the child may be reluctant to report positive feelings toward him or her out of loyalty toward the absent biological parent. Descriptions of common activities and questions about what kind of treatment the child receives from the substitute mother or father provide a more accurate impression of such relationships. When absent parents are not available to the child, his views, hopes, and fantasies regarding them must be investigated and his sources of information ascertained.

Functioning. The child's functioning includes his health, appetite, sleep pattern, academic standing, peer relationships, hobbies, and interests. The child's report of his health must be substantiated by a statement from his pediatrician or a physical examination requested or performed by the child psychiatrist. Statements about academic performance may be checked by asking the child to read from a book or do some arithmetical operations. The psychiatrist asks the names of best friends and the frequency of shared activities, and he uses the occasion to ask the child about how he settles his disagreements with his friends and how he tries to cope with various situations involving other children. Discussion about school must be broadened to include the child's view of his teachers and his relationships with them.

Presenting Symptoms. Questions regarding the presenting symptoms may be asked anytime after the child seems relaxed and engaged in the interview situation. Adolescents expect such inquiries to be made early, while children may not feel any need to talk about them. Some issues may be embarrassing to the child and have to be raised tactfully; other subjects are discussed with little hesitation. The affective responses of the patient; his explanations and guesses regarding the cause of the problem and the circumstances that engender the particular symptom; and his degree of unease and unhappiness with the behavior or its consequences must be noted. The strength of the child's motivation to rid himself of the problem behavior is evaluated by both direct questioning and an impression of the realistic and unrealistic attempts that he has made to alter his behavior.

Fantasies. The patient's fantasies cannot be strictly separated from his verbal and nonverbal activities during the session. However, questions regarding the child's wishes, hopes for the future, pleasant and unpleasant dreams, worries, and daydreams are an important part of the psychiatric interview. It must be noted that the child's play and drawings, although expressive of some aspects of his inner feelings, cannot be viewed as significant diagnostic tools without regard for the context in which they appear.

Estimates of the child's intelligence, his degree of freedom from unpleasant feelings, his competence in establishing a relationship with the interviewer, his manner of coping with limits and questions, his efficiency in learning, and his insight into his own behavior and the behavior of those around him are components of the child's mental status that will determine an evaluation of psychological health or disturbance.

Although the purpose of the psychiatric interview remains unchanged, modifications are needed according to the child's age.

Preschool Children. In these examinations, verbalization plays a small role. The interview must record the youngster's reaction to the novel situation, his relatedness to objects and people, his ease or difficulty in separating from the mother, and his response to the psychiatrist's verbal or physical overtures. Handling of objects and the level of understanding of their functions, as well as the amount of time that a child spends in playing with each toy, give information about his attention span and awareness of the nature of objects. Presence or absence of imitative behavior is noted because of its possible implication for learning, while comprehension of simple directions reflects the child's familiarity with language. Speech production provides an indication of the mental age, while gross and fine motor activities reflect other aspects of developmental status. The child's responses to tactile, visual, and auditory stimuli are noteworthy because they may shed light on the behavioral problems that concern the parents. The psychiatric interview must be conducted with the goal of arriving at a developmental status that includes information regarding the adaptive, motor, and verbal age of the child and evaluation of deviant behavior in a developmental frame of reference.

School-Age Children. Although play activities may provide significant clues as to the child's thinking, fantasies, and fears, it is the verbal interchange that allows the psychiatrist to assess the patient's mental status and his ability to cope with his environment. Some children may resist the psychiatrist's inquiries by engaging in solitary play. Others use toys as a means of indirect communication. Sometimes the psychiatrist's comments about the child's activities give the patient an opportunity to break his self-imposed silence. At other times, more than one interview is necessary to make the child sufficiently comfortable to talk. Interpretation of the child's negativism usually leads to stronger resistance, while acknowledgment of the child's anxieties and anger may be all that is needed to establish rapport.

Adolescents. Most adolescents view the psychiatric evaluation as imposed on them by their parents. However, they are usually willing to voice their opinions and discuss the possible reasons that may have led their parents to draw erroneous conclusions. The task of the psychiatrist is to convince the patient that as an interested and impartial professional he is willing to hear views contrary to those of the parents. The extreme sensitivity of adolescents requires that the psychiatrist avoid projecting an image of undue familiarity or paternalistic condescension toward the youngster.

Inquiries into such subjects as sex, use of drugs, or other socially unacceptable behavior must be made with the forthrightness and nonjudgmental attitude with which all other information is sought. The patient's desire to remain silent or to give answers that appear less than candid must be accepted without further questioning. The adolescent needs to feel that he can guard his privacy against the psychiatrist's probing without being made uncomfortable by it. Most adolescents, having been allowed to establish a social persona, are willing to engage in discussion of their private concerns and worries and to acknowledge their difficulties in coping with their own feelings or the demands placed upon them.

At the end of the psychiatric interview with adolescents, the psychiatrist must review the problem areas with the patient and give him some indication of the conclusions that are drawn and the recommendations that will be presented to the parents.

Conveying the Psychiatric Evaluation

Upon completion of the psychiatric evaluation, conclusions and recommendations must be conveyed to the parents and through them to the child. The informing interview must address those questions that prompted the parents to seek psychiatric opinion. While the psychiatrist may be more concerned about the child's total functioning, he must remember that the parents want to know the reasons for the child's behavior and the manner in which they can handle and manage the situation. Diagnostic labels are of little value to the parents and, in fact, may be quite unacceptable to them unless they are convinced of the relationship between their child's behavior and what is implied by the diagnosis. Vague statements about the child's emotional disturbance or his developmental lag in certain areas of functioning do not constitute useful information for parents.

Explanations must include a cohesive system in which the parents' report, the child's history, and the results of tests and observations are all taken into consideration and made meaningful for the parents. Time must be allotted for the parents to seek additional information and clarification, and a course of intervention must be detailed with an overall view of what is hoped to be gained, the length of time over which intervention may be necessary, and the prognosis for eventual adjustment. Professional cautiousness and conservatism should not leave the parents with an overwhelming sense of pessimism about the child's future, nor should a desire for implementation of a certain treatment strategy blind the psychiatrist to the uncertainties of psychiatric intervention.

PSYCHOLOGICAL TESTING

Psychological measurements are inferences made from the observable behavior of an individual in response to a defined set of stimuli called *psychological tests*. These inferences are based on the assumption that there is a lawful relationship between the observed behavior and the underlying psychological state or personality traits of the individual. The orientation, or conceptual frame of reference of the observer, influences both what is observed and how it is interpreted. Questions about what it is that psychological tests measure or in what way such measurements facilitate our understanding of the individual cannot be answered directly. Instead, psychologists try to ascertain the reliability of the tests and seek validating evidence from the individual's past, present, or future behavior outside the testing situation.

The reliability of a test depends upon its consistency over time in test/retest measurements, while its validity is assessed by the degree to which it can be correlated with significant aspects of the personality organization or other behavioral variables.

When a test is considered valid and reliable, the inconsistencies of an individual's performance over time are said to be due to extraneous factors such as variations in the administration of the test or response variations by the subject due to differing states of motivation, fatigue, anxiety, moods, or a disorganizing process affecting the personality.

Some psychological tests, such as the sentence completion test, are direct in that the manifest content of the response is the basis of interpretation. Other tests, such as the Rorschach, are indirect in that the categories utilized for interpretation are inferred from the manifest content and differ from the respondent's actual statement, although the psychologist may also analyze such directly observable behavior as the child's style of responsiveness to the test material or the quality of his cognitive organization and problem-solving strategies.

Objective tests, such as those concerned with attitudes and intelligence, have structured questions evoking replies that are viewed behavioristically. Projective tests involve free response to and associations with a series of stimuli that are then interpreted according to several assumptions and hypotheses regarding the psychological processes of apperception, projection, and personality organization.

In the following discussion only those tests that are widely used in child psychiatry are examined.

Intelligence Tests

Concept of Intelligence. Intelligence is a hypothetical concept and its existence can be inferred only from the way individuals behave. Spearman (1923) conceived of a general factor of intelligence (g factor) that is manifested in different degrees in various mental activities. For example, according to Spearman, finding similarities and differences among two concepts or discovering relationships between two categories has a higher loading of g factors than such mental activities as reproductive memory or arithmetic computation. It is therefore possible to hypothesize a hierarchy of mental functions and thus assess an individual's degree of intelligence according to which mental functions he can perform. Other theorists consider Spearman's notion inadequate and instead view intelligence as a multifactorial construct, with or without an underlying g factor.

More recently, intelligence has been operationally defined as the individual's ability to meet the demands of his environment. In this definition, no differentiation is made between the cognitive processes and the observable behavior. Chein (1945) stated, "Intelligence is an attribute of behavior not an attribute of a person." Therefore one may speak of an individual consistently behaving in an intelligent manner under various circumstances rather than identifying whether or not he receives a high score on a particular test. According to this view, a farmer or a construction worker can be considered as intelligent as a university professor if in his area of competence he can be shown to be equally effective. It is obvious that any test based on this theory must begin by sampling the criteria for effective performance under various conditions and should make provision for reflecting the increment in competence that occurs as the result of learning and experience. Tests of academic achievements, such as reading ability, meet such specifications.

Tests of intelligence based on Piaget's theory are constructed with the purpose of identifying the age at which a child has acquired a particular concept and the level of logical operation in which he is engaged. These tests give a better indication of the child's current status than a prediction of his future performance.

The historical roots of tests of intelligence can be traced back to two independent developments. The first is the early oral and written examinations of general information used to test the qualifications and competence of applicants for civil service positions. These were used first in China and centuries later were introduced in Europe and the United States. Examinations for entrance to and graduation from universities have also been used in the West.

The second root of intelligence testing is the studies of individual differences in sensory perception, sensory discrimination, memory association, and so on, which were constructed in the second part of the 19th century in Europe and America. Differences between children and adults, both normal and abnormal, were diligently detected and compiled by psychiatrists and psychologists, although the meaning and the application of such findings were not immediately apparent.

Stanford–Binet Test. In 1904 Alfred Binet, who had been actively involved in the research of individual differences and was well acquainted with the work of other researchers in this field, was appointed to a commission set up by the French minister of public instruction in order to provide guidelines and recommendations to the ministry to assure that all children, specifically abnormal children, would benefit from public education. Binet, in collaboration with Simon, selected 30 items from various sources and administered them to a group of normal children of ages 3, 5, 7, 9, and 11 and to a group of institutionalized children who were considered retarded. This battery of tests was first published in 1905 and was later on revised to include 58 items arranged in age groups from 3 to 13. Terman, in 1916, developed a new battery using the 1911 revision of Binet and adding more items so that the Stanford–Binet included 90 items. The much-revised battery comprises such tasks as naming the days of the week, detecting incongruity in pictures, copying geometrical forms, and reordering scrambled sentences. The test has been standardized and provides a mental age and IQ score from ages 2 to 18. The Stanford–Binet test is most frequently used with children whose IQ scores are expected to reach the lower or the upper limits of the IQ curve, namely, the retarded and gifted groups.

Wechsler Intelligence Scale. David Wechsler, in 1939, devised an intelligence test for adults and later on a scale for children: the Wechsler Intelligence Scale for Children (WISC), which has been revised several times by the author. The Wechsler Preschool and Primary Scale of Intelligence now provides a measure of IQ for the preschooler and thus supplements the WISC. Functions tapped on the WISC are divided into two categories: verbal and performance. Therefore the child receives a verbal score, a performance score, and a full score of intelligence quotient. Differences of more than 15 points between verbal and performance IQ are indicative of depressed functioning in respective areas and are in need of further clarification as to the reason for the depressed abilities in various task performance. The verbal part is comprised of six subtests: information, comprehension, similarities, arithmetic, digit span, and vocabulary. The performance part has five subtests: digit symbol, picture completion, block design, picture arrangement, and object assembly. The purpose of the test is to assess receptive and expressive language skill; computation ability; attention and recall; construction praxis; concept formation; and graphomotor skill. Some subtests are particularly sensitive to specific malfunctioning. For example, disturbances of attention can interfere with performance on digit span, arithmetic computation, and digit symbols. Language problems can be detected by difficulties in the comprehension, vocabulary, and information subtests.

Mental Age and IQ. Mental age was defined by Binet as the age at which the child passes all except one test on the scale for that age group. Later investigators divided the mental age by chronological age to arrive at a "mental quotient," which proved to be more constant during the child's intellectual growth. Terman introduced the concept of "intelligence quotient," which was derived by dividing the mental age by chronological age (up to 16 years), multiplied by 100 in order to remove decimals. The method of computation of the IQ score and mental age has undergone various revisions and is currently based on more sophisticated notions of statistical distribution of the raw scores on subtests and the year/month scores for basal and ceiling levels of performance.

Large-scale application of the intelligence tests has resulted in finding the mean IQ at each level and the standard deviation for each group. Plotting the IQ of a random population of children on a curve has provided a bell-shaped curve on which the mean IQ score is 100, with 50% of each age group falling between two standard deviations (85–115 on WISC).

Application of Intelligence Tests. Intelligence tests are used in child psychiatry as an aid in diagnosis and prognostication, particularly in relation to future academic performance. The IQ score plays an important part in the diagnosis of mental retardation, although a low score on intelligence tests without concomitant impairment in adaptive functioning does not fulfill the criteria for diagnosis of mental retardation set by the American Association on Mental Deficiency. Various subtests of intelligence tests may provide significant diagnostic clues regarding the child's development. For example, a depressed verbal IQ score may point to disorders of communicative language, while low scores on the performance part could be the result of disturbances of visual–motor perception. The diagnosis of psychosis on the basis of certain patterns of response on IQ subtests has not been validated. Impaired functioning on the performance portion may be due to brain damage, although the results with children are not as valid as with adults.

The style of a child's performance when confronted with specific demands, his willingness to participate, his fear of failure, and his need for feedback and encouragement—in short, his behaviors during the test situation—are sources of valuable information for evaluating his mode of functioning vis-à-vis the demands of the environment. These pieces of information must be incorporated into the data received from other sources and interpreted in the light of all that is known about the child. In the profile of assets and liabilities that is compiled for the purpose of diagnosis and treatment of each child, the IQ score is only one of the many factors under consideration. The fact that the IQ score is the result of responses to a series of structured stimuli plotted against a statistical norm does not endow it with any magical significance. When the IQ score is used as a factor in class placement or a prognosticator for future potentials, it is important to remember that the personality of the child and his level of emotional and social maturity are significant variables that will affect the outcome.

The most consistent relationship between IQ score and other performance has been found in the area of scholastic achievement. Some resarchers have questioned this relationship, and also the validity of the IQ score, on philosophical, methodological, and theoretical grounds. McClelland (1973) believes that the correlation between IQ score and school success is based on the similarities between the tests of intelligence and school examinations. In Terman's (1959) group of gifted children, the comparison between the most and the least successful subgroups revealed that factors such as freedom from emotional disturbance, high motivation, sociocultural background, and high achievement need play parts in whether or not a child with a high IQ score will effectively use his intelligence.

Some psychologists claim that general-intelligence test scores are correlated with job success. This contention has been criticized on the basis that factors unrelated to intelligence are operative in selection for various jobs and that the criteria for promotion and effectiveness on any job are not fully clear. For example, while Terman's study of gifted children showed that as a whole the gifted group were more successful as adults than the general population in areas such as occupational standing, income, and scientific and artistic productivity, the women in the group fared less well than their male counterparts. Therefore sex seemed to be a variable operating independently of IQ in occupational standing and related matters. A similar situation exists when the IQ score places an individual in the retarded or borderline range but, because of the nature of a local industrial pattern and the overall demands of the economy, he is accepted for job training and promoted to supervisory functions. The test/retest reliability of the intelligence tests, though statistically proven, does not hold for individual cases. Increments and decrements of up to 50 points have been shown to occur in individual children (Moriarty, 1966).

Infant Intelligence Tests. A variety of developmental tests have been devised to assess the developmental status of children under 4 years of age. These batteries are made up of subtests that assess fine and gross motor coordination, object manipulation, social skill, imitative behavior, and finally, language development. According to Bayley (1958), these scales assess "clusters of abilities which are age specific," and since there is little continuity between the child's performance at various stages, the developmental quotient cannot be considered a forerunner of the IQ score. In fact, during the first two years of life the predictive value of the developmental score is negligible, and only when verbalization becomes an important factor in the final score does the developmental quotient begin to show correlation with future IQ test results (Lewis and McGurk, 1972).

The most widely used scales of infant development are those developed by Gesell, Bayley, and Cattell. The most useful clinical application of such tests is in assessing developmental status and identifying infants who are at risk of future lags in development and therefore in need of periodic evaluation for the purpose of appropriate planning.

Projective Techniques

The projective method or technique is based on the psychological assumption that the various properties of stimuli are not the only determinants of our perception of, response to, and relation with external reality. The individual's level and style of cognition, attitudes, needs, wishes, and moods—or, in short, his personality characteristics—also influence the outcome of any interaction with the environment. This conviction that internal factors are projected or externalized and that reality is colored by intrapsychic hues has led psychologists to devise various instruments by which the responses of different individuals to a uniform series of stimuli are analyzed and compared in an attempt to obtain information and gain understanding of the personality characteristics of the respondent or group of respondents.

Not only have a wide variety of tests been constructed and used as projective tests, but at times the concept of projection has been extended to interpret the results of nonprojective tests and other human activities. Attempts have been made to use the Bender–Gestalt test as a projective instrument. Play activities of children, their choices of toys, and their statements about their future occupations or other make-believe situations have all been thus analyzed. In fact, the logic of projective techniques has played an important part in assigning meaning to and interpreting behavioral data in psychiatry. Research studies in projective techniques have focused on developing normative data, comparing various tests, and validating the results as well as the more basic questions about the nature of stimuli, the reliability of responses, and the usefulness of the instruments in diagnosis and prognostication.

The results of these studies so far have failed to clarify the issues. The normative data and the statistical computations give only a crude measure of what is to be expected at various ages among groups with different socioeconomic and cultural backgrounds. The reliability of the tests is to a large extent affected by the examiners' orientation, their degree of experience, and the extent of their familiarity with the subjects' background. Predictions based on the test results have been disappointing. While most studies have shown that groups can be differentiated in some categories of responses, the significance of any single sign in an individual protocol is less clear. The use of projective tests in children is further complicated by such issues as the paucity of normative data, uncertainty about the level of personality organization that is being tapped, and the relationship between fantasy and overt behavior. Furthermore, such situational factors as the length of the testing session, the style of the tester, and the events preceding the testing situation are more likely to influence a child's than an adult's behavior.

The most widely used projective tests with children are the Rorschach, the Thematic Apperception Test (TAT), and, to a lesser extent, the Children's Apperception Test (CAT), as well as children's drawings.

Rorschach. A Swiss psychiatrist, Hermann Rorschach, introduced a series of 10 inkblot pictures in 1921 as a method for the study of association and imagination. The cards are given to the subject one by one and he is instructed to give his impression of each card. The instrument has been used with various groups of patients and normal subjects. The scoring system has been based on responses elicited by the physical dimensions of the stimuli, such as form, color, and shading, and the content of the associative elements, such as presence or absence of human movement, the perseveration of a theme, and the degree of conventionality of a response. Rapaport *et al.* (1968) described the process by which the Rorschach responses come about in terms of three phases:

> In the first phase the salient perceptual features of the blot initiate the associative process; in the second, this process pushes beyond the partial perceptual impressions and effects a more or less intensive organization and elaboration of the inkblot; in the third, the perceptual potentialities and limitations of the inkblot act as a regulatory reality for the associative process itself.

The quality of responses is therefore a reflection of the individual's ability to analyze and synthesize perceptual cues and to integrate these impressions into a structured unit and of the flexibility and freedom of his associative processes within the boundary of a common reality.

The underlying hypotheses in the interpretation of a Rorschach protocol are as follows:

* Responses indicating conventional human movements represent an awareness and acceptance of one's inner urges and feelings, and their presence reflects degrees of emotional maturity and health. In conditions in which there is a paucity or an inhibition of ideation, these responses are decreased. Chil-

dren's protocols may show movements of inanimate objects and animals and only later show human movements.

- Popular responses are indications of an individual's conformity to, and awareness of, common reality and depend upon the socialization and acculturation of the subject.
- Texture and shading responses signify the sensitivity of the respondent, although extreme sensitivity may be the cause or the product of anxiety.
- Color responses are reflections of the respondent's handling of affects, impulses, and actions.
- The location of the percept and its clarity are other indications of the level of personality integration displayed in the child's protocol.

While in interpreting the meaning of Rorschach protocol and, in fact, most projective tests, the tendency has been to use the psychoanalytic theory as the basis for the delineation of motivating forces of personality and the defense structure, ego psychology has had a great impact on the theory of projection. Rapaport *et al.* (1968) stated; "In these tests, the ego, the carrier of conscious thinking, demonstrates its bent and its proclivities. The unconscious makings of the thought process will occasionally become palpable, especially when thinking is disorganized." The influence of ego and developmental psychology is particularly apparent in the use of the Rorschach test with children and adolescents. Efforts have been made to collect normative data for various age groups (Ames *et al.*, 1974). Developmental trends are emphasized, so that the child's immature reality testing, his limited association, and his magical thinking are taken into consideration. Furthermore, it is believed that no Rorschach protocol can be properly interpreted without a knowledge of such facts as the child's "socioeconomic level, his religious and racial background, the number, age and sex of his siblings, whether or not he comes from an intact home . . ." (Halpern, 1960). In discussing the use of the Rorschach with adolescents, Hertz (1960) concluded, "We may and do find certain imbalance in the records of adolescents—tenuous ego controls, regression to and resurgence of primitive thinking, immature affect, perhaps 'unhealthy' defensive operations and the like." According to Hertz, these deviations in the protocol are not always indicative of serious pathology; rather they "may represent temporary experimental and protective forms of adjustment."

It is clear that although the Rorschach test provides a wealth of information regarding the developmental stage and the style of problem solving and coping of children and adolescents, this information must be considered only as an additional element in the total evaluation of the child and the adolescent rather than a definitive indication of their mental health or illness. Furthermore, reciprocal communication between the psychologist and the clinician is necessary if the test results are to be appropriately interpreted and evaluated. The clinician's knowledge of the child's history can shed light on his responses to the test, and, in turn, the knowledge gained through the testing reveals aspects of his personality organization that may not be easily accessible in a clinical interview. The responses of the child on the Rorschach may point to certain diagnoses, but basing the diagnosis solely on the Rorschach protocol is an unwarranted acceptance of a single aspect of the behavior as the determinant of personality organization.

Thematic Apperception Test. The Thematic Apperception Test (TAT) consists of pictures of human figures of recognizable age and sex in ambiguous situations. They are presented to the subject one by one with the instruction that he tell a story about the people, their motivation, and their feelings. Further inquiries by the tester are designed to elicit elaboration on the stories relating to the background or the future course of events confronting the individuals in the stories. These fantasy productions are believed to reflect the child's perception of interpersonal relationships in his environment, his expectations with respect to other people's behavior toward him, and his needs, wishes, and conflicts. Normative data are lacking and the results of various research studies have failed to validate the test in more than a few selective tasks and situations.

The assumptions underlying the interpretation of the TAT protocol are, first, that the central figure, or the children in the picture, represents and reveals the subject's personality attributes. Therefore the motivations, feelings, and perceptions assigned to the central figure correspond to, or are identical with, what the child himself feels and thinks. Second, the attitudes, wishes, and behavior attributed to various characters in the stories are the respondent's views of his interpersonal relationships and conflicts with his environment. And third, the child's responses are not dependent solely on the strength of either his motives or his defensive strategies but rather are the outcome of the interaction between these two processes.

The TAT protocol, when interpreted in the context of other behavioral data by an experienced psychologist, provides valuable information regarding the child's present concerns and his attempts to deal with his environment. However, the relation between fantasy and overt behavior cannot be reliably predicted. Some subjects who produce a great number of aggressive responses on the test do not engage in overt aggressive behavior; therefore aggressive fantasies may reflect compensatory defense mechanisms. Furthermore, as the child becomes more socialized, his responses tend to show his awareness of what is thinkable within his culture, rather than what he spontaneously thinks. The role of such factors as socioeconomic background, religious affiliation, and ethnic group membership in fantasy production has not been broadly investigated. Therefore the value of an interpretation of any protocol is by and large dependent upon the psychologist's sensitivity to and awareness of the subject's life circumstances and his ability to identify the unique individuality of the child from this record of his fantasy production. Young children's protocols may be limited by such factors as their inability to identify with any central character in the TAT cards or by their lack of sophisticated knowledge regarding other people's motives. Differences among boys and girls on such dimensions as aggression or the need for nurturing may be more the result of the situations depicted on the TAT cards than of the personality variables between the sexes. The verbal facility of a child is reflected in the length of the stories and thus influences the content of the responses to the test.

Children's Apperception Test. This test, the CAT, is a series of 10 cards depicting animals in humanlike interactions. The test was designed with the idea that young children may find it easier to identify with animals and to describe with less inhibition their views of the interpersonal relationships. The range of application of the test was said to be from about 3 to 10 years of age, though some schoolchildren find the test silly and refuse to tell stories, since scenes of animals behaving like people do not correspond with reality as they have come to know it. From the results of research studies, it has not been conclusively proved that animal figures are superior to human figures in eliciting fantasy material, though this assumption had been based on the observation that children's Rorschach protocols show a high percentage of animal responses and that children tend to accept tales about animals without any reservation.

When the CAT is accepted and responded to, the findings are interpreted according to the criteria set for each card by Bellak (1950), who devised the test with the specific purpose of investigating such themes as sibling rivalry, relationship with parents, fears of desertion and punishment, and other themes that are directly related to psychoanalytic theory, such as fear of the primal scene or oral aggressive themes. Ballak believes that a CAT protocol allows the psychologist to describe "The psychic structure and unconscious needs of the subject," as well as "his conception of the world and significant figures around him." However, he warns against using the CAT as a diagnostic test and considers the data only suggestive of a particular clinical diagnosis.

Children's Drawings. Children's drawings have been the subject of naturalistic studies for at least a century, although it was not until 1926 that Goodenough published her scoring system for the measurement of intelligence by human figure drawing. At the present time, drawings by children are used as an aid in psychotherapy, as a projective technique, and, of course, as a means of intellectual assessment.

The young child's earliest graphic production is scribbling, which is largely dependent upon the movement of the whole arm, shoulder, or hand on the paper. The child may assign names to his scribbles—at first as an afterthought and later on as an intentional act.

Around age 3 or 4, the child begins to draw a primitive circular design with lines and loops inside or outside of the circle, and this is his first attempt to represent the human face. Shortly thereafter, more details are added, although arms or legs may come out of the head or

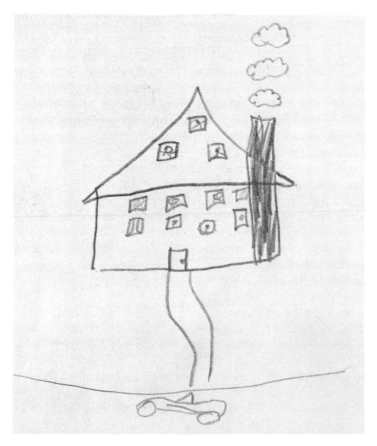

FIGURE 1   *Drawing of a house by a 7-year-old boy of average intelligence.*

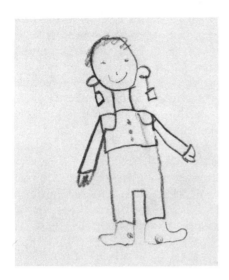

FIGURE 2 *Drawing of a "young lady" by a 7-year-old girl who would like to become a movie star.*

the child may draw only legs or arms and forget about the other extremities. In the face, the eyes are the earliest and the most frequent features, while the nose and mouth are sometimes forgotten. The nose may appear as a circle, a straight line, a triangle, or a rectangle. The mouth may be one big line going straight across the face, or an oval, or two parallel lines. Teeth are points or zigzag lines. Ears appear much later and are shown as two circles. The neck is a straight line or a rectangle between the head and the body. The body at first is an open space between the legs. Later, it is marked off by a cross stroke, or an oval, circular, or rectangular shape. The legs are at first simple lines; later on they are shown in outlines. The feet appear as oval, circular, or simple lines at right angles to the legs. The arms are shown as lines going upward, downward, horizontally, or alongside the body. At first, they are frequently joined to the head and are too long in proportion to the rest of the body. The fingers are drawn as a loose bundle of lines or are added to the arm as cross-strokes. The hands may be represented as a cross-line at the end of the arm, with fingers added like the teeth of a rake or spread in all directions. Later on, the hand is added as an oval form and the fingers are given an outline. The fingers may be too many or too few.

The proportions of various parts are at first quite unrealistic; the head is usually too large, the arms are long, and the legs may be too short. It seems that while drawing a part, the child cannot keep the whole image in mind and thus the relationships are lost. Children's attempts to put clothes on their drawings may be an afterthought;

transparencies are frequent findings in early drawings. Movement comes very slowly. At first, all drawings are expressionless and similar, though the child is able to give stories about how the people whom he has drawn feel or what they are doing. Later on, motion appears as lines of connection between the figure and the object of action. The child draws a person next to a tree, and a line going from the arm shows the person picking fruit from the tree. Drawings of seated figures are infrequent and come much later. Going from full face to profile is not a sudden accomplishment; rather, single parts of the body are turned sideways at different times. Profile drawings between the 6th and 9th year of age usually show a mixture of profile and full face. The head, feet, nose, eyes, mouth, arms, and finally the body are reproduced in profile.

Sex differentiation is not clear in children's drawings at first, although the child may assign a sex to his figures. As children grow older, clothing, hairdo, or makeup are used to represent sex. Around adolescence, physical characteristics such as breasts are added to signify the sex of the figure. Children may draw some parts of the body more prominently because of their particular concern with the functioning of that part; for example, ears may appear early on the drawings of a young child who is deaf, and often a hearing aid is included.

In scoring children's drawings for assessment of intelligence, the number of details on the drawings, the proportion of the various parts in relation to each other, the accuracy by which various parts are

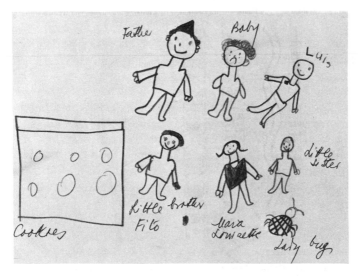

FIGURE 3 *A family portrait by a 10-year-old child who feels "lonely."*

reproduced, and finally, the quality of execution are taken into consideration. Goodenough's scoring system, by which the mental age of the child is calculated and compared with his chronological age, has remained a reliable system for obtaining a rough estimate of intelligence by a simple clinical procedure. The fact that such an estimate is largely, though not completely, independent of the cultural background and the amount of schooling that the child has received makes the test extremely helpful. However, a low score on the Goodenough cannot always be taken as an indication of low intelligence. Children with perceptual motor disorders or those who, for various causes, have not developed a well-articulated image of the human body do not produce well-detailed drawings that would reflect their intellectual abilities. In a series of clinical investigations of

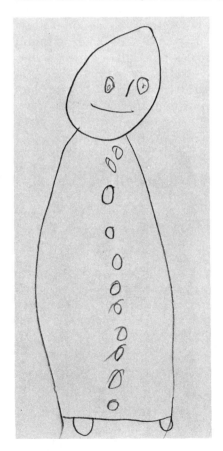

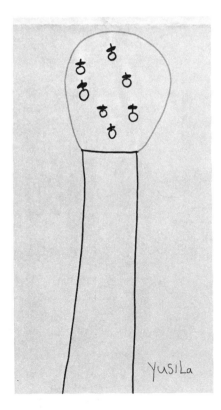

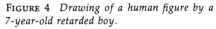

FIGURE 4 Drawing of a human figure by a 7-year-old retarded boy.

FIGURE 5 Drawing of an apple tree by a 6-year-old normal child.

the drawings of normal children between ages 5 and 12, Koppitz (1968) compiled a list of expected developmental items that characterize children's drawings of human figures at each age level. According to Koppitz, 5-year-old boys are expected to include six items in their drawings: head, eyes, nose, mouth, body, and legs. On the other hand, 5-year-old girls draw at least seven items; for example, arms are also included. At age 7, feet and two-dimensional arms are to be expected. By the age of 10, about 13 scorable items appear. Extremities are now shown in two dimensions, hair and neck are drawn, fingers are commonly present, and from then on smaller details such as nostrils, two lips, elbows, and ankles are added to the picture. Koppitz concluded that children's drawings can be used as a rough measure of their mental maturity and that at each age level the drawings of girls

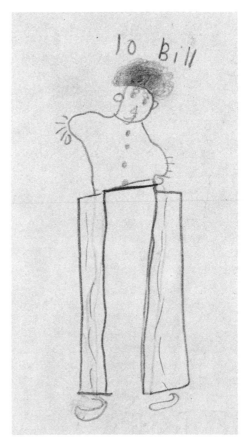

FIGURE 6 *Bizarre drawing of a human figure by a 10-year-old schizophrenic child. "Bill—he's walking to the store—going to buy food for his mother then he's going to bring it home."*

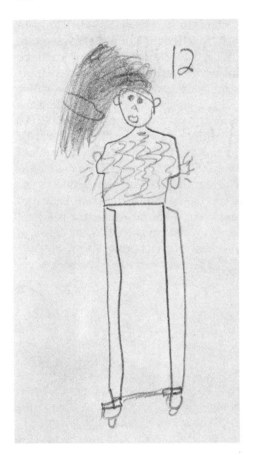

FIGURE 7 *Bizarre drawing of a human figure by a 10-year-old schizophrenic child. Jeanie—has cuffed pants—walking to play handball—and friend.*

show more scorable items than those of boys. She found the score on the drawing of the human figure to be independent of drawing ability and the amount of training. The medium used, whether crayon or pencil, does not affect the number of developmental items present in the figure.

Drawing as a Projective Technique. Like any other piece of observable behavior, drawings can be expected to express some of the feelings and thoughts of the person who made them. The meaning and content of the drawings of children and adults have been analyzed and guessed at by various clinicians according to their own orientations and expectations. However, such speculations can be verified only by supportive data from other statements by the person or other observations made in the process of clinical evaluation. When the picture is used as a projective test, the meaning that the psychologist may assign to it is not necessarily the meaning that the subject has set out to convey, though it is logical to assume that with or without intention, the person's anxieties, prevailing moods, and preoccupations are reflected in his drawings. Most experts in children's drawings do not believe that there is a one-to-one relationship between a sign on the drawing and a definite personality trait of the child. Rather, each child may express his concerns and anxieties in a different manner on different occasions.

Koppitz (1968) has tried to develop a list of "emotional indicators" by studying the drawings of a group of normal and disturbed children. Of the 30 items on her list, 12 items were found to differentiate between a clinic population and normal children; 4 items were statistically significant at a .01 level of confidence. These items are poor integration of parts in girls above 6 and boys above 7 years; shading of the body and/or limbs in girls above 7 and boys above 9 years; slanting the figure by 15 degrees or more; and drawing a tiny figure. A big

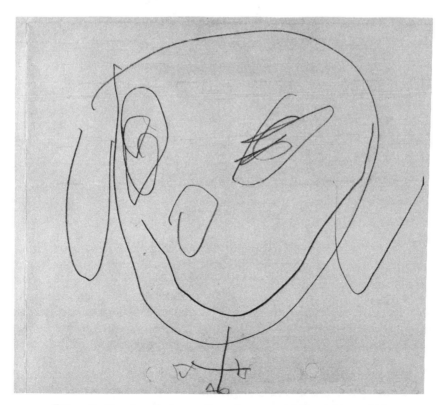

FIGURE 8 *Drawing of a human figure by a very intelligent 3-year-old boy.*

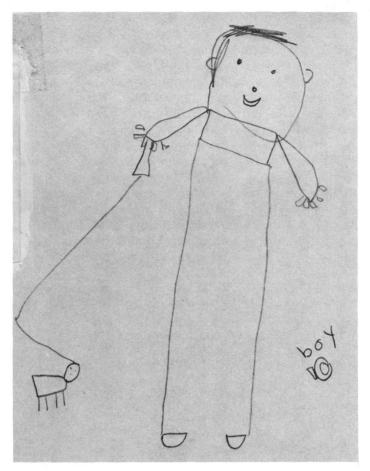

FIGURE 9   *Drawing of a boy with a dog by a 12-year-old retarded child.*

figure, short arms, cut-off hands, and the omission of the neck after 10 years of age were found to be significant at a .05 level. An additional four items—shading of the hands and/or neck, asymmetry of limbs, transparencies, and big hands—were statistically significant at a .10 level. In addition, the author reported that certain signs, such as the omission of the arms, the omission of the body, and grotesque figures, in drawings of school-age children were so rare that though they are always pathological, no statistical computation could be carried out. Three-quarters of the clinic group showed two or more emotional indicators on their drawings, while only 4 of the 76 normal children did so.

The interpretation and meaning assigned to various emotional indicators depend upon the orientation of those who analyze the drawings, although the following broad consensus of opinion exists. Among school-age children, poor integration of the parts is associated with such factors as developmental lag or deviation, poor impulse control, neurological impairment, or any severe emotional disturbance that hinders the child's ability to integrate and synthesize his thinking, sensations, and movements. Shading of the body, face, or neck in older children denotes anxiety and concern about the functioning of the parts or the whole of the body. Machover (1953) considers the shading of the neck to reveal the child's struggle to contain and control his impulses. It should be noted that in the current period black children often express self-identity by shading—in such cases, this cannot be correctly noted as a sign of anxiety. Koppitz stated that the drawing of a slanting figure by a child "suggests that the child lacks secure footing." Machover concurred. The sense of imbalance may be due to an unstable personality or an impaired central nervous system. Tiny figures represent feelings of insecurity, inadequacy, and depression. Shy and withdrawn children tend to draw small figures, though the finding is by no means universal. Big, expansive figures are frequently drawn by aggressive children who despite a tough exterior are in fact emotionally insecure.

Transparencies may be quite normal when the child decides to add clothing to a finished figure and therefore draws an outline around his naked drawing. However, transparencies of specific parts of the body reflect the child's anxiety and concerns related to that part. Koppitz stated that "children who draw such specific transparencies are in effect asking for information or reassurances concerning their impulses or experiences." According to Machover, omission of the hands reflects the child's guilt feelings over his activities or, like short arms, indicates his sense of inability to act. Harris (1963) reported that in his experience only very bright and highly imaginative children draw monster figures. Other researchers do not share this view and consider such drawings an indication of the child's poor self-concept or his desire to avoid exposing himself by producing a figure that is grotesque and unrealistic. Drawings of genitals are extremely rare and are usually associated with serious emotional distress about the body. Children with physical defects may represent their defective body image in their drawings, although it is not the presence of the defect that is the decisive factor in the representation but rather the child's awareness, anxieties, and preoccupation with the defect that loom large in his perception of his own body. It has already been mentioned that children with impairment of the central nervous system may produce drawings of human figures that are not well integrated and that may indeed lead to an underestimation of their intelligence.

While it is probably true that the child's drawings of the human figure frequently reflect the way in which he perceives himself and represents himself, it is erroneous to think that this is always so. In fact, the child may explicitly or implicitly draw another person who for various reasons has come to occupy a central position in his mental life. Some children draw the image they wish to have rather than the one that they know themselves to possess. In this respect, it is of interest that several authors have found a change in the drawings of black children during the past decade in that there is a definite increase in identifiable black features in the drawings of human figures (Fish and Larr, 1972).

The principle that the child's drawing need not represent himself also explains the findings that the sex of the figure is not always in accord with the sex of the child. Machover has hypothesized that such discordance is due to confused sexual identification on the part of the subject, but other normative studies have failed to sustain this hypothesis.

Children's family drawings and drawings in which children are asked to draw their whole family doing something reveal the child's perception of his own place within the family or what he wishes his family to be like. Burns and Kaufman (1972) used kinetic family drawing as a projective test in which various elements of the drawings are interpreted according to psychoanalytic theory. The objection to such an approach is the fundamental question of whether the associations of various symbols by the investigator can be accepted as identical with their symbolic significance for the subject.

After human beings, the most frequent subject that children choose to draw is a house. The drawing of the house at first is a simple rectangle without doors or windows. As the child grows older, other features are added. Perspective is usually not taken into consideration until much later, so that two or three sides of the house are shown on the same plane as the front side. A view of the interior is indicated by drawings of a chair, table, or other objects. People are shown as standing next to the house or floating in midair within the house. Interestingly, even urban children living in apartment houses usually add a chimney on the roof with smoke coming out to indicate that the house is occupied.

When the child first chooses to draw animals, the face of the human figure is retained, while the body is placed horizontally with legs and tail added. Animals are always shown sideways. Either four legs are placed equally distanced under the body or there are only two because, the child explains, one cannot see the other two. In drawings of a tree, leaves at first are usually not differentiated and a circle or a bundle of lines represents the leaves on top of the trunk with fruit placed on the same plane. Roots are shown because children know that they are there. This transparency as well as the view of the inside of the house through the walls is normal for younger children.

Like other expressive acts, drawings are used as an integral part of psychotherapy with younger children. Some children use drawings as their main mode of communication and expression. Others try to articulate their fears and anxieties through their drawings, and yet another group looks upon drawing as an activity to be enjoyed for its own sake or as a chronicle of their experiences of the discovery and synthesis of reality. In all instances, the experienced therapist attempts to understand and accept the child's manner of self-expression and to use this understanding to help the child.

Bender–Gestalt Test. This is a paper-and-pencil test in which nine cards with various geometrical configurations are presented to the child one by one and he is asked to reproduce them. The ease with which the test can be administered has made the Bender–Gestalt the third or fourth most frequently used test by psychologists, although it does not meet the standards of validity set by the American Psychological Association on test construction.

The configurations used by Bender (1938) in devising the test are adaptations of forms that were originally used by Max Wertheimer (1923), a classical gestalt psychologist, in his investigation of the gestalt principles of visual perception. Wertheimer asked the subjects to describe what they saw, while Bender asked for the reproduction of the figures. Hence the test came to be known as a test of visual–motor gestalt, and, at least in young children, the two functions—the perception of the forms and their motor execution—cannot be clearly differentiated.

Furthermore, while the classical gestalt psychologists believed that in perceptual experience whole structuralized patterns are the primary form of biological response, Bender considered this to be a static concept and set out to prove that biological response in perception evolves from maturation and is under the influence of the integrative state of the central nervous system and even the psychological state of the individual. The test was thus devised to discover the principles underlying perception across ages and in neuropsychiatric conditions. The principles postulated by Bender to account for the differential functioning of children and adults and normal and neuropsychiatric patients have not been, so far, proved or disproved by other investigators.

Bender stated, "There is a tendency not only to perceive gestalten but to complete gestalten and to reorganize them according to principles biologically determined by the sensory motor pattern of actions." The biological principles, according to her, are that vortical movements are the earliest formations; foreground–background differentiation is the first step in the construction of the perceived object; the maturation of the body schema gives rise to vertical reproduction of horizontally perceived objects; and the last level of maturation occurs when corner formation, crossed lines, and diagonal relationships are reproduced.

As can be noted from the above principles, the question of whether a subject perceives the design accurately and distorts it in the process of reproduction or misperceives the design and makes an accurate reproduction of his own perception cannot be answered. According to some clinicians, children who have perceived the designs accurately and reproduced them incorrectly are usually able to say so when the question is put to them, while children with difficulties in perception insist that their reproduction is a faithful copy of the figure.

Regarding the administration of the test, Bender did not approve of attempts to formalize it. She thought there should be no time limit on the individual taking the test, no attempt to prevent him from looking back at a card that he has already finished, and no denial of permission for multiple trials. However, any rotation, whether of the card or of the paper, should be discouraged, though if the child persists in rotating, he should be allowed to reproduce the design, but note should be made of the angle at which the design was reproduced.

Applications of Bender–Gestalt. The test has been used as an aid for diagnosing many different conditions and for assessment of the maturation of visual–motor patterns. Bender's original application of the test showed that children between 2 and 4 years of age can only scribble, while between 4 and 7 children's performance on the test gradually becomes more differentiated and more closely resembles the figures, although they may verticalize the horizontal designs. By age 11, most children can reproduce all of the Bender figures, and from 12 years into adulthood, only the quality of lines and proportions becomes more perfect.

Koppitz (1964) developed a scoring system for the Bender test production of children between 5 and 10 years of age and concluded that until about age 8, the test can discriminate those with extreme immaturity of the visual–motor system as well as those with outstanding functioning in this area. Although Bender herself considers the test to be corroborative of the performance part of the IQ tests, the assessment of intellectual ability or mental age through the use of the Bender–Gestalt test is an unreliable procedure.

The most important features of Bender test performance in patients with clinically proven brain pathology are rotation (more than 75 degrees in axis), distortion of the gestalt, collisions in which the designs run together, fragmentation of the designs, oversimplification of complex configurations, use of angles or straight lines for curves, and perseveration. The location of the lesion, the extent of brain involvement, the size of the lesion, and its relationship to the premorbid personality of the individual are factors that cannot be differentiated on the basis of the Bender test performance. The use and interpretation of the Bender test as an aid in the diagnosis of "minimal brain damage" are an extrapolation and extension of the findings in cases of clinically proven neurological damage in adult patients and can therefore be considered only suggestive rather than pathognomic. Bender test recall has been used by some investigators to distinguish between normal and brain-injured subjects, but the results are not satisfactory. In studying groups of children and adults with known organic brain pathology, more rotations (45 degrees) are found as compared with groups of normal subjects, but the individual performance varies.

Bender considers the test performance of schizophrenic children to be characterized by the following: an overabundance of vortical movement, which gives the pattern a certain "fluidity"; loss of boundaries between forms; and destruction of the original gestalt by elaborations that are ideational. It is as if the child is not able to limit his response to the reproduction of the stimuli and embellishes the designs by adding elements from his own thoughts and associations. However, all psychotic children do not respond in this manner to the test, and some nonpsychotic children choose to turn the Bender figures into imaginary forms that are more pleasing to them.

Given the ability to perceive and reproduce the designs, deviations in performance may reflect the unique interpretation of each individual. This has resulted in a series of investigations and attempts to use the Bender test as a projective device. The results have so far been quite disappointing. When the clinician knows enough about the patient, the meanings read into the Bender test are superfluous, and when the subject is unknown, the interpretations have little value.

After an exhaustive review of the 30 years of research on the application and standardization of the Bender–Gestalt test, Tolor and Schulberg (1963) concluded that although it is popular and easy to administer, the amount and the validity of information obtained by its application are disappointingly limited. Furthermore, the efforts at standardization and the development of several scoring systems have not significantly added to the validity of the overall subjective judgment of an experienced clinician.

Tests of Specific Functions. A variety of tests have been devised as research instruments or aids in the diagnosis of specific functions. Among those most widely used with children are tests of language ability, auditory and visual perceptual tests, nonverbal tests of abstract thinking and concept formation, and scales of social maturity.

The Auditory Discrimination Test (Wepman, 1958) consists of 40 pairs of words that evaluate the child's ability to distinguish between various phonemes in the English language. It is used with children with articulation problems and other disorders of spoken and written language.

The test of auditory perception is devised to assess the accuracy of the child's reception of sounds and words, his comprehension of the spoken language, and his integration of auditory and visual stimuli. The degree of retention and accurate reproduction of the sounds and words gives information regarding the child's ability to comprehend and use language.

The Frostig Developmental Test evaluates five areas of visual perception by a battery of tests graded by their degree of difficulty. Eye–*hand* coordination is revealed by the child's ability to draw straight and curved lines between increasingly narrower boundaries. In figure–ground perception tasks, the child is expected to discriminate between various geometrical figures superimposed on each other. To test the perception of form constancy, the child is asked to find squares and circles among other figures on the paper. The detection of rotated figures tests the child's perception of position in space. And the reproduction of various forms tests the perception of spatial relationships. Frostig (1963) stated that the subtests are independent of each other and related to school learning and possibly behavior problems during the first two to three years of school.

On the Peabody Picture Vocabulary Test, the child's verbal intelligence is assessed by the use of pictures requiring naming of objects, description of actions, understanding of positions, and so on.

The Illinois Test of Psycholinguistic Ability (ITPA) was devised for children from 2 years and 4 months to 10 years and 3 months of age and gives the level of the child's communication ability in various areas. The type of tasks in the ITPA are specifically designed to evaluate receptive and expressive language and the level of organization between receptive and expressive processes. This test is particularly useful in evaluating children with central language disorder.

The Ravens's Progressive Matrices is a nonverbal test, standardized for children between 8 and 14 years of age, in which 60 designs, or matrices, have been arranged in five series of increasing difficulty. Each design has a part missing. The subject is required to identify the missing part from six to eight alternative forms on a card. Although the test has been constructed as a test of general intelligence, such factors as visual scanning and visual discrimination affect the outcome.

In the Vineland Social Maturity Scale, the source of information is the detailed report requested from the child's caretakers. The items are categorized under such headings as self-help in dressing, eating and general care, socialization, participation in games, ability to amuse self, and ability to be helpful to others. Comparison with expected behavior at each age level gives the child a score of social maturity in relation to his peer group. The scale is particularly useful in assessing the degree of social handicap and adaptational problems of children with low intelligence and those with various physical defects. However, the findings on the test cannot be evaluated without reference to the child's environment and the parental expectations of him. For example, parents in unsafe urban areas may hesitate to allow the child to go unattended to various locations, or they may be reluctant to send him to do shopping errands. Overprotective mothers may discourage a handicapped child from trying to dress or bathe himself, or they may find the child's performance below their demanded standards and take the responsibility away from him. The tests of social competence do not give a realistic assessment of the child's potential, although they may accurately reflect his present status.

NEUROLOGICAL EXAMINATION

Neurological examinations in infancy and childhood differ from those given to adults in that maturational factors as well as clear deviancies have to be assessed. Certain signs are always pathological, such as paralysis of legs or arms. On the other hand, delayed walking may not constitute an indication of damage to the nervous system. The early neurological assessment is a neurobehavioral evaluation of the state of arousal, responsiveness to sensory stimuli, muscle tone, the level of integrative behavior such as sucking, successful coordination of swallowing and breathing, and finally, presence of any abnormality such as hydrocephalus, spina bifida, and so on. As the child grows older, certain reflexes normally present at birth are expected to disappear within varying periods of time. For example, the plantar reflex (Babinski) is usually present till 1½–2 years of age, while the sucking reflex diminishes within the first few months and is not present after a year. Furthermore, the growing infant is expected to achieve various developmental milestones with age: to be able to sit, stand, walk, and climb; to drink from a cup and hold and manipulate objects; to comprehend language and begin to verbalize. The posterior fontanel should be closed by 6 weeks, and the anterior fontanel should remain open at least up to 9 months of age. The neurological examination thus encompasses the developmental assessment.

In older children, not only should the presence or absence of gross neurological defects be established, but for the child psychiatrist, the mild, diffuse, nonfocal signs may provide information regarding the child's total ability and areas of significant difficulty in adjusting to the demands of his environment. While the existence of mild deviations such as poor fine or gross motor coordination are noncontroversial, their significance in terms of actual damage to the central nervous system or their etiological role in the causation of various behavioral disorders remains hypothetical. In fact, in anterospective neurological studies of infants born after pre- and perinatal problems, Corah and Pantera (1965) found no correlation between the newborn neurological examination and the incidence of neurological, intellectual, and behavioral problems at age 7. On the other hand, a variety of nonfocal signs have been reported among children with hyperkinetic syndrome, learning disability, and schizophrenia. A subgroup of schizophrenic children, distinguished by the presence of such signs of "organicity" as impairment in gross and fine motor coordination, poor muscle tone, and subtle problems with posture and balance, were described by Goldfarb (1974). While these children showed improvement in these functions over the three-year period during which annual assessments were made, even their best performance fell short of those of younger, normal control subjects. Nonfocal neurological signs are not indicative of morphological damage and cannot give localizing information regarding the central nervous system. Whatever has happened to the brains of these children has happened to an organism in the process of formation; therefore it may be the rate of maturation and integration that has been affected. The influence of dysfunction and lag in development can be judged only by the degree of interference with the acquisition of the basic skills and the psychological reactions to the handicap by the child, so that the same degree of clumsiness that may be looked upon as a handicap by one family may go unnoticed by another. The poor handwriting of a child may be accepted as a trait that he shares with his father, or it may be taken as a sign of his sloppiness and unwillingness to make the effort required to form letters. Furthermore, while a child of superior intelligence may easily compensate for his minor weaknesses in coordination or confused directionality, a child with more limited ability is unable to do so.

Depending on the purpose and orientation of the examiner and the presenting problem of the child, the search for indications of maturational lag or disturbances in the integration of the higher nervous system focuses on eliciting dysfunctions in particular areas. For example, when disorders of communication and articulation are under study, it is important to assess the child's ability to perform skilled movements of the facial muscles or fine movements of the hand following verbal commands or visual demonstration (praxis). Thus the child is asked to do such things as pretending to cough, yawn, whistle, blow, snap his fingers, comb his hair, and wave good-bye. It is known that praxis is a maturational process that is totally acquired by approximately 6 years of age, when normal children are able to perform on verbal command or following a demonstration by the examiner. Such ability is necessary for successful acquisition of communicative skill and may be delayed in children with developmental aphasia or other speech problems.

Dyslexic children may show difficulties with visual–motor perception, poor memory for shapes, confusion between right and left, and an inability to integrate visual with auditory stimuli. They may also have difficulty with spatial concepts, such as up and down and in and out. These chidlren are asked to reproduce geometrical forms, as in the Bender–Gestalt test; match symbols and numbers; tell right and left on themselves and on the examiner, and point to parts of their bodies on the left side with their right hands or vice versa. They are asked to differentiate between two words with similar but not identical sounds or to match the sound of a letter with its written form. Children with hyperkinetic syndrome may have difficulty performing all of the above tasks. In addition, they may show hyperactivity, short attention span, distractibility, and perseveration. Clumsiness may be evident in performing such acts as buttoning, tying shoelaces, holding a pencil, and imitating fast alternating movements with the fingers (dysdiadochokinesis). Jerkiness; tremor; minor choreoathetotic movements of the upper extremities; face, and trunk; disturbances of conjugate movement of the eyes; nystagmus; and/or dyskinesia (finger to nose or heel to knee) may be also present. The muscle tone may be increased or decreased. Symmetrical hyperreflexia may be noted.

In schizophrenic children, hypotonicity of the muscles is manifested by lack of resistance to passive motion and limpness or flaccidity. These children may show an inability to dissociate the movement of the eyes from that of the rest of the body, so that when asked to look in various directions without moving the head and neck, they cannot do so, although with age, this function improves. Whirling as a test of postural adjustment has been emphasized by some authors. In this test, when the child is standing with feet together, arms at his side, and eyes closed, the examiner rotates the head—first only gently with slight pressure of the finger and later on more forcefully, so that the head is at first a 30-, then a 45-, and finally a 90-degree angle from the original position. Children above 6 years of age usually accommodate these movements of the head without moving their bodies. When the child is too young or misperceives the purpose of the test, the movement of the body following the change of the position of the head cannot be taken as a pathological finding. Only when an older child shows this tendency over a period of time and following several examinations can one consider positive the result of a passive head rotation experiment. Even then, the finding cannot be construed as a diagnostic test for a particular psychiatric entity; rather, it is another possible indication of maturational lag or disturbance in central nervous system function, the psychological significance of which is a matter of conjecture.

Fink and Bender (1952) have reported on perception of simultaneous tactile stimuli by normal children below 6 years of age. In this test, the child's ability to perceive two simultaneous tactile stimuli on the back of both hands, on hand and cheek, on both cheeks on the same or opposite sides, and with eyes closed or open is appraised. In normal children below 6 years of age, with closed eyes the cheek stimulus is reported correctly, while the hand stimulus either is not located or is falsely located. As children grow older, the errors diminish. In some children with other signs of cerebral dysfunction, performance is more accurate with closed eyes, contrary to what is seen in normal children. This observation has prompted some authors to speculate that these children are not able to integrate their visual stimuli with tactile ones. The double simultaneous stimulation test is therefore used as a test of intersensory integration and organization.

Neurobehavioral examination has been used in an attempt to shed light upon the possible etiology of psychiatric disorders in children. When defects in performance have been causally related to dysfunctions, remedial programs have been designed to provide the child with intensive training. Some authors have speculated that children with signs of cerebral dysfunction and neurological immaturity may be more vulnerable to the effects of stressful environments since they are not able to organize and integrate the avalanche of stimuli to which they are exposed. Therefore, to maximize their functioning, care must be taken to protect them from overstimulation. In some theoretical discussions of childhood schizophrenia, such as the one by Bender (1958), the neurological dysfunctions manifested as disturbances of posture, muscle tone, and so on are considered a cause of extreme anxiety that is then expressed by various psychological manifestations.

While patients with obvious signs of neurological disorders are not expected to be referred to child psychiatrists, behavioral abnormalities may be the early manifestations of some neurological diseases. For example, children with neuromuscular disorders that have an insidious onset may be considered lazy, negativistic, or malingering or may even be diagnosed as showing hysteric neurosis. Or patients with progressive damage of the nervous system may be brought to a child psychiatrist because of their deteriorating school performance. A careful history and progression of symptoms and, finally, a neurologic examination may clarify the source of the patient's problem and prepare the way for appropriate referral and treatment.

In performing a neurologic examination, systematic attention must be paid to evaluating the motor and sensory systems, cranial nerves, reflexes, mental status, and special symptoms such as headache, vomiting, and vertigo.

Disturbances in motor function are manifested as difficulties in balance, ataxia, abnormal involuntary motor movements, or muscle weakness. Disturbances in sensation may appear as congenital indifference to pain, hypersensitivity to pain, and loss of tactile or proprioceptive sensation. Disorders of the cranial nerves are manifested by loss of hearing, vision, disorders of ocular movements, and facial weakness. Reflexes may be absent, hypoactive, or exaggerated. The presence of some reflexes is always pathological after certain ages. Evaluation of mental status during neurological examination includes assessment of the patient's memory, level of consciousness, global intellectual ability, and orientation. Presence or absence of convulsion and the history of headache, vertigo, and vomiting must be noted in detail.

Consistent, localizing neurological signs are usually referred to as *hard signs*, while a variety of findings that are present occasionally and inconsistently and do not signify the localized involvement of certain parts of the nervous system are called *soft neurologic signs*. Because of the uncertain nature and equivocal import of such signs, the presence of two or more of these soft signs is needed as an indication of generalized dysfunction of the nervous system. The most commonly encountered soft signs among psychiatric patients are as follows.

Motor impairment is seen as clumsiness reported by a history of frequent falls, bumping into things, and breaking objects. Poor coordination is manifested by poor handwriting and difficulty in tying shoelaces and fastening buttons. Upon examination, the child may show tremor on intentional movement, trembling of extended fingers, inability to bring his or the examiner's index finger to touch his nose, or inaccurate rapid movement of the hands.

Muscle tone may be poor and choreiform movements and/or tics may be present. The child's balance may be impaired, particularly when visual cues are absent. Gait may be broad-based, or the child may walk mainly on his toes. Poor tandem walking or poor hopping on one foot may give other indications of poor balance and underdeveloped coordination. Apraxia may be elicited after demonstration of the movements required for execution of certain functions such as combing the hair or whistling or by a request for their performance.

Sensory impairment in visual perception, graphomotor reproduction, or auditory discrimination and sequencing is demonstrated by special tests. Stereognosis is the ability to perceive objects or form by touch. The child is asked to close his eyes and identify a small object that is placed in his hands.

In examining the cranial nerves, one may observe horizontal nystagmus, choreiform movements of the protruded tongue, or inequality of the pupils. Speech defects and misarticulations are other signs of neurological dysfunction.

Reflexes may show bilateral hyper- or hypoactivity in the absence of related upper or lower motor neuron damage characterizing the hard neurologic signs.

In eliciting the neurological signs, one must assure oneself that the patient comprehends the meaning of the request made of him and is willing to cooperate. Furthermore, soft signs elicited when the child is tired, irritable, or in ill health may not be valid, since fine, coordinated movements are adversely affected by generalized malaise, particularly in younger children. Psychotic children or children who are under acute psychological stress may be unable to cooperate or may consider the doctor's requests irrelevant to their problems and be unmotivated to comply with such an examination.

ELECTROENCEPHALOGRAPHY

The bioelectric activities of the brain were first recorded in 1929 by German psychiatrist Hans Berger, who was attempting to find a measurable physiologic property of the brain representing mental activities. Since the time of its discovery and the subsequent refinements of the recording techniques, the EEG has become an indispensable tool in the practice of neurology. Psychiatrists have attempted to use the EEG as a research device in studying the electrical activities of the brain in various psychiatric disorders.

The EEG electrodes do not directly pick up the activity of any particular cell or combination of cells. Rather, the signals recorded on the EEG are a summation of the electrical charges of all the cells underlying the electrodes, which are a few millimeters in size. Cortical activities are prominent on a scalp EEG record only when the area covered by an electrode is large enough (at least 6 cm²). The lesions of the deeper structures of the brain may not show on a tracing taken from the scalp. Furthermore, because the summation of all electrical charges is reflected in an EEG record, such clear impairment as the atrophy of the cortex may not change the EEG at all.

Present EEG apparatus has between 8 and 16 channels, although machines with more electrodes are used in electroencephalographic research. EEG records are usually read by visual scanning, and the degree of accuracy is to a considerable extent dependent upon the skill and experience of the electroencephalographer. Recently computer quantification has been developed for more precise reading. Records are taken during both sleep and waking states, since abnormal manifestations may appear in either. Furthermore, various methods such as photic stimulation or hyperventilation are used to activate a dormant abnormality. In very young children or in those who are extremely agitated, sedation may be necessary before a record can be obtained. Secobarbital or chloral hydrate (secobarbital from 8 to 24 mg rectally for infants; chloral hydrate 0.25–1.5 g orally in children) may be administered to induce light sleep so that a tracing may be secured. The norm for EEG is empirical in that it has been determined by studying the records obtained from samples of subjects who do not show any clinical symptoms of functional or structural damage of the brain. The norm for EEG in children is more difficult to assess because maturational factors and fluctuations in state of arousal, particularly in very young children, are operative.

Alterations of the bioelectrical activities of the brain may be due to structural damage; disturbances in cellular metabolism, such as uremia, hypoglycemia, or disequilibrium in acid–base balance; or physiological variables, such as state of awareness or abnormal moods like anxiety and excitement. When abnormalities are due to structural damage, the changes on the EEG reveal only that a certain number of brain cells are functioning in an abnormal manner. The EEG gives no information regarding the condition of the remaining normal cells, nor can one make any assumption as to the prognosis for the abnormal ones. The malfunctioning cells may regain their normal activities or they may be destroyed and become electrically silent. In both conditions, the subsequent EEG will show lesser degrees of abnormality. The EEG signals form a series of waves that consist of a positive and a negative charge above and below a base line. These waves have a waxing and waning quality that usually forms a sinusoidal pattern. The amplitude and the frequency of the waves, as well as the rhythmicity and organization of the pattern and their location on the scalp are the diagnostically significant elements in an EEG record. The amplitude of a wave is measured from the baseline to the highest point of the positive peak or the lowest point of the negative valley and is expressed in microvolts (mV). The frequency is the number of waves or cycles per second (cps). The waves are divided into four categories according to their frequencies:

- Delta waves: less than 3.5 cps.
- Theta waves: from 3.5 cps to 7.5 cps.
- Alpha waves: from 7.5 cps to 13.5 cps.
- Beta waves: more than 13.5 cps.

Cycles with very high amplitude and a frequency of more than 12 cps are called *spikes*. Paroxysmal abnormalities may appear in the form of bursts of sharp waves and spikes or slow waves such as delta and theta with an amplitude at least twice as high as the background activities.

Abnormalities on the EEG may be diffuse or localized. They may appear on homologous parts of the two hemispheres or they may be unilateral. Focal abnormalities may appear on a background of well-organized electric activities or they may be accompanied by poor organization. These abnormalities are graded as mild; mild to moderate; moderate to marked; and marked. Rare theta activities are considered mild, while increased delta activities of low frequency are markedly abnormal. For sharp (epileptiform) waves, the mild category usually refers to less than three bursts of spike and sharp waves during 20 minutes of recording. Marked abnormalities refer to discharges appearing every 10 seconds. The dominant wave in a normal EEG of adults in resting wakefulness is the alpha wave of about 10 cps. It has been known since Berger's time that the alpha wave in children is of slower frequency. It has also been shown that in geriatric populations alpha waves tend to be less than 10 cps. The EEG in children shows a variety of characteristics that are considered due to immaturity of the brain, such as predominance of low-frequency waves, presence of spike foci in a high percentage of nonepileptic children, and increase in frequency, amplitude, and the amount of alpha waves with age. Because of maturational factors and the high incidence of individual variability, the interpretation of EEG records of children requires great skill and experience.

Epilepsy. The basic EEG phenomenon in epilepsy is the spike discharge of various forms and amplitudes. The diagnostic value of these discharges is particularly high when spikes are found during seizure-free intervals. In young infants, rhythmical spiking begins in one area of the brain, shifts to other locations in the same or the opposite hemisphere, and may be followed by a period of electric activities of very low amplitude. Sometimes spiking begins in several foci concomitantly, and high voltage, abundant spikes, and waves dominate the EEG tracing (hypsarrhythmia). These patterns are usually present during the interictal period. In older children, numerous spike foci may be seen on the EEG, with various degrees of epileptogenicity. For example, spikes in frontal areas may lead to clinical seizures in 80% of children, while in those with occipital foci, only 40% may have convulsive episodes. The spike foci on the EEG may change location over a short period of time.

In a follow-up study of 242 children with spike foci over a period of 3–15 years, Trojaborg (1968) reported a localization change in 85% of the subjects. In more than two-thirds, the original focus multiplied with migration to contralateral or other areas of the ipsilateral hemisphere. At times, the EEG becomes normal and the foci completely disappear, so that in about one-third of children with EEG abnormality of spike and wave nature, over a period of a few years the tracing may become normal. The EEG record of children with petit mal epilepsy may not show any abnormality during the interictal interval; however, hyperventilation usually can trigger the appearance of the characteristic abnormalities.

Diagnosis of temporal lobe epilepsy in children is difficult because while in adult patients the sharp waves and spikes are seen in the anterior region of the temporal lobe, in children diffuse spiking of midtemporal or central areas is more frequent, and about one-half to one-third of these foci disappear with age. In some adolescents with hysterical seizures, a mild to a moderate degree of EEG abnormality may be present, and the differential diagnosis is thus more complicated. The so-called abdominal epilepsy and other episodic disorders such as headaches do not show a characteristic pattern on the EEG. In fact, the tracing may be normal, and although these disorders may respond to anticonvulsive medications, the positive response cannot be construed as affirmation of the diagnosis. In children with febrile convulsions, the EEG is normal in about 80–90% of the subjects. When the EEG is abnormal, the likelihood of future nonfebrile epileptic attacks is higher.

Infections. Newborns with acute intra- or extracerebral infection show mild abnormalities on the EEG record. In subacute encephalitis, periodic bursts of mixed slow and sharp activities dominate the record. Sometimes these episodes are accompanied by grand mal seizures, but more frequently the EEG abnormalities are associated with myoclonic jerking or atonia of the extremities. Chronic noninfectious encephalopathies, such as lead poisoning, may produce focal or diffuse changes on the EEG with seizures.

Tumors or Abscesses. The EEG in space-occupying lesions may show foci of slow activities with clinical seizures. In subdural hematoma, the area over the site of the lesion may be electrically silent, or it may produce waves of very low amplitude. Cerebral malformations and severe perinatal anoxia give markedly abnormal tracings.

Mental Retardation. The EEG of even severely retarded individuals may be quite normal. In Lennox–Gastaut syndrome, retardation is associated with a multitude of seizures, usually nonresponsive to medication and with very slow (1–2.5 per second) spike and wave complexes. EEG abnormalities in the form of various foci of sharp waves or slow activities have been reported in about 50% of the child psychiatric clinic population (Aird and Tamamoto, 1966). These foci may appear on a background of well-organized alpha rhythm or may be associated with poorly organized background activities. In a study of 102 children in whom the EEG revealed a focus of spikes or sharp waves, Lairy and Harrison (1968) found that the control group of children from the same psychiatric clinic and without EEG abnormalities tended to have higher IQ scores; however, the difference between the two groups was not statistically significant. They also found that children with excessive clumsiness and poor motor coordination had proportionally more foci of abnormality unilaterally in the parietal area or had multiple foci. Temporal foci were more often associated with affective disorders, while occipital foci were accompanied with a higher incidence of poor performance on the Bender–Gestalt test. Follow-up studies of half of the group (56 children) from one to several years later failed to show any significant relationship between these EEG abnormalities and the future appearance of epilepsy. In some children, the foci persisted; in others, they disappeared; and still others showed a decrease or accentuation of amplitude or a shift to a new location. When the background activity was well organized and rhythmic, more foci disappeared. The authors concluded that since a large portion of these foci disappear with age, their presence is a sign of immaturity and plasticity of the brain, and that because no correspondence has been found between these abnormalities and concomitant or future epilepsy, the use of anticonvulsant drugs is not justified.

"Minimal Brain Dysfunction." Capute *et al.* (1968) found EEG abnormalities in 50% of 106 school-age children diagnosed by clinical evaluation as hyperkinetic, while only 15% of a matched control group without any behavior problems had abnormal tracings. Of the 50% with an abnormal EEG, 14% had paroxysmal abnormalities without seizures. Other investigators have arrived at more or less the same conclusion, though the nature of EEG abnormalities varies in different samples. Shetty (1973) considers the absence of well-organized alpha in age-appropriate proportion to be the most consistent finding, while others (Wilker *et al.*, 1970) have noted the excessive amount of slow-wave activities in EEG tracings of these children.

Dyslexia. Abnormal EEG records have been reported in a considerable percentage of children with dyslexia (Hughes and Park, 1968), although the specific nature of these abnormalities differs in various reports. Comparisons of dyslexic children with and without abnormal EEG have failed to show any significant difference in their clinical status or performance on psychological tests.

Aggressive Behavior. In clinically normal adult samples, between 5 and 15% have been found to have nonspecific abnormalities on EEG, particularly in the posterior temporal areas. Among adults with histories of aggressive and antisocial behavior, a higher incidence of such abnormalities has been reported. However, no direct relationship has been found between these abnormalities and aggressive tendencies. Up to the present, there is no solid basis for assuming any relationship—least of all a causal one—between EEG abnormalities and various conduct disorders of childhood and adolescence of the antisocial or aggressive types.

Other Psychiatric Disorders. In groups of adult schizophrenics, various quantification procedures have revealed differences in the amplitude of various EEG waves in comparisons with a normal population. However, this research is still in preliminary stages and no etiological interpretation is yet possible. In states of acute anxiety, decreases in rhythmical activities and amplitudes have been noted. In anorexia nervosa, background activities are slower. This change may be due to the metabolic consequences of self-imposed malnutrition.

Effects of Psychoactive Drugs. Tricyclic antidepressants and phenothiazines change the EEG pattern. The alpha rhythm may be reduced following the administration of tricyclics, while phenothiazines increase the percentage of theta and delta waves. Barbiturates or benzodiazepine derivatives produce low-voltage beta rhythm in the frontocentral area of the cortex. Diazepam (Valium) causes lowering of the voltage of the alpha rhythm, decreases the quantity of the alpha, and produces beta activities. Withdrawal from alcohol, barbiturates and benzodiazepine may be accompanied by paroxysmal abnormalities or other changes in the EEG. If an accurate EEG tracing is to be obtained, all medications should be discontinued at least 72 hours before the recording. When large doses of phenothiazine are used over a long period of time, the EEG changes may remain for periods up to nine weeks following discontinuation of the drug.

As has been noted above, EEG changes in various behavioral disorders of childhood are nonspecific and not of significant help in diagnosing "minimal brain damage," aggressive behavior, dyslexia, and mental retardation. On the other hand, the EEG is a valuable tool when the clinical picture raises the possibility of various forms of epilepsy. Although brain tumors are not as frequent in children as among adults, questionable symptoms that may point to a space-occupying lesion, such as abscess or brain tumor, are indications for obtaining an EEG record.

III
SYNDROMES IN CHILD PSYCHIATRY

7

Issues in Classification

Ideally, the diagnostic classification of childhood and adolescent psychiatric disorders should indicate the nature of the individual's pathology; the severity; the etiological agent or agents, if known; and the prognosis, if known.

An official classification, used in accordance with its accompanying definitions and descriptive examples, has a threefold purpose. With respect to the individual patient, the classification makes it possible to tap the accumulated knowledge regarding natural course and prognosis, the treatment and management strategies that have been employed, and the success of various strategies in altering natural course and prognosis. The child psychiatrist can compare his patient to these data and design an individualized plan of intervention.

A second reason for using a generally accepted nosological scheme is that it provides an objective base for comparisons of group trends over time and between geographical regions. This base is of extensive or limited use, depending on the breadth of the scheme's acceptance and on the frequency and nature of alterations in official terminologies. Thus an idiosyncratic scheme used only in one country or by one theoretical persuasion limits comparability between patient populations. When disease descriptions and titles are altered, comparability prior to and after such change becomes questionable, as from a past century to the current period.

A third purpose for an official classification has arisen as a result of such factors as third-party remuneration of physicians and hospitals, as well as the need for peer review of handling of cases. The identification of diagnosis by official name and statistical number is required by many health insurance forms, and treatment that is appropriate or unusual for a given diagnostic entity can be identified in cases whose handling has been questioned.

The demands of diagnostic accuracy and comparability sometimes appear to be mutually exclusive. In medicine in general, as well as in psychiatry, as knowledge increases, general diagnostic groupings are found to consist of descriptively similar but etiologically divergent syndromes. Conversely, it may be demonstrated that hitherto apparently unrelated complaints are in fact aspects of the same underlying disease process. If maintaining old terminology for the protection of comparability results in official categorization with little relevance, it then fails to meet the basic purpose of nomenclature.

Nosology in child psychiatry has had more than its share of the problems noted above. At this time, both the *Diagnostic and Statistical Manual* of the American Psychiatric Association (DSM II) adopted in 1968 and the eighth version of the *International Classification* (ICD 8, 1968) are under active revision. In general, most of the past and current utilized diagnostic classifications are unsatisfactory for the purposes noted above. There are several reasons.

The diagnoses of psychiatric disorders of childhood and adolescence have been derived from adult nomenclature. While this is a satisfactory approach in the case of disease processes found in adulthood that may also occur in childhood and adolescence, some behavioral deviations specific to the childhood period have been unrecognized in current classification lists or have been given terms that are imprecise. Actual detailed observations of children are relatively recent in psychiatric history. Infancy, for example, has only recently been examined intensively. Studies have shown many long-accepted concepts of age-specific capacities to be inaccurate. Hence diagnostic nomenclatures based on obsolete data require modification.

A number of nomenclatures are related to specific theoretical orientations and consequently each employs terminology unique to its given theory. Terms such as *latency period child* cannot easily be applied by psychiatrists whose theoretical orientations are in disagreement with the concepts inferred from this and other theory-bound terms.

Some diagnostic terms in DSM II have their derivation from conclusions about states of feeling, such as "overanxious reaction of childhood or adolescence," while others have been purely descriptive, such as "hyperkinetic reaction of childhood." The diagnostician may be confused by the mixed basis of terminology. Often he places a behavioral deviance in a category that appears to do least violence to his actual opinion. Where a diagnostic term implies greater pathology than he believes exists, the tendency has been to use a grab-bag category. "Adjustment reaction of childhood" (or adolescence) or "passive–aggressive personality," for example, have been overemployed in this manner and hence have limited value either for conveying the nature of the behavior disorder or for providing comparability between groups of patients.

The solution to these dilemmas by some has been to develop individual schemata. Cameron (1957) devised a symptom classification for child psychiatry. In simplified outline, this classification is as follows:

Developmental
- Physical handicap or ill health
- Intellectual handicapping
- Variant of personality type

Reactive
- Primary habit disturbance
- Secondary habit disturbance
- Motor disturbance
- Education or work disturbance

Individual
- Minor symptoms
- Psychoneurotic syndrome
- Established psychosomatic entity
- Organic brain damage syndrome
- Psychotic syndrome

In the first American textbook on child psychiatry, Leo Kanner did not employ a specific classification. Dr. Kanner (1948) commented upon the many problems of diagnostic accuracy in attempting to use the Kraepelin nosology for childhood. While this nosology served to provide statistics for institutionalized mental patients, he felt it had the defect of ignoring the dynamic processes involved in cases of individual child patients. Kanner presented Adolph Meyer's tentative groupings. Dissatisfied with a disease concept of pathological behavior, Meyer conceived of patterns of performances or "ergasia." Thus he grouped patients as follows:

- Anergasia: loss or deficit due to brain damage
- Dysergasia: disturbed functioning, such as delirium, stupor, or coma, due to metabolic malfunction
- Parergasia: schizophrenia and paranoid behavior
- Thymergasia: mood elevations and depressions
- Oligergasia: feeblemindedness
- Merergasia or kakergasia: nonpsychotic disorders, mainly anxieties or neurotic behaviors

These are groupings aimed at adult patients, and Kanner has not advocated their use with children but rather suggests the employment of diagnostic word pictures that indicate both the behavior noted and a dynamic explanation of its cause, particularly with relation to parental attitudes.

In a later textbook, Chess (1969) suggested a simplified categorization that was consistent with DSM II:

- Normal
- Mental retardation
- Organic brain disturbance (includes temporary maturational lags)
- Reactive behavior disorders
- Neurotic behavior disorders
- Neurotic character disorders
- Neurosis
- Childhood psychosis and schizophrenic adjustments
- Sociopathic personality

An intent of the above schema was to provide broad categories that would permit comparison between groups of child patients who come from differing ethnic and socioeconomic origins or whose sources of stress are diverse.

The Group for the Advancement of Psychiatry (GAP, 1966) suggested a nosological grouping that arose out of the clinical experience of its Committee on Child Psychiatry. They proposed 10 major categories, with subheadings under each, and provided detailed discussion of the rationale for their definitions. The overall classification is:

- Healthy responses
- Reactive disorders
- Developmental deviations
- Psychoneurotic disorders
- Personality disorders
- Psychotic disorders
- Psychophysiologic disorders
- Brain syndromes
- Mental retardation
- Other disorders

A major premise of the committee that formulated this report was that its organization and the definitions must not be wedded to a single theory. Its intent was to provide a workable nosology that included phenomenology and also took into account a developmental framework.

Since the International Classification of Diseases of the World Health Organization was made official in 1968 (ICD 8), a series of studies have been sponsored in different countries by the World Health Organization to establish a useful psychiatric classification and to identify problems of variability in the use of terms in different countries (Rutter *et al.*, 1969). With regard to child psychiatry, the evaluation of a multiaxial classification has been the focus. Case histories of child patients were sent to the participating child psychiatrists, and the diagnostic variations of the replies were used for further refinement of the instrument. Essentially the strategy has been to regroup the categories of ICD 8 into separate axes, adding new factors not previously contained in the classification. ICD 8 suggested 11 categories, in form suitable for statistical handling:

0. Normal variations
1. Reactive disorders
2. Specific developmental disorders
3. Neurotic disorders
4. Personality or character disorders
5. Psychotic disorders
6. Somatic disorders of presumably psychogenic origin
7. Disorders directly due to demonstrable acute or chronic organic brain condition
8. Mental retardation
9. Antisocial behavior not classifiable elsewhere
10. Disorders not classifiable under 0–9

The concept of a multiaxial scheme is that it can provide symptom description, developmental data, biological concomitants, and relevant environmental factors. Since concepts of etiology may change with the acquisition of new knowledge or advances in organizing already established facts, the axis descriptive of the functioning of the child at the time of diagnostic study provides for continuing comparability. The use of terms such as *associated factors* in two of the axes indicates that while these may in fact be causative, at the present time this has not yet been scientifically established. The five axes under consideration as of 1973 (Rutter, 1973) are:

Axis 1: Clinical psychiatric syndrome
Axis 2: Developmental disorder
Axis 3: Intellectual level
Axis 4: Associated biological factors
Axis 5: Associated psychosocial factors

Each axis is to be coded in accordance with a list of terms and their code numbers. A glossary defining all words employed is intended to ensure comparability.

Because of the close relationship between the American official classification and the World Health Organization's nomenclature, the final adoption of a multiaxial approach is likely to influence future revisions of the *Diagnostic and Statistical Manual* of the American Psychiatric Association.

The initial draft of DSM III, prepared by the Task Force on Nomenclature and Statistics (Spitzer *et al.*, 1977), as of May 1975 to be considered for official adoption by the American Psychiatric Association, does contain some important revisions along the lines of the revisions being worked on by the World Health Organization and responds to the major complaints about DSM II. Prominent among the new features are the accounting for developmental disorders as such and a clearer identification of other emotional and behavioral difficulties. Overall the section of the new classification dealing with childhood derives more closely from the clinical pictures encountered in practice than the two previous versions.

As was pointed out by Veith (1957), from the time of Hippocrates on attempts to classify mental illness have reflected the etiological concepts of particular periods. The current emphasis on including both current and historical symptom description was originally the contribution of Thomas Sydenham in the 17th century, but it is only now being recognized as useful for identifying childhood disorders.

Dissatisfaction with the use of the medical model has been expressed regarding some of the terms included in various classifications. Such opinions stem from a belief that these are not in fact diseases and that their inclusion improperly preserves the ascendancy of the physician in dealing with them. These points have been raised particularly with respect to mental retardation. For example, there is a high percentage of mentally retarded children for whom there is no known organic etiology and whose major needs are educational, recreational, vocational, and/or custodial. None of these services lies within the expertise of the psychiatrist.

No classificatory scheme, however encompassing of the knowledge of its time, will be forever accurate and complete. Nor can any diagnostic term describe the unique aspects of each individual patient. But the use of uniform nomenclature is necessary to identify the nature of the deviant behavior in a language that can be comprehended by all those providing psychiatric care for children and those involved in research. It can further extend our knowledge of psychopathology, etiology, prognosis, and effective treatment and management of behavioral disturbances in childhood.

8

Adjustment Reactions

The term *adjustment reaction* denotes a combination of the stress response and compensatory adaptive mechanisms that characterize the behavior of an individual who experiences disruptive life events, usually of an unpleasant nature. While the initial impact of stress *per se* is expected to decrease with the passage of time, the coping mechanisms employed to reestablish the previous internal and external equilibrium may become incorporated into the structure of personality and be resistant to further modification. An acute situational reaction is the transient outcome of the interplay between the severity of the disruptive elements and the child's intellectual level and emotional maturity at the time. To a large extent, the child's cognitive stage determines his perception of stress, while the nature of his response is dependent upon the level of behavioral organization that he has achieved. For example, in very young infants, hospitalization or surgical procedures may be tolerated without any observable behavioral changes; or their disruptive influence may be manifested in such areas as the patterning of the biological functions of sleep, feeding, and elimination. On the other hand, when the child has begun to differentiate between his customary caretakers and other people, hospitalization is experienced on a higher psychological plane, and stress response is expressed as a suspension or diminution of active exploratory behavior and as withdrawal and apathy.

When disruptive elements block the normal process of development, the organization of behavior and structuring of the personality must proceed along alternative pathways, and the outcome depends upon a multitude of factors, such as the degree of incapacity, the basic intellectual endowment, and the temperamental quality of the child, as well as environmental variables such as the parents' attitudes and adequacy, their aspirations for and expectations of the child, and their own adaptive capacities.

Psychological reaction to stress in children may take various forms, such as aggressive and antisocial activities, withdrawal and depression, increased preoccupation with morbid fantasies, decreased interest in the environment, loss of previously acquired functions, accentuation of preexisting deviant behavior, or the appearance of a new set of symptoms. While the disorganizing influence of stress may be conceptualized as causing regression in the child's level of functioning, the particular form of behavioral manifestation cannot always be foretold. A dependent child may become clinging following a period of unexpected absence of the mother, although he may continue to attend school with no reluctance. On the other hand, a poor scholar may develop school phobia following a minor illness. The severity of a reactive behavior disorder is not a direct reflection of the intensity of disruptive forces. Other factors, such as the child's previous level of competence, his vulnerability, and the availability of environmental support and understanding, all play a part in whether aberrant behavior will be pervasive or isolated and the speed with which preexisting organization is reestablished (Newman, 1976).

When the noxious stimuli cannot be removed, the child must be helped to accommodate to the new situation. Such help may take the form of providing an opportunity for the child to express his feelings of resentment, anger, and fears; to receive clarification and assurances; and to discover and appreciate the possible positive aspects of the changes that have taken place. While it may be impossible for any adult to perceive and interpret reality as a child does, it is often sufficient to understand and clarify those concerns that are articulated by the child. Most parents are intuitively capable of providing the necessary support for their children's distress. On these occassions, the child psychiatrist's role is that of diagnosing the problem and counseling the parents. When the parents cannot tolerate the frank expression of the child's anxieties or are unable to provide the necessary support, short-term individual treatment for the child is indicated. At times, certain behavioral symptoms that have originally appeared in stress situations are inadvertently reinforced or achieve such symbolic importance that they become a part of the child's habitual coping strategy long after the initial impact of the stressful situation has passed. Treatment of this chronic maladaptive behavior requires a change in interactional patterns between the child and his family as well as the strengthening and encouragement of adaptive behavior.

Reactions to Illness and Disability. In infants and young children, physical illnesses are usually preceded and accompanied by irritability, feeding problems, sleep interruptions, and lack of sustained interest in the environment. High fever may be accompanied by confusion, delirium, and a variety of fears and apprehensions. When the illness requires hospitalization, the necessary medical and surgical procedures and removal from the home are additional sources of distress with psychological implications. At times, neglect or ignorance of the hospital staff and parental inability or unwillingness to prepare the child for the therapeutic procedures leave the young patient at the mercy of his own limited knowledge and morbid fears of physical injury and annihilation. Some children express their fears by becoming physically or verbally combative, others refuse to cooperate, and yet another group become helpless and sullen and exhibit regressive behavior.

In a study of the effects of cardiac catheterization, Aisenberg and co-workers (1973) found negative behavioral and psychological changes in 70% of their 50 child patients, although none of the children was incapacitated by their illness nor had any complications related to the catheterization. The authors concluded that even though in some children the negative changes were transient, their influence on the later social adjustment of these patients should not be ignored. The report of Galdston and Gamble (1969) provides a contrast to Aisenberg's findings and sheds further light on the subject. In a study of 16 children with implanted cardiac pacemakers necessitating frequent operative procedures (an average of 4.8 operations over a 30.6-month period), the authors were impressed by the absence of psychopathological reactions related to the physical illness among the children and their families. The factors that seemed to have contributed to the successful adjustment of patients and their families were (1) they identified with the action-oriented, positive medical attitudes; (2) they searched for and acquired information regarding the illness and treatment procedures; and (3) they denied the affect surrounding the illness and its implication. Similar psychological coping mechanisms were found among well-adjusted hemophiliac children studied by Mattsson and Gross (1966). In both studies, denial of affect helped the patients and their families to function normally within the limitations imposed by the disease and to cooperate in the medical regimens. On the other hand, when the fact of illness or the necessity for treatment was denied, patients were maladjusted and self-destructive. Some children who had accepted the medical regimens during childhood became uncooperative during adolescence, some refusing to follow treatment, others actively engaging in hitherto forbidden activities.

The clinical experiences of most authorities in the field reveal that children's adjustment to chronic physical illness depends on factors related to the nature of the illness, the adaptive capacity of the child, and the quality of the parent–child relationships. Some chronic illnesses may reduce the child's functioning by their direct deleterious consequences on the central nervous system, such as hypo- and hyperglycemic episodes in juvenile diabetes or intracranial hemorrhages in hemophiliacs. Medical treatment, although necessary, may have undesirable side effects, such as the sleepiness due to some anticonvulsive drugs. The age at which the illness appears and the length and frequency of hospitalization and convalescence may interfere with the acquisition of particular sets of skills or may interrupt and impair opportunities for normal socialization and peer interaction. Parental attitudes may vary from guilt, sorrow, and overprotection to acceptance and encouragement. Some children find it easy to play the role of invalid and, with subtle feedbacks, invite overprotection, while some guilt-ridden parents impose such roles on their children. Other parents are so disappointed in their progeny that they refuse to acknowledge their limitations.

Children's responses to catastrophic injuries and accidents such as burns or loss of limbs are at first stress reactions with withdrawals, regressive behavior, or hostile and belligerent attitudes. Later on, they become more cooperative and hopeful about their eventual recovery and the restoration of their physical integrity. Depressive mood and hopelessness set in once the youngster realizes that scars are permanent or that the amputated leg will not grow back. During this stage, the support and understanding of the staff members and of family and friends is particularly necessary for the patient's adjustment to his new body image. In discussing the role of child psychiatrists in a burn treatment unit, Bernstein et al. (1969) pointed out that at times the attitudes of caretakers within the hospital may be nontherapeutic for the patients in that they foster regressive behavior or tacitly approve the child's and the parents' magical beliefs in total recovery and absence of any disfigurements. Patients thus come to mistrust further reassurances, and their apprehension and fear of the world outside the hospital become refractory.

Handicaps and disabilities that are present from early infancy may have specific influence over personality formation; however, no personality type can be said to be associated with a certain kind of handicap. Although various aspects of motor, cognitive, or social development may be delayed as a result of handicapping conditions, at times minor modification in the environment is enough to assure the maximum growth of the handicapped child. Parental attitudes are of utmost significance in whether a child learns to use his potentials or remains in a state of crippling dependency. "Organ inferiority," as conceptualized by Adler, is a part of a general insecurity of some children who have sensed parental rejection and disappointment because of their less-than-perfect body or performance. While some children are driven to overcompensate for their inadequacies in one area, others are left with a sense of deep dissatisfaction and bitterness, which blocks their normal development.

Psychiatric interventions for children with chronic physical illnesses and disabilities are most helpful as preventive measures directed at the child, the family, and the patient's caretakers. Preparation for surgical operations, particularly those that will have visible sequelae, requires enough time to allow the patient to absorb the information and its implications. Parental fears, whether rational or irrational, are conveyed to their children and need to be aired out and discussed. Issues such as the possible implications for future academic, vocational, and reproductive adequacies or inheritability of a disease must be raised whenever indicated or when the physician detects concerns regarding them. For the patients themselves, immediate problems of acceptance by peers, freedom from discomfort, and ability to move and play are more important than long-term outcomes; however, their fear of physical injury may be intensified by parental apprehension for their future.

Psychotherapeutic encounters with parents must provide an opportunity for them to express their feelings as well as positive guidance regarding their handling of the child. Psychiatric advice may be sought when the child has developed behavioral problems that may or may not be directly related to his physical illness but that interfere with his maximum functioning or the implementation of treatment procedures. The child psychiatrist must be sensitive to the anxiety and depression that may be masked by a facade of physical and verbal aggressiveness. Sometimes inclusion of these patients within a group of well-adjusted children with similar disabilities may be advised in order to provide the youngster with examples of a more hopeful outcome. School placement for a child with a visible handicap requires special attention because these children's self-consciousness and extreme sensitivity about their imperfection may be aggravated by the teasing, ostracism, intolerance, and outright cruelty of their nonhandicapped peers. On the other hand, attempts must be made to reintegrate these children within the mainstream of normal academic and social programs as soon as possible in order to prevent their eventual isolation.

Psychological reactions of children with terminal illnesses and of their families have received some attention during recent years. While earlier writers had maintained that up to about 9 or 10 years of age dying children do not show specific awareness and anxiety regarding their impending death (Richmond and Waisman, 1955), more recent investigators (Spinetta, 1974) have questioned this assumption, pointing out that the child's inability to express, articulate, or conceptualize his fear of death cannot be taken as an indication of his lack of concern and awareness on a biological level. Furthermore, studies of adaptational processes and psychological reactions of families with a dying child have revealed the intensity of parental emotional struggles with the threat of the loss. Therefore it seems logical to assume that a dying child is not only aware of his biological disintegration but is also sensitive to his parents' moods and their varied emotional responses to him. Although it is a herculean task to become or remain emotionally involved with a child when one must at the same time be prepared for his death, the psychiatrist may be called upon to help not only the family or the caretakers but also the child himself. Whether the child is only barely aware of others' emotional withdrawal and thus is left with a deep sense of loneliness or, as an adolescent, understands the nature of his predicament and is terrorized by it, it is important to remember that even though the psychiatrist cannot postpone death, he can try to improve the quality and the richness of the patient's remaining days through attempts at encouraging the patient's involvement with his environment and the exercise of his mental faculties of perception and cognition.

9

Disorders of
Biological Functions

EATING DISTURBANCES

The need for food is such a basic survival requirement that one would hardly expect to encounter numerous problems associated with feeding in childhood. From early infancy, children's appetites can be adversely affected by physical illnesses, overexcitement, fatigue, and emotional factors, but the majority of eating disturbances in early childhood are caused by the child's reaction to the regulatory demands of his caretakers. The process of regulating the child's intake begins with birth. The interval between feedings, the amount of food, and later on the nature of the nutritious material allowed or forbidden are all matters of parental choice and cultural norms. Thus the battle between rigid parents and difficult infants may begin with the feeding preferences of the child and the regulatory demands of the mother. Child care manuals have reversed their earlier advocacy of rigid timing and duration for infant feedings and ideal ages for weaning. Parents are now advised to observe their infants for cues and to allow them to regulate their own intake. However, there are general expectations as to when a child should begin to imitate the eating habits of his family and community.

Kanner (1972) stated that about 25% of parents complain of the eating habits of their children. Some children refuse food, others are extremely selective, some take a long time to eat, and others eat at intervals that parents do not like. Eating problems may be primarily due to the child's idiosyncrasies or may have their origin in parental handling. Some children cannot sit still for the length of time required to finish their meal. They may be hyperactive and distractible, and since they are not satiated in the time that is allowed, they are hungry later and request food between meals. Other children are slow eaters because they are preoccupied with their fantasies and daydreams. Some children have a low sensitivity threshold and may find certain tastes, consistencies, smells, or temperatures unacceptable. For other children, any novel stimulus may be at first aversive, so that they prefer to eat familiar foods and do not accept an expanded diet. A particular food or a category of edible materials may become associated with unpleasant sensations or occurrences for a child and may thus be avoided. Parental oversolicitousness and the degree of attention paid to the child's eating can provide him with an easy strategy for attracting attention or expressing anger, or he may receive other secondary gains.

Case History

Cheryl, a 6-year-old girl, was brought to the psychiatrist because of the very limited number of food items that she would eat. Cheryl was a premature baby, weighing 3 lb 5 oz at birth. She had been breast-fed for three months, with supplementary formula. The parents remembered that she had refused the bottle when the nipple was changed, so that the old nipple had to be used until it was practically torn to pieces. The parents had tried to introduce Cheryl to solid foods several times before she finally accepted them. As a toddler, she had started to eat dry cereal of a certain brand and this had become her staple diet. At the time of referral, Cheryl ate one brand of cereal, two kinds of ice cream, two brands of crackers, potato chips, apples, and oranges, and she would drink only milk. The parents had tried to coerce and bribe her to eat at various points in her life, but they had refused the advice of their family physician to starve her. Cheryl was to start school in three months, and the parents were concerned that her eating habits would be a subject of teasing and ridicule by other children.

During the interview, Cheryl was shy and cooperative. She said she did not believe her parents should be concerned about her eating because her current friends did not tease her. She explained that she could not eat meat because "It is too soft, it tickles my throat." Cheese and eggs had a "funny smell" and chocolates were "too sweet." She said she ate only things that were "crisp and hard." She reluctantly accepted a roasted salty peanut from the psychiatrist, but after eating a very small piece, she asked for more and declared that she would add them to her diet.

A long period of behavior modification and desensitization was necessary before Cheryl could add a dozen items to her diet. Follow-up contact with the family when Cheryl was 9 years old revealed that she had managed to expand the variety of food that she ate but her mother said, "I don't expect her to become a galloping gourmet."

In managing eating problems, it is important to obtain a clear picture of the eating habits of the family and the pattern of interactions between the parents and the child surrounding the meal. A series of counseling sessions with the parents may modify those aspects of their behavior that maintain the child's particular reaction. When the problem is primarily due to the child's style, the parents can be helped to understand and readjust their demands and thus avoid the subsequent emotional responses that create tension within the family. Some children may need psychiatric intervention because their eating habits are limiting their opportunity for normal participation in the activities of their peer group. In other cases, food may have acquired such a central role in the child's mental life that there is very little room for other experiences. On these occasions, psychiatric treatment should be directed toward expanding the child's options for interaction with his environment, with the view that personal preferences in diet, in and of themselves, do not need modification even though they may inconvenience the parents.

Pica

During the first 12 months of life, infants bring everything to the mouth as an exploratory maneuver, though they do not eat these materials. It is between 12 and 18 months following birth that some children begin to eat nonnutritious material. In some children this becomes a selective, purposeful, and habitual act that is called *pica*. Pica is most frequently seen in children living in rural areas or in those whose parents or older sibs have had the habit. While at one point pica was considered a possible outcome of various nutritional deficiencies, evidence supporting such contentions has not been found. In children with average intelligence, the incidence of pica decreases with age, so that by 5 years of age most children give up the habit. In older children, pica may be maintained as an attention-getting device, or the habit may acquire anxiety-reducing properties and may therefore be engaged in when the child is under stress. Retarded and severely psychotic children may continue with the habit well into their middle childhood. Most authorities believe that pica is a learned behavior pattern. On the other hand, once pica has become habitual, parental handling may play an important part in maintaining the behavior. Children coming from neglected homes may never have been properly supervised or taught that particular substances should not be consumed. Lead poisoning is the most common and most harmful side effect of pica. In any child with a history of pica, assessment of blood lead level is a necessary part of medical and psychiatric evaluation. Lead encephalopathy and the neurological sequelae of lead poisoning in children are associated with behavioral problems of varying severity.

Obesity

Obesity is excess weight caused by an increase in the number of fatty cells of the body. Accurate estimates of the prevalence of obesity in childhood and adolescence is lacking; however, it is known that obesity in childhood and adolescence is the forerunner of obesity in adults. About 80% of obese children will become obese adults, and studies of obese adults and adolescents have revealed that in at least half of the group, the onset of obesity dates back to the age of 6.

Etiology. A multitude of causative factors have been shown to be operative in the genesis of obesity.

Genetic factors are implicated because 60–70% of obese children have obese parents. When one parent is obese, between 40 and 50% of children develop obesity. The weight of adoptive children has been shown to correlate more with that of their natural than of their adoptive parents, and identical twins raised apart have closely similar weight.

Constitutional factors are also at play. Longitudinal studies of the development of fatty tissues in children have revealed that the number and size of fat cells in nonobese children approach adult value between the ages of 9 and 12, while obese children obtain adult values around 5–7 years of age. In fact, in some children, the deviation from normal development can be observed as early as 2 years of age (Knittle, 1972).

Studies in animals have shown that early nutritional experiences also have an important role in the development of fatty tissues in animals. However, the role of feeding practices in early infancy and their relationship to obesity in children have not been fully investigated. Studies of the caloric intake of obese and normal children and adolescents have failed to show a significant difference between the two groups, but it must be noted that these observations are made when the obesity has already set in and therefore cannot rule out the possibility of earlier overeating. The low caloric output and reduced activity level of obese children may be the result rather than the cause of obesity.

Evidence of deviations in the metabolism of carbohydrates and insulin in obesity has been reported. However, since weight reduction has at times caused a normalization of these disturbances, some researchers believe that these deviations are secondary to obesity. The results of hormonal studies are also inconclusive.

Mother–child relationships and style of child rearing in regard to obesity have been subjects of psychiatric interest. Hilda Bruch (1963) considers obesity to be the outcome of disturbed communication between the child and the mother. According to her, the insecure mother has a tendency to overfeed the child, and the compliant–passive child accepts the mother's direction. Other authors have theorized that these parents overvalue food and have a tendency to use candies and sweets as reinforcers for good behavior.

Early-onset obesity is associated with problems with body image, a sense of inferiority in relation to peers, difficulties in interpersonal relationships, and, in adolescence, concern over acceptability to the opposite sex. Mayer (1966) believes that psychopathology is the effect rather than the cause of obesity and has pointed out the similarity between psychological problems of obese and other minority groups in society. In one subgroup of obese children and adolescents, the eating pattern is extremely deviant. These are children in whom eating is associated with intrapsychic cues, so that they eat when they are depressed, angry, or anxious. In this form of eating, satiety does not depend on the cessation of hunger; rather, eating binges are responses to psychological factors. In some patients, obesity is due to excessive intake, but the overeating is symptomatic of the emotional state of the child. Feelings of emptiness, worthlessness, and self-loathing are openly described. For some patients, being unacceptable and ugly on account of their obesity is preferable to feeling unloved and unwanted because of what they consider to be their basic worthlessness.

At times, these patients become convinced that losing weight will solve their psychological problems, and they go on a reducing diet, only to become ambivalent and return to their previous eating habits with a considerable amount of guilt feelings and a stronger sense of helplessness. They accept the derogatory cultural statements about their lack of will power and the flaws in their character. They are scapegoats in their extra- and intrafamilial milieu, and although depressed, they feel that they deserve such treatment. In some patients, weight reduction aggravates the underlying psychological problems in that it removes a psychological defense and brings the patient face to face with his intrapsychic conflicts.

Treatment. The prevention of obesity must start in early life, particularly in those families in which the parents are obese and the children are therefore at a higher risk of developing obesity. The simplest and safest manner of weight reduction is through decrease in caloric intake. In limiting the intake of a child, sufficient knowledge of nutrition and the physiological requirements of a growing child is necessary in order to assure continuous normal development. High motivation on the part of the family is necessary in order to limit the child's intake of food. Without the cooperation of all members of the family and their help in monitoring the child, the effort is doomed to failure. Furthermore, the child is in need of support and encouragement during this period in order to sustain his efforts, to start him participating in those areas of activities that will be rewarding to him, and to reinforce his desire to remain within the normal weight group. Once the ideal weight has been achieved, the maintenance of weight is a lifelong project. Eating habits may have to be modified and caloric intake must remain somewhat limited. This seems to be the most difficult part of dieting.

The role of psychiatrists in the treatment of obesity, in the majority of cases of children and adolescents, is motivating and supporting the child and his family. In the subgroup in which obesity is caused or maintained by psychological factors, the underlying problems must be treated and the association between overeating and emotional cues must be broken. Behavior modification techniques have been tried with adults and reports so far have been encouraging. These techniques may be used as part of psychotherapy with obese children and adolescents. Appetite-reducing chemical agents do not have any place in the treatment of childhood and adolescent obesity.

Anorexia Nervosa

Anorexia nervosa is a constellation of symptoms that includes persistent refusal to eat in spite of good appetite, extreme weight loss, and malnutrition, sometimes leading to death from starvation. The majority of reported cases are teenage girls, although some boys also develop the disorder.

When the child is prepubertal, the menses do not start on reaching puberty. Those who have begun menstruating develop amenorrhea. The onset may be as early as 9 years of age, and the illness may continue over several months to several years. In some patients, the disease is transitory. Others have one or more relapses. The weight loss may range from 15 to 50% of pre-illness weight. In some patients, there is a history of feeding problems in early childhood, and some children are overweight before the onset of the illness.

Physical examination reveals varying degrees of weight loss, generalized hirsutism, hypothermia, bradycardia, and bradyphea. Almost all parents report constipation. Metabolic and hormonal studies may reveal the expected disturbances associated with malnutrition. The findings of various hormonal imbalances have been nonconclusive, and so far no etiological significance can be attached to them.

Etiology. Psychiatric studies of children and adolescents with anorexia nervosa have revealed disorders ranging from neurosis to schizophrenia, so that no particular personality characteristics or psychiatric disorders can be said to distinguish these patients. Profound disturbances relating to body image, obsessional rumination about foods, and high suggestibility are found in the majority of the patients. While some patients are alert and unusually active, others may be withdrawn and depressed. The patient's interpersonal relationships are usually unsatisfactory. There may be indications of poor relationships with both parents, especially the mother or other female relatives. Although most authors have commented upon the patients' reluctance to discuss their feelings, some patients have revealed their concerns about growing up and accepting the role of sexually mature adults.

In a series of 20 cases of anorexia nervosa, Warren (1968) reported the following findings. The age of onset was between 10 years and 6 months and 15 years 9 months, with a mean age of 12 years 3 months. Of the 20 girls, 8 were prepubertal, 4 had reached puberty but had not menstruated, and the remaining 8 had developed amenorrhea following the onset of their illness. Depression of moderate degree was found in 17 patients, while 3 were judged to be severely depressed. In comparison with other children in the inpatient adolescent unit, the anorexic group came from a higher socioeconomic class and had a higher incidence of physical or mental illness in their families. Shyness, timidity, and limited social contact were the most common personality traits, although obsessional traits were found in 35% of the sample. Follow-up study of one to nine years for 11 patients who had recovered showed that 2 were psychiatrically normal, 4 had required repeated psychiatric hospitalizations for conditions other than anorexia, 1 had been diagnosed as schizophrenic, and 5 others showed various degrees of neurotic disturbances, although they were not receiving any psychiatric care. Of this group of 20 patients, 2 had died of starvation. In all the patients who had recovered from anorexia, no stunting of growth had taken place and menstruation had been established.

CASE HISTORY

Katty was 14 years old at the time of referral. She had lost 35% of her weight over a period of six months. She reported that sometime in the last week of the schoolyear, a friend had teased her about her protruding stomach and had jokingly asked if she were pregnant. A week later, her older sister had bought a book about dieting and showed Katty the book without any suggestion that she should or needed to go on a diet. However, Katty had begun to worry about her weight and her looks. She had decided that her weight of 105 pounds was too much for her height of 5 feet 4 inches and began to limit her intake. When she had lost 20 pounds, her parents became concerned, but Katty could no longer stop the dieting. She believed that she would look better if she became still thinner in some parts and put on weight in other parts. What was disturbing to her was her constant rumination about food and her inability to stop insisting that all other members of the family consume a large quantity of food. This was the source of constant tension at home. She had become withdrawn and isolated from her friends, though she rationalized this by saying that she could not be in their company at lunchtime since she did not eat and could not take the bus home with them because she wanted to walk in order to burn more calories. Somewhat embarrassingly, she gave the measurements of a famous movie star and "sex symbol" as the ideal measurement for herself, although she could not explain how by refusing to eat she hoped to attain this goal. She believed that before reaching this ideal image, she could not hope to attract the attention of any boys and therefore tried to avoid them.

Treatment. In the treatment of anorexia nervosa, the first important consideration is the fact that excessive loss of weight, unless stopped, can cause death by starvation. Therefore hospitalization may become the only option at some point in the course of treatment. Since the patient's refusal to eat is a voluntary act, the goal of treatment of anorexia is to motivate the patient to agree to eat (Lucas *et al.*, 1976). Some authors believe that the goal is best achieved away from the family in a hospital setting. However, some patients gain weight rapidly in the hospital and insist on being discharged or convince their parents to terminate the treatment, and the underlying psychiatric disorder remains untreated. In some patients, the threat of hospitalization is enough to mobilize the patient to begin to eat. Therefore, before hospitalization becomes absolutely necessary, the psychiatric treatment necessitates a planned, flexible strategy of removing the symptom and concurrent exploration and modification of the underlying disorder.

DISORDERS OF SLEEP

Sleep problems of children can be broadly divided into two categories: physiological disorders and psychological–environmental disturbances. This division does not imply that physiological disorders are impervious to the vicissitudes of the child's life experiences. On the contrary, it has been shown that a physiological disorder such as sleepwalking can be brought about by anxiety in individuals who have had long periods free of the symptom.

Psychological–Environmental Etiology. Although newborn infants do not show nocturnal preference for sleeping and diurnal wakefulness, most infants begin to establish this rhythm between 3 and 6 months of age, so that a period of uninterrupted sleep between midnight and early morning is expected during the second part of the first year of life. Unregulated sleep may be due to parental mishandling or the infant's chronic discomfort brought about by hunger, cold, or physical illness. Infants with high sensitivity, irritability, or biological irregularity are slow to develop patterned behavior. The tension and dissatisfaction created in the parents by the infant's behavior, in turn, decrease their effectiveness in rational handling and may aggravate the situation. Once the infant's sleep pattern has been established, sleep may still be interrupted by various environmental factors, such as temporary separation from home and changes in sleeping arrangements. However, most of these disturbances are of transitory nature. During childhood and adolescence, interrupted sleep and difficulty in falling asleep are the two major complaints.

Interrupted sleep due to bad dreams seems to be a part of the normal development of toddlers. The expanding world of childhood and the limited conceptual ability to deal with the new reality give rise to anxieties and fears that do not stop when the child goes to sleep. Refusal to go to sleep in this age group may be due to the child's concern about loss of control over his newly acquired functions, such as bowel and bladder control, or it may reflect the child's worries that people and places that are associated with his feelings of security may vanish when he loses contact with them. Because young children do not differentiate between dreams and reality, after having awakened with a bad dream they may be reluctant to allow themselves to fall asleep again. Parental reassurance and understanding are all that is needed to help the child during this period. However, for some children parental behavior may inadvertently provide the kind of secondary gain that tends to maintain the disturbed sleep pattern. These children learn to use their sleeping behavior as a device to attract parental attention and to manipulate their environment. They beg or demand to postpone their bedtime and insist on having their parents in their bedroom before they fall asleep, and when they awaken during the night, they call for their parents or go to sleep in their parents' room or bed. Parental counseling and suggestions for a change in their response to the child's behavior will improve the sleep problem and relieve the parents.

The restless sleep of children may be due to their general high activity level, and any modification or treatment should be addressed to the child's total behavior. As children grow older, their unarticulated fears and anxieties regarding interpersonal relationships within and outside the family are sources of bad dreams, nightmares, and sleep disruption. Among older children and adolescents, difficulties in getting to sleep are due to concerns and preoccupations with emotional conflicts. Obsessive thoughts, sexual arousal, and depressive moods are among the most common causes of insomnia in adolescents. While engagement in various activities may absorb the child's attention during the daytime, fears and desires occupy the child's mental energy when he is in the state of inactivity that must precede sleep. In some children anticipation of various events may temporarily cause sleeplessness.

Children's dreams are simpler than dreams of adults. They are recreated from fragments of their daily experience and activities, including their impressions of people and events and even the television programs or movies they have seen. The child's ability to describe his dreams and his level of comprehension of the dream events determine his willingness or his ability to recall a dream. Disturbances in the child's personality and his pathological preoccupation may introduce bizarre and unpleasant elements into his dreams. Fears of the unknown and concerns over personal and parental safety may be expressed directly in the dream or may be seen as threatening monsters, mysterious destructive forces, kidnappers, and so on.

Hypersomnia in children and adolescents is usually of psychological origin. For some children, sleep is an easy escape from the demands of an environment with which they cannot or do not wish to comply. Disturbances of sleep pattern, when not directly related to parental handling, should always be treated as one aspect of the child's total emotional problem. Hypnotic drugs are usually not indicated in dealing with children's sleep problems since they are either unnecessary or only of symptomatic value.

Physiological Etiology. Sleep polygraphy has provided an objective tool by which the differences between organization, rhythm, and proportion of sleep in adults and children can be observed and abnormal sleep patterns that are clearly of physiological origin can be identified. In adults, a sleep cycle, as defined by the neuronal activities on the EEG, begins with NREM (no rapid eye movement) sleep, descends from Stage 1 to Stage 4, and then emerges in reverse order to end in a REM period, after which a new cycle begins. In early infancy, the sleep record cannot be so clearly defined; only an indeterminate period is distinguishable between REM and NREM sleep. REM sleep in adults occurs during the last third of the night, while children may enter sleep with a REM period. Also, while in adults the REM sleep constitutes 20% of all sleeping time, in infants and younger children,

REM is about 35–45% of the total sleep. The significance of this developmental shift is not as yet clear, though some authors have hypothesized that REM sleep in infants and young children is a reflection of autostimulation of the central nervous system and may serve the purpose of differentiation and organization of the neuronal structure of the immature brain. Differences between adults' and children's sleep disappear during the first two years of life except for the higher proportion of REM sleep, which shows a steady decline with age and approaches normal adult values in the early teens.

Sleepwalking and Sleeptalking. Sleepwalking consists of a sudden sitting in bed, which may or may not be followed by actual walking and moving about. The child's eyes are open, though he does not appear to see. The child's walking may appear purposeful in that he opens doors and avoids obstacles. Some children may talk during this period, though their responses to questioning are unintelligible. The episode lasts between a few seconds to 30 minutes and ends with the child's returning to bed to continue sleeping. The child is totally amnestic about the sleepwalking. Episodes of sleepwalking occur during the transition between NREM and REM sleep and are not associated with dreaming. The EEG record during the episode reveals paroxysmal, high-voltage, slow-frequency waves, which, according to some authors, are an indication of immaturity of the central nervous system. Somnambulism is more frequent in boys than in girls and the incidence decreases with age. In some cases, sleepwalking is associated with enuresis. Some children talk in their sleep in association with a dream and, if awakened at the time, can recall the dream.

Pavor Nocturnus. Night terrors are episodes of distressful awakening, during which the child abruptly sits in bed and screams. He is obviously frightened, may be perspiring, and breathes heavily. Although some fragments of dreams may be reported at the time, the child is usually too distressed to give a coherent account. After a few minutes, the child calms down and returns to sleep. There is no memory of the event the next morning. Attacks of night terrors are differentiated from nightmares and anxiety dreams by their occurrence during sudden arousal from NREM sleep, while nightmares appear during the stage of rapid eye movement.

Narcoleptic Tetrad. Most patients with this constellation of symptoms are diagnosed during adolescence or young adult life. It is possible that a less intense form goes unnoticed during childhood. The narcoleptic tetrad consists of narcolepsy, which is sudden episodes of sleepiness during daytime; catalepsy, which is the abrupt loss of muscle tone resulting in a fall while consciousness is maintained; sleep paralysis, the awareness during sleep, or while falling asleep, that one is unable to move; and hypnogogic hallucinations, vivid auditory and visual imageries at the onset of sleep. Patients may show all or some of these four symptoms (Zarcone, 1973).

The sleep record is diagnostic in that while in normal adults and adolescents a sleep cycle always begins with NREM sleep, in these patients the cycle is reversed and the patient begins sleep with a prolonged REM period. The etiology of the disorder is unknown. Anxiety and emotional factors can precipitate an attack. The nonepileptic nature of these attacks is now firmly established. Drugs that suppress REM sleep, such as amphetamine and MAO inhibitors, have been used in the treatment of the narcoleptic tetrad with varying degrees of success.

ENURESIS

Enuresis is defined as involuntary incontinence of urine after the age of 4. In the course of normal development, bladder control is first established during the day and later on for the night. Epidemiologic studies have shown that by 6–7 years of age, 80% of children have full bladder control, while 20% have diurnal or nocturnal enuresis or both. Boys outnumber girls, and diurnal enuresis is more frequent in girls. Social class and family status are unrelated to presence or absence of enuresis; however, children living in institutions have a higher percentage. The incidence of enuresis declines steadily with age, so that by the age of 14 only 2–3% of adolescents are so affected. Some children, having established sphincter control, remain fully continent; in others, the control is so tenuous that after a period of dryness, the child loses the function. This is called *secondary enuresis*.

Etiology. Psychiatrists do not see all children who are enuretic, and some parents do not consider the symptom of such a deviant nature that medical advice should be sought. Others refer the problem to pediatricians. However, among the children seen by psychiatrists, there seems to be a high percentage of concomitant behavior disorders, particularly among girls. The nature of the behavior disorder differs in various reported samples. Some authors believe that in children with aggressive behavior, enuresis is another aspect of poor impulse control. Others report that enuresis is usually seen among overinhibited and shy children. In some children, once bladder control is established, psychiatric symptoms disappear. In others, the behavior problem is said to antedate enuresis and the treatment of enuresis does not lead to disappearance of the psychological difficulties. Some psychoanalysts state that enuresis as a symptom has erotic significance. Others stress the revengeful and hostile nature of the act, which inconveniences the parents.

Gerard (1939) reported 72 cases of enuresis. Of these, 7 cases were said to be due to physical causes (epilepsy and other neurological disorders). In 4 cases, the training had been faulty, and in 61 cases, no etiology could be found. In this group, Gerard considered "sexual trauma" etiologically significant. Fathers of enuretic girls were said to be seductive to their female child, while in boys a significant number had rejective mothers. There is little evidence for the conclusion that child-rearing practices may be responsible for enuresis, though in families of enuretic children, other members may have been enuretic. Oppel *et al.* (1968), in epidemiologic studies of Baltimore area, found some relationship between maternal attitudes and enuresis in girls. But subsequent to studies on the Isle of Wight, Rutter (1970) has suggested that the nature of enuresis in boys and girls may have to be conceptualized along different lines; that is, enuresis in boys as a developmental lag and in girls as a behavioral deviation secondary to emotional factors.

The role played by external or internal stresses in failure to achieve bladder control, or in the loss of function once control has been achieved, has not been fully investigated. In some children, enuresis appears after parental separation, divorce, or hospitalization. Neurological studies of children with enuresis so far have failed to provide any consistent evidence of neurologic abnormalities. Incontinence associated with loss of consciousness in epilepsy or interruption of the reflex due to damage to the nervous system is of a clearly defined pathological nature and is accompanied by other signs of disturbed functioning due to the original illness. Studies of bladder capacity have not shown a "weak" or "small" bladder in all children with enuresis. Furthermore, it has been pointed out that any decrease in the capacity of the bladder may be the consequence rather than the cause of enuresis.

When it was assumed that enuresis occurred during the deep stage of sleep, some authors had theorized that unusually deep sleep or the difficulty in rousability might account for these children's failure to respond to the stimuli coming from a full bladder. However, recent studies of the polygram of sleep in enuretic children have shown that bed-wetting is associated with emergence from the stage of deep sleep and does not occur during the deepest period of sleeping. It seems reasonable to assume that enuretics are not a homogeneous group and that in each child a different set of circumstances may be responsible for the symptom.

Treatment. As was noted earlier, in the majority of children enuresis is a self-limiting disorder and the successful treatment of an enuretic child may be due to the fortunate timing of intervention. Current treatments can be divided into two major categories: retraining and chemotherapy. Children may be highly motivated to stop bedwetting and open to retraining at a particular time, such as before summer camp. The common practice is to decrease the amount of liquid intake a few hours before sleep and to awaken the child every two to three hours to empty his bladder. Some parents report success with this schedule. Behavior therapists have devised a "bell-and-pad" method in order to condition the sphincter to resist relaxation when it receives a signal from the bladder. In this method, relaxation of the sphincter and the presence of the first few drops of urine on the pad electrode activate a buzzer that interrupts the child's sleep. To avoid such interruption, the child learns to contract rather than relax his sphincter in response to the stimulus to urinate. The theoretical explanation is not strictly scientific, though the method is reported to be highly effective in older children. Some children relapse when the treatment is discontinued. The length of time for the treatment and the frequency of sleep interruption have been changed to avoid the recurrence of the enuretic pattern, and the recommended schedule depends upon the experiences of the individual practitioner (Lovibond, 1964).

Some clinicians recommend the use of stimulant drugs in order to interfere with the depth of sleep and to make the child more responsive to the biological signals emanating from the bladder. The effectiveness of such a regimen has not been established. Recent reports indicate that imipramine in a low dosage may stop enuresis. The reason for the effectiveness is not quite clear, and there is a high rate of relapse following discontinuation of the drug. Psychotherapy has not proved to be of value in the treatment of enuresis *per se*, though one can expect the treatment of underlying emotional factors to be helpful in the cessation of enuresis in those children whose symptoms are clearly of psychogenic origin.

Encopresis

Bowel control is commonly established before bladder control, so that by the age of 4 almost all children are trained except for a minority in whom the training has not been achieved because of parental neglect or indifference toward all standards of cleanliness. Soiling beyond the age of 4 is a deviant behavior. In some children, toilet training is at first established, only to be lost months or years later; this variety is called *discontinuous encopresis*. When bowel control has never been achieved, the soiling beyond 4 years is referred to as *continuous encopresis*. Encopresis is further differentiated into two distinct groups: the retentive and nonretentive types. In the retentive type, the child is continuously leaking fecal material, while in the nonretentive type, defecation is a formed stool deposited in an inappropriate place (the child's own clothing, various parts of the house, etc.).

Etiology. In the retentive type of encopresis, both sexes are equally represented. The child has long periods of constipation, during which the fecal material is collected and hardened in the rectum, and subsequently the rectum becomes enlarged. When the child finally has a bowel movement, it is of great quantity. No physical symptoms other than constipation and distention of rectum and leakage of fecal-stained fluid is present. Most pediatricians believe that the problem starts as constipation in infancy with pain and discomfort on defecation, leading to reluctance on the part of the child to defecate, which, in turn, aggravates the constipation to the point that the normal defecatory reflex is extinguished. For these clinicians, the emotional problems associated with encopresis of the retentive variety are secondary to the child's physical symptoms. Psychiatrists, on the other hand, consider this type of encopresis the outcome of a disturbed mother–child relationship, particularly during the crucial period of toilet training.

Regardless of the etiology, children who are encopretic show a variety of emotional and psychological symptoms that, although at the beginning they might have been limited to eliminatory functionings, are soon generalized to other areas of their interpersonal relationships. Their image of themselves is that of an unacceptable and unwanted playmate, and they feel the weight of parental disapproval and disappointment. They may compensate by being extremely docile and eager to please, only to puzzle their parents with their insensitivity and stubbornness in matters relating to their toilet training. Some mothers try to prevent the constipation by the administration of laxatives and are then disturbed by the ensuing diarrhea, which does not help the soiling. Soon the child's bowel movement comes to be the most time-consuming part of her functioning, with little opportunity for pleasurable interactions between the parent and the child. The embarrassing symptom also limits the child's interaction with his peers, and although he tries bravely to keep a facade of indifference or actually denies being concerned about the teasing of others, he tends to become isolated and depressed.

In nonretentive encopresis, boys outnumber girls. Anthony (1957) considers coercive toilet training the etiological factor in this type. According to this view, the circumstances surrounding training have induced great anxiety in the child, so that the function, even when controlled, remains susceptible to the effect of later stress and is easily lost. The child thus tends to defecate as soon as he feels the urge without any regard for the proper location. These children try to hide their clothes or other soiled objects, fearing parental reprisal. In this group, soiling may be an indication of various internal or external stresses, and therefore a thorough investigation of intrafamilial factors is necessary for an understanding of the child's symptom. Prugh *et al.* (1954), in a study of 100 cases of encopresis, concluded that the fecal incontinence in these children is an immature way of handling tension and does not seem to have any symbolic significance. Other reports have tended to agree with this assessment.

Treatment. Encopresis tends to disappear with age, so that no cases have been reported in adolescents over 16 years of age. The treatment of encopresis is important, as the symptom may interfere with the normal socialization of the child and may create sources of tension and dissatisfaction in the family. Motivating the child and decreasing the environmental pressure on him are the first steps in treatment. In the retentive type, pediatricians have claimed a high rate of success with laxatives and enemas, provided that the emotional struggle between the child and his parents is kept to a minimum. In the nonretentive type, psychotherapy may be of considerable help in decreasing the anxiety and the hostile interaction between the parents and the child. Behavior modification may be useful in the earliest stage of encopresis, when parental resentment and the child's sense of demoralization has not intervened (Halpern, 1977).

PSYCHOSEXUAL DISORDERS

The characteristics of adult sexual behavior are the end result of the interplay between biological, social, and psychological factors operating during the course of development from early infancy to late adolescence. Biological sex is dependent upon chromosomal, gonadal, and hormonal factors as well as the structure of the internal reproductive system and the external genital morphology. The most important factor in the sex assignment of an infant is the appearance of the external genital organs. In cases where the external morphology cannot be clearly differentiated, an infant may be assigned to the wrong sex. This leads to the unsettling experience of "abnormal" secondary sexual characteristics at puberty, such as breast development in a child raised as a boy or the deepening of the voice and the growth of facial hair in a girl.

The onset of puberty is ushered in by an increase in hormonal production of the gonads. In both boys and girls, the level of androgens in the blood shows a sharp rise, and in girls, there is a substantial increase in the level of estrogens. Puberty in girls begins earlier than in boys. Breast development and the appearance of pubic hair are followed by the onset of menarche. For the majority of girls, menstruation begins around the age of 12–13, though in some, menarche may start as early as 9 or as late as 17 years. In boys, with puberty there is an increase in the size of the genitalia, a deepening of the voice due to the growth of the larynx, and the appearance of pubic and, later on, facial hair. Ejaculation usually occurs around 14, with an age range between 10 and 17 years. The intensity of sexual desires in both sexes is partially related to the level of androgens excreted by the gonads. Fluctuations of the sexual appetite in women during various stages of the menstrual cycle are reported. The estrogens have thus been implicated as playing a part in female sexuality.

Children come to regard themselves as boys or girls during the first four years of life. Gesell and Amatruda (1940) found that about two-thirds of 3-year-olds could correctly identify their sex. Other studies have shown that 5-year-old children can correctly differentiate the sexes of other people. This differentiation seems to be based on subtle perceptual clues. Now that long-haired men and unisex clothes have deprived children of the gross dissimilarities in the appearance of the two sexes, they have found other ways to tell men and women apart. A 5-year-old boy with a fine auditory discrimination said he knew how to differentiate little boys from little girls by their voices. A girl claimed that boys and girls walk differently, like men and women. Sexual identity in children seems to be remarkably independent of the biological sex. Hampson and Hampson (1961), in a series of studies of patients with biological sexual disorders, found that the majority of patients in whom gonadal sex differed from the assigned sex identified with their assigned sex. Even in hermaphrodites in whom the external genital morphology was in gross disagreement with their assigned sex, only 2 out of 25 patients expressed doubts about their sexual identity.

Another aspect of sexual identity is the preference for one's own sex. In answer to direct questions and through a variety of projective techniques, children indicate their satisfaction with their own sex from early childhood. This preference is strengthened with age, especially in boys. Kagan (1964) stated that the reason that fewer girls than boys prefer their own sex is the cultural overvaluation of masculinity and the greater power and prestige enjoyed by men in our society. Sexual differences in children's attitudes and behavior are a socially determined phenomena, though some authors have argued that higher aggressivity in boys precedes the efforts of acculturation. The process by which sexual identity is established and the sexual role accepted is a complex learning experience. Sex typing by parents begins at birth. The culturally prescribed sex-appropriate behavior receives reinforcement within and outside of the family. Even in theories such as psychoanalysis, the genital stage of psychosexual development can be conceptualized as a series of complicated sexual-role learnings by such processes as imitation and modeling (Birns, 1976).

While sex role identification is a necessary condition for the development of adult sexual behavior, its achievement does not guarantee that adult sexual relations will be a satisfactory experience or result in heterosexual orientation. Sexual competence is learned through practice. Studies of sexual activities among adolescents have revealed that a large number of boys and girls find their first sexual experience unrewarding. Precocious children of both sexes, while easily aroused, do not show mature sexual behavior. Furthermore, an individual's ability to relate to another person without undue anxiety or anger is an important component of satisfactory sexual activity.

Sexual Behavior in Childhood

In male infants, penile erection can be detected a few days after birth. This erection seems to be a physiological reflex associated with urination and defecation. As the infant begins to explore his own body, genital manipulation in the form of pulling of the penis acquires a particularly pleasurable quality. Most mothers report such genital manipulation around 1 year of life, though earlier occurrences of the activity have also been noticed. Genital manipulation in infant girls is seen less frequently. In a study of 2- to 5-year-old middle-class children, Sears *et al.* (1957) found that about 50% of the children engaged in genital manipulation.

During early school years, sexual games involving exploration or peeking at boys' and girls' genital areas are quite common. In middle childhood, it is now clear that, contrary to Freud's assumption, sexual interests and masturbatory activities do not cease; rather, the child comes to realize that such activities are not well tolerated by adults and therefore does not display them in public. In fact, the process of socialization requires that children control overt sexual activities as they enter school, and teachers and parents are in agreement on the inappropriateness of such behavior in public. Ramsey (1943) reported that the incidence of masturbation in boys shows a steady rise with age, so that while at 7 years only 10% of boys masturbate, the figure is close to 80% by 13 years. The incidence of masturbatory activities in girls is lower than in boys, though the same trend of increased incidence with age holds true. The same study shows that heterosexual interest and play also increase with age.

Masturbation and sexual play may become a cause for parental concern when the behavior occurs in inappropriate settings or with high frequency. Although there is no rule by which the normal frequency can be judged, a child who engages in repeated daily auto-stimulation or prefers sexual games to all other activities is in need of a psychiatric evaluation. Preoccupation with sex and excessive masturbatory activities may be the result of a child's failure to participate in social interchanges and to derive pleasure from other kinds of interaction with his environment. Withdrawn and depressed children may try to lift their mood or alleviate their anxieties by self-stimulation. Sexual themes may occur as obsessive thoughts in spite of the child's attempt to avert his attention from them. Some children are exposed to the sexual activities of adults at home and fail to develop the socially required control over their sexual impulses, engaging in such activities in public. Predelinquent children or those who have difficulty in controlling their impulses are unable or unwilling to conform with the behavioral expectation of the environment. Psychotic and retarded children may fail to appreciate the inappropriateness of their behavior and may display sexual activities long past the age that other children learn to stop them in the presence of other people. In very young children, genital manipulation may be due to a local irritation and infection that the child cannot describe.

Interest in the process of birth and how children are made is a normal curiosity. Questions in this regard, though seemingly repetitive, are asked with different degrees of cognitive sophistication during the child's mental development. While parents may assume that they are answering the same questions each time, the child's understanding of their responses is limited by his cognitive ability at each stage, and his curosity is satisfied only when he manages to comprehend all aspects of the issue and its implications. Sexual jokes and sexual stories may interest children partly because of their meanings and partly because of the kind of response they elicit from their peers or from adults. Boys or girls may consider sharing sexual jokes and stories a means of forming friendly groups with "secrets" that are not given out to the nonmembers. The sexual activities of adults are particularly fascinating subjects in those years during which children view their own sexual behavior as primitive and colorless.

During early adolescence, boys may engage in group sexual play such as showing their genitals or touching and feeling the genitals of their friends. This form of behavior is not a precursor of later homo-sexuality, though children who become homosexuals as adults may also engage in these activities. Girls also engage in homosexual games, though genital exhibition is rare. Children in boarding schools and in-stitutions are more likely to engage in sex play.

The long-term effects of children's sexual experiences with adults have not been fully explored. Most reports in the literature are based on adults' memories and descriptions of these incidents. In a follow-up study of a small group of children who had been engaged in inces-tuous relations, Bender (1954) did not find any lasting influence on the sexual adjustment of her subjects during their adulthood. Small chil-dren who have been victims of rape react to the experience as they would react to any other physical injuries, and it is usually the re-sponses of parents or other adults that give the child the feeling of the particular nature of the incident. In older children and adolescents, the experience is extremely disturbing and the victim of rape is in need of psychological support, reassurance, and other protective measures to enable her or him to overcome the traumatic event and to prevent psy-chological sequelae.

Homosexuality. The choice of a sexual partner in adult life is the final outcome of multiple factors operating during childhood and adolescence. Studies of adult homosexuals have revealed that child-parent interactions, early sexual experiences, and other environmental circumstances may play a part in the development of sexual orienta-tion. However, no single etiology can be said to underly the eventual choice of sexual partners. Fear or hatred of the same-sex parent may result in a boy's inability to use the father as an identification model; or a close, overpowering relationship with the mother may turn the child away from any close relationship with women. In a study of homosexual female adolescents, Kremer and Rifkin (1969) found that the attachment to the mother and fear and hostility toward an absent father were important determinants of these adolescents' homosexual-ity. Other authors have pointed out that homosexual activities may begin as the only possible sexual activities in such environments as boys' or girls' boarding schools and may remain as preferred activity by virtue of the person's familiarity with his or her own sex and anxi-ety in relating to the opposite sex.

Studies of adult sexual behavior have provided ample evidence for the observation that sexual arousal and sexual satisfaction may be-come associated with a variety of situations and individuals, and in a high percentage of these cases, such association dates back to middle childhood or early adolescence. However, in some children, such be-havior does not continue into adulthood, while in others, the preference becomes a part of adult sexuality. The intrapsychic and environmental factors that determine the extinction or continuation of childhood sexual behavior are not as yet fully understood, and this area is in need of longitudinal exploration.

Transsexualism. Transsexualism is a rare disorder of sexual identification in which the child, though biologically normal, fails to develop a sense of same-sex identity and indicates a desire to change sex. In a study of three transsexual boys, Stoller (1968) reported that these children had manifested a desire to be girls, dressed like girls, and displayed feminine gestures and mannerisms as early as 2 years of age. According to Stoller, the disorder was caused by the total symbiosis of these infants with their mothers, who themselves had not developed a well-differentiated sexual identity. The fathers were described as "dynamically" absent, in that their presence did not provide a counterbalance to their wives' feminizing influence on their sons. Transsexualism must be differentiated from young children's occasional cross-dressing or isolated imitation of opposite-sex mannerisms. Effeminate boys or tomboy girls do not wish to change sex, though they may show a preference for what they consider to be the privileges of the opposite sex. Gender identity in adolescent homosexuals is firmly established, and avoidance of a heterosexual relationship is not coupled with a desire for a change of sex.

Treatment. Parents' complaints and concerns over the sexual behavior of their children always require a full evaluation of the child and a thorough exploration of parental opinions and attitudes about their expectation of the child's sexual development. When the child's behavior is clearly within the normal range of sexual activities of the age group, reassurance and explanation suffice. On the other hand, the child's sexual activities may be symptomatic of other psychological problems or disturbed interactions between the child and his or her parents. These situations are in need of vigorous intervention. Conjoint treatment of the parents and the child and/or individual psychotherapy for the child may be needed to rectify the situation (Newman, 1976). Adolescent boys or girls may seek homosexual or heterosexual interactions as remedies for their sense of loneliness and depression or as a replacement for the loss of emotional support from their families (Money and Dalery, 1976). Others may accede to adults' sexual advances in order to secure feelings of protection and desirability. Psychotic adolescents may find sexual stimulation and relationship their only assurance of their sense of identity. The treatment in these patients should be directed at the underlying emotional disturbance and the control of the unplanned and unwanted consequences of the sexual behavior, such as pregnancy and venereal disease.

Treatment of transsexualism should begin in early life, and both parents should be involved in the treatment along with the child. When a child has been assigned to the incorrect sex because of the ambiguity of the external genital morphology, all attempts at biological identification must be made during the first three years of life, and sexual reassignment must be accomplished before the age of 4. In children who are in need of sexual reassignment later on, supportive psychotherapy before and after such change is necessary, particularly when the child has already entered puberty. In these children, identity confusion is compounded by the inevitable loss of the previous peer group and the close emotional ties that have already been made. Long-term psychotherapy may be necessary to assure the normal development of the personality and to provide clarification of and encouragement in the acceptance of the new role.

Fears of homosexuality in adolescent boys and girls may be due to anxiety over their acceptability to the opposite sex or their intense feelings toward members of their own sex. Exploration of the nature of these feelings and clarification of the meaning of these reactions are usually enough to reassure these adolescents.

Other Sexual Disorders. Adult sexual disorders, or those identified in adolescence, are generally assumed to have their origin in pathologic experiences that have occurred during childhood. In psychoanalytic theory, such deviances as fetishism or voyeurism are explained as due to fixation of or regression to a stage of normative infantile sexual development (Freud, 1905). In fetishism, sexual pleasure is attained through the manipulation of some object that does not ordinarily possess a sexual connotation but that has such significance for a particular individual and has been endowed with such significance because of unusual childhood experience (Wulff, 1946). Such an object creates sexual arousal and orgasm.

In voyeurism, similarly, gazing at the unclothed body of an individual, usually of the opposite sex, not only leads to sexual pleasure but is sufficient in itself to lead to orgasm. Exhibitionism, in which the individual's own naked body is shown—usually to strangers—is a similar sexual perversion that is a preferred mode of achieving sexual satisfaction.

Each of the above-described behaviors is usually a compulsive, repetitive behavior. They are significantly more frequently reported during adolescence for males than for females. However, neither longitudinal nor follow-up studies have demonstrated either a relationship between atypical childhood sexual experience and later sexual aberration (Bender and Blau, 1937, 1952) or between adolescent sexual offenses and perversions and adult marital difficulties (Robins, 1966).

While individual case reports of an anecdotal nature have asserted that the appearance of adult perversions is explained by experiences in the individual's childhood, there has not been any conclusive study that supports this theoretical position.

A common complaint is that of little boys looking up the skirts of girls or women. This can usually be identified as teasing behavior that has been reinforced by a selectively strong response on the part of adults as compared with other teasing actions of children. Voyeurism is not uncommon in adolescence, particularly among boys. It is difficult, in a society that not only condones but actively promotes the exhibiting of the nude female body, to distinguish in the adolescent period between a normal heterosexual curiosity and the beginnings of pathological voyeurism (Offer and Offer, 1971; Schofield, 1971).

Similar problems exist in the attempt to correlate childhood and adult sexual sadism and/or masochism. Both Krafft-Ebbing and Freud considered sadism to be an exaggeration of the normal aggressive component of masculine sexual instinct (Bieber, 1966). Masochism has been explained in Freudian theory as representing punishment deriving from a sense of guilt over forbidden Oedipal wishes. However, these theoretical formulations have not been demonstrated in controlled studies and cannot be verified.

10

Psychophysiological Disorders

Psychophysiological disorders are physical illnesses in which psychological factors are presumed to be of etiological significance. The concept of a psychophysiological disorder, or psychosomatic illness, has undergone important changes during the past two decades. The current emphasis is away from investigating the particular psychic conflict or personality configuration of the patient. Rather, efforts are made to discover the necessary physical conditions that will, under the influence of aversive emotional factors, give rise to a psychosomatic illness.

Studies in psychophysiology have shown that emotional responses such as anger and anxiety are concomitant with such physiological events as increase or decrease in heart rate, blood pressure, perspiration, and hormonal activities. Under normal circumstances, the autonomic system restrains the degree of physiological response associated with intense emotions and re-creates the internal homeostasis of the organism. When this restraining mechanism fails, however, and/or the intense emotions become chronic or repeatedly aroused, the physiological responses of the body can cause tissue pathology. Repeated, intense, aversive emotional states and an imbalanced autonomic system are, therefore, two necessary conditions for the development of psychophysiological disorders.

Psychosomatic illnesses involve various bodily organs or systems, such as the digestive tract and the respiratory system. The responses of individuals tend to be stereotyped—that is, they are usually expressed in the same manner and in the same system. This observation has led to the hypothesis that the particular organ or system is predisposed to responsiveness when the other two necessary conditions are present. This predisposition may be constitutional or it may be acquired through sensitizing life experiences (Minuchin *et al.*, 1975). Sternbach (1966) conceptualized a psychosomatic episode as a series of events beginning with an aversive psychogenic stimulus that elicits physiological responses from a vulnerable organ or system when the homeostatic mechanism of the body has failed to neutralize the overactivity of the physiological responses. The aversive psychological stimuli may be a series of objective external stresses or the individual's perception and interpretation of events that are uniquely stressful to him. Therefore an individual's attitudes and personality play a role in the causation of psychosomatic illnesses. The role of constitutional factors or early conditioning in producing organ sensitivity and autonomic dysfunction are not as yet clear. Of the long list of presumed psychophysiological disorders, a limited number can be unquestionably identified in childhood. However, psychiatric and psychoanalytic studies of psychophysiological disorders have usually been carried out among adult patients, and only few of the resultant hypotheses have been tested in children.

We have chosen to discuss asthma as an example of psychophysiological disorder because asthmatic children have been the subjects of more psychological studies than children with other psychosomatic illnesses.

Asthma

Asthma is an episodic bout of breathing difficulty caused by overactivity of the parasympathetic system involving the bronchial tubes. The incidence of asthma is about 2% of the child population, and boys are more frequently afflicted than girls. Allergy and respiratory infections play an important part in bringing about an attack of asthma and, according to some authors, create the basic vulnerability of the respiratory system. Psychological investigations of asthmatic children have developed along the two lines that follow.

Parental Pathology. In a study of the parents of 100 asthmatic and 100 physically disabled children, Fitzelle (1959) did not find any qualitative or quantitative differences in psychopathology among the two groups. When the parents of 71 asthmatic children were studied on a variety of psychological tests and during psychiatric interviews, Dubo et al. (1961) found no relationship between the severity of asthma in the children and the type or extent of psychopathology in their parents. Block (1966) tried to identify the concept of the "asthmatogenic" mother by using a forced-choice 100-item Q-sort technique administered to 14 clinicians who worked with asthmatic children. The agreement among clinicians as to the maternal attitudes precipitating or causing an asthma attack in children proved to be disappointingly low. Of the three clusters of maternal characteristics that emerged from this study, only one set of responses could be used to differentiate between the mothers of asthmatic and physically handicapped children. The asthmatic mothers were found to be overprotective, controlling, guilt-ridden, and doubtful about their own adequacy in the maternal role. It should be pointed out that these characteristics may have been responses to the child's illness in a cultural milieu that considers the disease to derive from the parents' relationship with the child.

Psychological Studies of Asthmatic Children. In a study of children with allergic reactions, including asthma, Miller and Baruch (1957) concluded that as compared to a normal control group, allergic children had more difficulty in expressing anger and hostility. The observation paralleled Alexander's (1950) view of asthma as a "suppressed cry for help." Other researchers, using more objective instruments, were not able to duplicate Baruch and Miller's study. Furthermore, reports from parents and children have indicated that aversive affects and negative feelings are perceived as precipitating an asthmatic attack and are carefully avoided by asthmatic children, so that the suppression of hostility and the reluctance to express anger may be the consequence rather than the cause of asthma.

Clinical features of asthma, such as the duration or severity of an attack, are varied among children, and, at least on clinical grounds, asthmatic children do not form a homogeneous group. Purcell *et al.* (1961) divided the asthmatic children admitted to the Children's Asthma Hospital and Research Institute in Denver into two distinct categories: the rapidly remitting group, who were free of asthma attacks within three months of hospitalization, and the steroid-dependent group, who could not be maintained free of attacks without steroid. Psychological studies failed to show any difference between the two groups. Interestingly, while the authors found the fathers of the rapidly remitting group to be punitive and authoritarian, the children viewed their fathers as passive and weak individuals.

Block *et al.* (1968) divided the children attending an asthma clinic into two groups based on high allergy potential score (HAPS) and low allergy potential score (LAPS). The LAPS group showed more signs of emotional immaturity on projective tests, and more parents reported these children as emotionally immature; however, the asthmatic group as a whole could not be differentiated from a group of physically disabled children on the basis of their psychological test results. In both the LAPS and the HAPS groups, the severity of asthma attacks was the same and attacks were precipitated by allergy, infection, and/or psychological factors. The authors reported a somewhat higher incidence of marital dissatisfaction and overprotectiveness among the mothers of their LAPS group.

In studies on the Isle of Wight, Rutter and his colleagues (1970) failed to find any significant psychological difference between asthmatic and nonasthmatic children, though they reported some relationship between the severity of asthma and the extent of the child's emotional problem. Block and Purcell have both concluded that studies of personality variables of asthmatic children and their parents are not likely to shed any further light on the disease.

Current research attempts are directed toward study of the mechanism by which the antecedent event(s) precipitates an asthmatic attack. Owen and Williams (1961) found that in a number of asthmatic children the sound of the mother's voice, irrespective of the content of the speech, elicited abnormal respiratory response. Comparing the autonomic responses of asthmatic and normal children, Hahn (1966) concluded that asthmatic children showed evidence of autonomic dysfunction.

These investigations, though still in preliminary stages, reveal that in at least one subgroup of asthmatic children, psychological factors may play an important part in eliciting abnormal respiratory responses and may precipitate an asthmatic attack in a predisposed individual. The psychological reaction to a disabling disease may be seen in all other subgroups and should not be mistaken for the primary causative factors. The role of psychiatrists in treating secondary reactions is a supportive one. However, for those children whose attacks are precipitated by psychogenic factors, investigation of the nature of the psychological stress and modification of the child's perception may be the most important part of his treatment (Sperling, 1968).

11

Childhood Neuroses

In psychiatric literature, neurosis is commonly defined in terms of presumed etiologies or by contrast to psychosis. In their book *Common Neuroses of Children and Adults*, English and Pearson (1937) fail to define neurosis even though the book is primarily addressed to general medical practitioners and medical students. In the *Diagnostic and Statistical Manual of Mental Disorders* (DSM II) of the American Psychiatric Association, neuroses are defined as etiologically caused by anxiety and further delineated by their differences with psychosis.

From the clinical point of view, a neurosis is a nontransitory constellation of subjective distress and objective deviant behavioral manifestations that appear in childhood, or at any time after that, and affect most areas of the individual's functioning. However, there are no lasting intellectual deterioration and no primary mood disturbance; the misrepresentation of external reality is not global, as in psychosis, and the overall personality remains intact.

The overall incidence of neuroses in the child population is unknown. Various surveys of the populations of child psychiatric clinics have reported prevalence rates ranging from 5 to 20%. These figures cannot be totally relied upon because of the absence of a clearly defined, universally accepted definition of childhood neurosis.

Etiology. The psychoanalytic formula regarding the etiology of neuroses postulates the presence of unresolved Oedipal conflicts, aggravated or reactivated by some external events: for example, the birth of a sibling, the death of a family member, and seduction. The excessive anxiety thus provoked cannot be adequately handled. Therefore a regression to an earlier level of psychosexual stage takes place and neurotic symptomatology appears. The symptoms are elaborated and exaggerated manifestations of defenses of the earlier era in psychosexual development and in symbolic manner express the patient's conflicts. The choice of symptom is determined by the level of regression—and this "fixation point" in turn is determined by the failure of the individual to master earlier phase-related conflicts (A. Freud 1965).

Other psychodynamic theoreticians have rejected various aspects of Freudian formulations, although the concept of conflict and anxiety generated by the conflict remains the core of the etiological hypothesis of neurosis.

The learning theorists have applied the principles of conditioning and learning theories to the development and generalization of the behavioral symptoms in neurosis and have devised techniques of therapeutic intervention based on these principles.

The issue of predisposition to neurotic development is implicit in both Freudian theory and the various schools of behaviorism. Constitutional or temperamental factors are invoked in order to explain the statistical fact that only a minority of any given population develops various neuroses, while the same set of circumstances and traumas is operative in the majority of families.

A synthesis of all the observed facts and elaborate hypotheses leads to the conclusion that neuroses are caused by many contributing factors. Each individual child's unique style of activity and reactivity is in continuous interaction with his environment. Fortuitous stimuli and unplanned occurrences are part of any child's environment. All of the variables in a field of human interaction cannot be identified, nor are we as yet able to specify all the principles by which normal and abnormal behaviors develop. It remains for future researchers to elucidate these principles and for the experimental psychologist to discover precisely how a particular trauma or a series of traumas can produce the neurotic symptoms.

Classification. It must be mentioned at the outset that the picture of any neurosis in childhood is less well defined than in adults. In fact, neurosis in childhood is usually a mixture of several kinds of symptomatology. It is not unusual for an obsessive–compulsive child to have various phobias or for a phobic child to use obsessive mechanisms. Anxiety, phobic obsessive–compulsive, conversion, dissociative, and hypochondriacal reactions are discussed in this chapter. Depressive neurosis was discussed in the section on depression in Chapter 5.

Anxiety Reaction

Anxiety is an unpleasant sensation that, in milder forms, is experienced by children as a feeling of apprehension and general irritability accompanied by restlessness, fatigue, and such visceral components as headaches, a "funny feeling" in the stomach, or heaviness in the chest. In an acute anxiety attack, the apprehension is intensified, the child is in terror, cries, looks frightened, is not easily reassured, and may believe that his death is imminent. He may complain that he cannot breathe, that his heart is stopping or going too fast, that people look different to him, and that he has changed into another person. He may be pale or perspire profusely, cling to whoever is around, ask for his mother, and altogether present a pitiful picture of a helpless child. An older child, in search of an explanation for his fear, may accuse people around him of wanting to harm him, strike out at peers, overthrow whatever is in his way, and behave as if he is having a temper tantrum. However, he may be crying while violent and may cling to the trusted person who tries to stop him. After the attack subsides, the child is perplexed as to what has actually happened to him. He may accept whatever excuse or explanation is offered him, or he may halfheartedly try to find a cause in what somebody else had done to him.

CASE HISTORY

Elizabeth, a 12-year-old, pretty, black girl, was brought to the hospital by her mother because she had been suspended from school following an incident in which she had thrown a book at the principal while he was trying to find out the reason she was crying in the classroom. Elizabeth was restless and confused and could not concentrate for more than a few minutes. She said that people did not like her, that everybody thought she was ugly. She believed that she had been justified in throwing the book at the principal: "He was bugging me; I was nervous." While Elizabeth's mother was being interviewed in another room, Elizabeth began to pace up and down, said that she was feeling hot, showed her clammy, perspiring hands, and began to cry, saying, "I am dying. Something in my throat does not let me breathe. My stomach is not pumping. People are trying to kill me. I will die if I stay here. I was normal before I came. Now I am dying . . ." During the next three days, Elizabeth had one or two severe anxiety attacks a day. In between the attacks, she was anxious, restless, and depressed. She did not show any sign of psychosis clinically or on psychological testings.

Her background history revealed that Elizabeth had been an insecure, timid, and friendless child since entering school. When Elizabeth was 7 years old, her father had been charged with attempting to seduce a 13-year-old girl neighbor, and though the charges had been dismissed, the family became alienated and ostracized. The father had then deserted the family, and Elizabeth, her 13-year-old brother, and her mother had been left with no source of income. Elizabeth's mother was a tense, depressed woman who felt harassed by the responsibilities of finding a job and caring for her children. Six months before Elizabeth's admission, her mother had found a job that kept her away from home from 8 A.M. to 6 P.M. She had not found time to go to school when Elizabeth brought a letter from her teacher reporting that she seemed very unhappy, her schoolwork had deteriorated, and she was frequently absent. The mother was now extremely angry at Elizabeth. She explained; "I knew she was sad and hypersensitive, but it was not causing anybody else any problem. Now she has become violent and I can't take that."

Clinical Pictures. In a chronic state of anxiety ("overanxious reaction," DSM II), the child is said to be generally unhappy, seeking an inordinate amount of reassurance, and reluctant to meet new people. He may tend to be sickly and overconcerned about bodily injury, which he uses as an excuse to avoid participating in group activities. He may have various fears and complain of nightmares and bad dreams. His anxiety may interfere with his learning ability because he cannot concentrate fully on a task. He may be restless, pull his hair, chew on his nails, or show tics.

An acute anxiety attack may develop in a child who has been suffering from mild chronic anxiety or may be seen in apparently well-adjusted children. The precipitating factor may be one major occurrence or a series of seemingly trivial incidents following closely upon each other. The attack is characterized by a feeling of panic, shallow breathing, palpitation, and trembling, and it may be accompanied by such phenomena as perceptual distortion, loose association, and feelings of depersonalization and impending death. The attacks may last for a few minutes to an hour. They may be repeated several times during the day. When the true nature of the attack is not diagnosed, the child may undergo various laboratory tests or unwarranted medical treatment. When anxiety attacks happen primarily at night, the child may have night terrors that frighten him so much that he becomes afraid of falling asleep. Sleepwalking may accompany night terrors. At times, children's anxiety attacks are triggered by hypnogogic phenomena as they enter deep sleep.

Physiologically, acute anxiety states are accompanied by an increase in adrenaline secretion, which causes such visceral symptoms as palpitations, sweating, queasy feelings in the stomach, dizziness, or lightheadedness. The awareness of visceral sensations increases the child's apprehension and accounts for strange statements, such as "My stomach has stopped pumping" and "My head is changing."

Etiology. In studies of infants, variations have been found in their reactivity to stress, their state of arousal, and the strength of their sympathetic and parasympathetic nervous system responsivity. Variability in children's intensity of reaction and their predominant style of approach to or withdrawal from novel stimuli have been reported from longitudinal studies of children's temperamental styles. These findings have been interpreted as indicating that proneness to anxiety may also depend on constitutional variables that are as yet uncharted.

There are also some indications that paranatal injury of the central nervous system may predispose such infants to higher degrees of anxiety. However, it must be noted that such vulnerability to anxiety is only one factor in the child's continuous interaction with his environment. In an "average expectable environment," such an infant may exhibit shyness, withdrawal, and high sensitivity and finally may develop an introvert personality. On the other hand, an inconsistent, rejecting, or neglectful household may tax the child's coping abilities and result in a chronic state of anxiety in the child. Such a child overreacts to an event such as the birth of a sibling, parental separation, and maternal tension with an acute anxiety attack. Sometimes the precipitating factors may be a minor illness, the expectation of a bad mark on an exam, or tense relationships with peers or teachers.

In children with high activity level and chronic anxiety, the clinical picture may resemble that of hyperkinetic syndrome. Children of insecure and anxious mothers may show contagious fearfulness, but unless the mother's anxiety is coupled with hostility toward the child, the latter learns to cope with the mother's anxiety and develops normally. During long states of environmental upheaval such as war, natural disaster, or violence in the community, a child may appropriately remain hyperalert and anxious. However, once the external situation stabilizes, the child becomes less anxious.

Differential Diagnosis. In all developmental disorders of childhood, some degree of anxiety is present, so in differential diagnosis one should carefully consider the possibility that anxiety may be secondary to another disorder. A child with a learning disability may be in a constant state of anxiety because of his inability to meet parental and societal expectations. Parents' hostile interactions with the child, or with each other, can result in a child's feelings of insecurity regarding the future stability of his home or his own safety. Feelings of irritability, fatigue, and apprehension may be caused by a variety of clinical or undiagnosed physical conditions such as anemia, hypoglycemia, or chronic malnutrition. Acute anxiety attacks may usher in an episode of psychotic breakdown. They may resemble episodes of psychomotor epilepsy or be the indications of such an underlying metabolic disorder as hyperthyroidism. A careful history of the child's early development and an investigation of the sources of stress in his environment are the prerequisite for making the diagnosis.

Treatment. Acute anxiety attacks usually respond to reassuring words and the presence of an adult. In severe cases, mild tranquilizer medications are necessary to lessen the anxiety and help with sleep. Environmental manipulation may be necessary to relieve the sources of stress. Remedial work with a child may help alleviate one source of insecurity and apprehension, and protective group activities may be necessary to allow the child to interact with his peers. Individual psychotherapy is indicated when the source of conflict is in the child's inter- or intrapersonal relationships.

Phobic Reactions

Epidemiological studies of normal children have revealed that they have a variety of fears that do not seriously interfere with their functioning and that decrease in the course of normal development. In a survey of 6- to 12-year-old children in Buffalo, New York, Lapouse and Monk (1959) reported that 43% of their population had seven or more fears. MacFarlane *et al.* (1954) reported fears in 90% of their sample, with a downward trend with age except for a slight increase around 11 years of age. The child's sex and socioeconomic background influenced the content of fears, so that lower-class boys more frequently feared direct violence with knives and guns while children from the upper classes were more concerned about car accidents and disasters. Lower-class girls were afraid of strangers and animals, whereas upper-class girls feared kidnappers and shipwrecks. Fear of darkness and being left alone in the dark was the most prevalent fear among younger children. Lapouse and Monk found no relationship between children's fearfulness and other behavioral symptoms such as tics, frequent temper tantrums, nightmares, or nail biting. MacFarlane reported a significant correlation between numerous fears and irritability, timidity, and overdependence in a group of 5-year-old girls. However, in no other age group could the statistical correlation be considered significant. Poznanski (1973) stated that childhood fears are a reflection of the child's limited comprehension of his environment, while psychoanalysts consider all fears to be a symbolic expression of the child's castration anxiety and a displacement of his own aggressive impulses.

When the childhood fears become so excessive that they dominate the child's feelings and external activities and persist over a long period of time, the term *phobic reaction* is applicable. Furthermore, as in all neuroses, the children find their fears illogical and distressing and want to be rid of them. Animals are among the most prevalent fears of younger children. Freud gave an example of such a phobia in a 5-year-old boy (Little Hans) and interpreted the child's fear of horses as a projected fear of his father. The source of this fear, according to Freud, was castration anxiety. The mother's "seductive behavior" was considered to have set the stage, and the trauma of a tonsillectomy was the precipitating factor. The case of an 11-month-old boy (Little

Albert) in whom Watson (1917) was able to produce a phobic reaction by conditioning is used by behavior theorists as the prototype of all phobias. According to this school of thought, associating a neutral object with a fear-producing stimulus results in a conditioned emotional response to the neutral object. Furthermore, this fear generalizes to other objects and situations resembling the original neutral stimulus. The principles of learning theory have been used by practitioners such as Wolpe (1963) and Rachman and Costello (1961) to devise various methods of treatment for phobias.

In older children, the phobia takes an ideational form, so that the child is afraid of dying, being drafted into the army and sent to war, and being at home when burglars break in. These fears have their peak around 8–9 years of age. They may follow a child's first experience with death or may develop in an overanxious child who has acquired the concept of death as an irreversible process and is overwhelmed by the idea of his own mortality. Phobic children seek reassurance from their parents and insist on having one parent around, usually the mother. The phobias do not completely disappear when the parents are around, but the child reports that he believes that his parents will not let anything happen to him. In the parents' absence, the child may have anxiety attacks, which act as a reinforcer for his reluctance to remain alone. Some children lose most of their fears with the passage of time, but in others, although the intensity of fears is diminished, the underlying anxiety continues into adulthood (Waldron, 1976).

School Phobia. A special form of phobic reaction is school phobia. Intense anxiety and outright refusal to go to school may appear at the beginning of a child's school career because of his reluctance to separate from his mother and leave the safety of his home. Timid children may find it extremely difficult to meet new people and to venture into new situations. Fearful children consider themselves at the mercy of unknown forces that they cannot hope to deal with on their own. The child's mother may not view him as quite ready to enter school; she may believe that he needs special handling that only she can provide. She may have found school a trying experience herself and may overtly or covertly side with the child's fears. For some young children, a visit to school in the company of their mother is enough to assure them of the safety of the school and the benevolence of the teachers. Others may need a few days during which the availability of their mother dispels any anxiety. For children with intense separation anxiety and overdependency upon the mother, such measures are insufficient. They develop somatic symptoms just before departing for school that are relieved when the mother accepts the validity of their distress and allows them to remain home, but symptoms return the next day. During early childhood, school phobia is a relatively uncomplicated symptom. Maternal overprotection has caused or intensified the child's feelings of vulnerability, and the mother shares the conflict with the child.

In older children with or without previous overt anxiety in regard to school, going to school may become the focus of anxiety and fears. The precipitating causes may be school-related, such as worries about exams, peer relationships, and interactions with the teachers, or they may be due to real or fancied fear of parental desertion. Fear of parents' disapproval and disappointment may produce a state of uncertainty in the child that could be manifested as soon as he prepares to leave home. Although separation anxiety has usually been regarded as a reaction resulting from child–mother interaction, the role of the father in these situations cannot be totally ignored. In fact, in a two-parent family, an intense emotional bond between an older child and the mother is always an indication that the father has actively encouraged or passively acquiesced in the development of such over-dependency.

Kahn and Nursten (1962) found that between 2 and 8% of the referrals to a child guidance clinic were school phobics. The true frequency is hard to come by because various agencies, such as schools and clinics, may deal with the same problem. In its severe form, particularly around adolescence, school phobia is a disabling disorder of childhood. The peak age is around 11–12.

Clinical Picture. The child usually begins to have vague complaints around breakfast time. He feels nauseated and has a headache, and his stomach feels "funny." He may begin to cry, cling to his mother, and beg to stay home. If forced to go to school, he may refuse to enter the classroom or feel miserable while sitting there. He worries about what is happening at home in his absence or about what has happened to his mother. He may call his home simply to ask if everything is fine, or he may want to be reassured that his mother will be home when he returns. He is seemingly relaxed when he is back but begins to worry at bedtime about the next morning. He may be forced to go to school, but he does not perform in the school. In the majority of cases, the child finally refuses to go to school, or the school decides that the child should be suspended until such time as he can attend and benefit from the school.

The child's willingness to study at home may persuade some parents that the problem does not need any further attention. However, the child soon becomes homebound, isolated, and fearful of venturing outside by himself. Other parents are totally frustrated and angered by the child's refusal to go to school, and this reaction, in turn, intensifies the child's anxiety. Some children find themselves the focus of parental dissension and arguments. Parents may blame each other for neglecting or spoiling the child, and he, in turn, becomes depressed and guilty within this mesh of strong conflicting emotions. There is very little that the child can do in order to overcome his fears. When these children appear in the psychiatrist's office, they present a mixture of anxiety, depression, anger, and low self-esteem. They may contemplate suicide or talk as if they feel that only with their death can they bring peace to themselves and their family. Argas (1959) has stated that severe school phobia may be a "part of natural history of depressive disorders," and Frommer (1967) has used antidepressant drugs in a group of children, some of whom showed school phobia along with depressed mood.

Etiology. While some authors have equated school phobia with separation anxiety, others have remarked on the multiplicity of factors operating in each situation. Among these factors is maternal dissatisfaction due to marital problems and depression, which can provide a particularly insecure ambience at home. In some cases, children are afraid of failure at school, expecting disappointment and rejection from their parents and other significant persons in their lives. School phobia in these situations takes the responsibility off the child's back: their failures are excused because of their illness. Some children perceive that their parents are disappointed by their incipient independence and cannot tolerate the danger of being rejected should they continue on the same course. Combinations of contradictory desires and conflicts make the adolescent's school phobia a complicated affair.

CASE HISTORY

Paul was 12 years old when he began to develop anxiety in relation to going to school. He was the younger boy in his family. His older brother was an exceptionally good student and an all-around athlete who was well known in their hometown. Paul's parents had divorced when he was 10 years of age. His father had been hospitalized because of depression and a suicidal attempt. His grandfather had killed himself before Paul was born. According to the mother, Paul had adjusted well to the divorce and did not seem particularly disturbed when his mother informed him that she intended to remarry. Paul and his brother accompanied the mother and the stepfather on a trip, during which Paul began to complain of headaches and seemed irritable and tense. He had wanted to go to camp but now went with little enthusiasm. After a week, his mother received Paul's first letter. He reported that he could not sleep and was not feeling well. At this point, Paul's father took it upon himself to go and see him. Paul began to cry when he saw his father and begged to be returned. He came back to his mother, and the rest of the summer went by with little change. Paul visited the pediatrician on account of his headaches and was assured that there was nothing wrong with him. The first week of school, Paul was tense, complained about the changes in the program, said that all the subjects were hard, and began to worry about not being able to perform. He began having more and more somatic complaints, lost his appetite, and remained home a few days at a time. After four weeks, he refused to go to school.

When first seen, Paul had been housebound for almost a month. He was depressed, anxious, and hopeless about his future, and he referred to his past as always miserable. He refused to talk to his stepfather but denied having any affection for his own father. He believed that he had a "brain tumor" that would eventually kill him. He was envious of his older brother's success and would become very angry when his brother was mentioned. The parents had received various recommendations regarding Paul. The mother did not want to send him to a residential treatment center, while the stepfather believed that this was the only thing that could work. The natural father blamed the stepfather and the mother for Paul's anxiety and his depressed mood. The father's psychiatrist had raised the question of possible depression, and the parents were worried about what would become of Paul.

Paul was seen in psychotherapy, and a course of an antidepressant drug was initiated. He was maintained on home instruction for four months. When he was free of depression and anxiety, his parents were informed that only their complete agreement could give Paul the final push to return to school. Paul gave various reasons as to why he should remain home and not risk having his symptoms back. However, faced with the firm resolution of all adults and reassurance from the therapist, he gave in. His return to school was uneventful, and he has continued to attend school and has spent two summers in camp.

Treatment. The principle of an early return to school is supported by the majority of child psychiatrists of all persuasions. Some psychiatrists have tried to involve the parents, the child, and the school in management of school phobia. Others believe that the mother–child dyad is to be treated. The return to school in some cases has to be done in stages; behavior therapists have been advocates of this regimen. The varying circumstances surrounding each case do not allow for rigid adherence to any dogma, though the goal of treatment remains the same.

In severe cases of school phobia, residential placement may be the only workable plan. In some cases, the mere threat of hospitalization may mobilize the child and the family to begin to work together. Mild tranquilizers and antidepressants in cases of older children may be necessary to alleviate the extreme anxiety or depressed mood and help along the psychotherapy. In treating the child, one must always consider the possible contributions of various academic problems and provide the child with whatever remedial help is needed to make the school experience more successful.

Prognosis. Follow-up studies of children with school phobia have revealed that for older children the prognosis for future adjustment is considerably poorer than for the younger age group. Prompt treatment has been correlated with better prognosis. Weiss and Burke (1967) found that in a group of 14 hospitalized school phobics, all had graduated from high school. Half showed good social adjustment, while half remained somewhat limited in their social interactions. Coolidge *et al.* (1964) did a follow-up study of 37 school phobics. They found 13 with good adult adjustment, 10 with only mild degrees of social maladjustment, and 14 severely limited and disabled.

Obsessive–Compulsive Neurosis

Obsessions are ideas, fears, or doubts that intrude into the child's awareness without any apparent external provocation and are felt as alien, unrelated, and undesirable. Compulsions are repetitive, stereotyped acts executed by the child in order to ward off some imaginary threat. *Obsessive–compulsive personality structure* refers to the child's tendency to be rigid, self-righteous, excessively orderly, and perfectionistic.

Obsessive–compulsive neurosis is believed to be relatively rare in childhood, though various studies have shown that a great number of adults with obsessive–compulsive neuroses date the onset of their symptoms to their preadolescence. Adams (1973) gave the figure of 1.2% for obsessive–compulsive neurosis among all referrals to the University of Florida Children's Mental Health unit. The onset of symptoms is usually around 6–10 years, although because the child is usually referred when the symptoms become disruptive, one may postulate an earlier appearance. Some parents, indeed, report symptoms as early as 18 months to 2 years of life. The onset may be sudden, in a previously well-adjusted child, or insidious, in a child with multiple difficulties.

In the United States, middle-class white families have contributed the largest proportion of obsessive–compulsive children reported in the literature. Some form of psychopathology has been present in more than half of the families of these children. Obsessive–compulsive traits or personality structures are usually present in one or both parents. Twins studies, though rare, have confirmed the presence of the disorders in both members of the pairs. However, because of the low frequency of the disorder in childhood, one cannot draw any firm conclusion regarding the genetic causation of obsessive–compulsive neurosis. In adults, men outnumber women in showing obsessive–compulsive neurosis, and this seems also to hold true for children. For example, in the Florida group, only one out of every four reported cases was a female. Most of these children have average or above-average intelligence, although mentally retarded children are by no means exempt from the disorder. The clinical picture of obsessive–compulsive neurosis in children may be mixed with various phobias, and this fact presents a problem in the assignment of a diagnostic label and therefore reporting of the prevalence.

Clinical Picture. Presenting complaints may be the child's incessant questioning, his fears and worries about his parents' health or safety, his frequent hand washing, and his ritualized dressing and undressing. Younger children involve their parents in their rituals, so the family is usually aware of the child's obsessive thoughts and has made unsuccessful attempts to stop his rituals. The child himself complains of ideas coming into his mind over which he has no control, or acts that he must carry out to keep some terrible thing from befalling himself or his family. Though mild depression may be present because of the child's frustration over his unwanted symptoms, most children show very little affect while describing their obsessional ideas.

Compulsive children may experience a high level of anxiety when they try to resist the execution of their compulsions. Thought content is pervaded by magic, although the thinking process in other areas is logical. The patient cannot explain how his acts could prevent something from happening or through what intermediary his thoughts may harm another person. This meaning of his obsessions completely escapes him despite his usually average or above-average intelligence. Some children may concede that they are angry at their parents or feel insecure and unwanted. However, these statements are uttered without concomitant feelings. They may have guilt feelings because they have a rigid moral code by which they strive to live. They consider themselves always, or nearly always, right and describe their peers or their teachers as being stupid or inferior to themselves. They are pedantic and argumentative, and demand to know why each question is asked of them or what possible relation the subject could have to their problems. They examine the therapist's statements and often reject them as not meeting their standard of clarity and exactness.

Acknowledging feelings, even those patently obvious during the therapy session, is very difficult, as if the child's concept of himself does not allow any "irrationality" and he considers feeling angry, annoyed, or embarrassed irrational. Some children may exhibit bizarre movements or tics that are conscious stereotyped maneuvers by which they try to rid themselves of some obsessive ideas. These children usually feel lonely, though they may have superficial contacts with a large number of peers during their daily activities.

Etiology. Psychoanalytic theory maintains that in obsessive–compulsive neurosis, the child has regressed from the Oedipal to the anal–sadistic stage and the psychological defenses that he uses to counteract his anxiety are isolation of affects, displacement, and reaction formation or undoing. Harsh toilet training is often held responsible for fixating the child on the anal–sadistic stage. A history of harsh toilet training has been obtained for some, but by no means all, obsessive–compulsive children (41% in the Florida group). Furthermore, prospective studies of child-rearing practices have failed to substantiate the relationship between toilet training and the so-called "anal personality."

The presence of obsessive trends and perfectionistic standards in the families of obsessive children has been repeatedly noted. Expectation of high regularity and conformity to the mother's standard is certainly operative in such a family during the child's toilet training. However, since all children of obsessive parents do not become obsessive, one must assume that the child's pattern of reactivity in interaction with parental expectation is responsible for the development of neurosis. Families that discourage or disapprove of affective expression provide breeding grounds for isolation of affects. When love and acceptance are contingent upon meeting strict standards, children may come to view their slightest infringements of the rules as possible causes for rejection and loss of love. They therefore strive for perfection and feel anxious and guilty over their failures. We still lack sufficient explanation of the circumstances under which a particular child adheres so rigidly and concretely to parental standards that even cognitive growth and expansion of social awareness cannot tear off the straitjacket that he has helped to impose on himself and his spontaneity.

CASE HISTORY

Barbara, the 10-year-old daughter of a professional father and a college-graduate mother, was brought to the psychiatrist because she had repeatedly told her parents that at times she found herself thinking that she should kill herself. Barbara was the middle child in her family, with a younger and an older sister. She believed that her father was very fond of her, though she herself felt closer to her mother. In describing her symptoms, Barbara stated that once or twice a week she got a strange idea that she should walk to the bridge near their house and jump off. She denied being sad or dissatisfied with anything, though she said she did not have any close friends because she did not think that any of her classmates were worthy of her friendship. She further revealed that whenever her parents were out of the house, she worried about their being in a car accident or fire. She graphically described how her parents would be multilated and drew pictures of how blood would be running all over them. In response to the question of how she felt while visualizing these scenes, Barbara said matter-of-factly that she was scared. She then took the drawing to the faucet and let the water run over it before she disposed of it. She explained that this would assure that such a thing would not happen.

Differential Diagnosis. Ritual activities in toddlers, excessive questioning in the 3- to 4-year-old preschooler, and ritualized, repetitive games in the early school years are all normal developmental phenomena. On the other hand, an obsessive desire for sameness and ritualized activities accompanied by a lack of interest in human interaction may be found in early infantile autism. Children with brain damage may exhibit stereotyped behavior, and some authorities have noted a higher incidence of obsessive–compulsive symptomatology in childhood schizophrenia.

Nonpathological, circumscribed interests in some specialized areas to the exclusion of all other leisure activities may have an obsessive quality and may isolate the child from most of his peers. However, the child himself does not consider his interest an imposition on him and is content with his own involvement. Therefore the element of subjective distress, which is common to all neurosis, does not exist.

Some psychiatrists have reported cases of transient obsessive–compulsive symptoms in preadolescence. Therefore, unless the particular behavior has become chronic, one should be cautious in labeling the child as neurotic. Some obsessive–compulsive children may be hoarders and frugal in spending money. However, frugality may be a much valued trait in a family, and hoarding various objects may have an individualized benign meaning for a child.

Treatment. Psychotherapy with obsessive–compulsive children is usually a long-term process. Paul Adams (1973) believes that 24 months of weekly sessions is the average length of time necessary for treatment. Eclectic therapists advise a more direct approach and less time spent on uncovering the symbolic meaning of the symptoms. This is the opposite of the analytic approach to the problem. Whatever the theory, the goal of treatment is to alleviate the child's suffering as soon as possible, since during the formative years of life any disability may have detrimental effects on the development of personality.

Prognosis. In treated cases of obsessive–compulsive neurosis, there is complete recovery in about 50%, worsening of the symptoms in 30%, and marginal adjustment in 20%. Of the 30% who do not improve with treatment, some have later been diagnosed as schizophrenics.

Conversion Reactions

Conversion reaction is a disturbance of voluntary motor or sensory systems that is the bodily manifestation of a psychic conflict. Zeigler (1967) gave three criteria for the diagnosis of conversion reaction. First, there is a prominent somatic symptom for which no anatomical or physiological basis can be found. Second, the symptom serves a psychological need. And third, the appearance of the symptom or its exacerbation follows an event of deep emotional significance. Looff (1970) described the conversion reaction as "shifting disabilities in various sensory and voluntary motor systems of the body." As can be noted from the above definitions, the relationship between the psychic need or significant emotional conflict and a particular constellation of symptomatology is not a simple causal one. The rationale behind the choice of symptom in conversion reaction, as indeed in all neuroses, remains hypothetical.

The frequency of conversion reactions in childhood is not easily established. Authors who have limited their reports to clearly defined clinical entities involving sensory and voluntary motor systems report somewhat lower rates than those who include the majority of suspicious and exaggerated reactions to physical illnesses as "hysterical" in nature. Proctor (1958) and Looff (1970) reported a higher incidence of conversion reaction in southern and midwestern rural areas of the United States. Rock (1971) reported 10 cases referred to the Walter Reed General Hospital in Washington, D.C., and the Tripler General Hospital in Honolulu during the period between 1967 and 1969. These children came from a variety of ethnic, national, and geographic locations.

Clinical Pictures. Conversion reaction is most prevalent among children over 7 years of age, though some cases of 2- to 3-year-old children with conversion reactions have been reported in the literature. A diagnosis of conversion reaction should be considered along with other diagnoses whenever a child presents disturbances of the sensory or motor systems.

All varieties of motor and sensory disturbances are seen during childhood. Looff's group of eight children showed the following clinical picture:

Astasia–abasia	1
"Seizures," tonic and clonic	3
Acute urinary retention	2
Hemiparesis	1
Aphonia	1

Rock's group of 10 patients presented as many as eight different clinical symptoms:

Coma, astasia–abasia	1
Flexion contracture of right leg—knee	1
Stiffness of leg and limping	1
"Seizures"	2
Aphonia	1
Scoliosis with deformity	1
Loss of vision	1
Hearing loss, total and partial	2

As is obvious from the above tables, conversion reaction in children can mimic a great number of diseases. In cases of hysterical blindness, children show a constricted visual field. Deafness may be shifting, total, or partial and may change from one situation to another. Contractures of muscles may lead to anatomical changes because of disuse.

The symptoms in conversion reaction do not correspond to any known pattern of physical illnesses, and they can be removed by firm suggestion or under hypnosis or sodium amytal interview. The child may show an attitude of nonconcern toward the symptom (*la belle indifférence*). However, with removal of the symptoms, the distress and anxiety are easily discerned. Symptoms may disappear spontaneously or through various therapeutic techniques. However, the chronic anxiety and vulnerability to distress may have far-reaching consequences for personality development. Boys with conversion reaction in childhood have been diagnosed as being overanxious neurotics or having personality disorders as adults.

Etiology. Children with conversion reaction are usually shy, unhappy, and insecure. Like all neurotic children, they harbor fears of parental rejection, worry about their own worth, have conflicting feelings regarding their dependence on their parents, and have a longing for more attention and acknowledgment from them. They may have average intelligence and normal physical growth; but their peer relationships are unsatisfactory and their academic performance suffers from their preoccupation with their internal struggle.

Psychoanalytic theory currently holds the view that these children regress to the oral–incorporative level. The sexual seduction theory of Freud's earlier writings has been revised. Freud wrote about a basic "constitutional disposition to hysteria." Proctor (1958), on the other hand, considers cultural factors to be of prime importance in the development of symptomatology. He described the cultural milieu of the rural South of the United States as denigrating all pleasures while providing a high degree of actual sexual stimulation. The ensuing psychic conflict sets the stage for conversion reaction. Looff (1970) considers conversion reaction body language or nonverbal communication among the members of an inarticulate subculture. In the majority of cases, some precipitating events can be identified. Injury, illness, or the departure of a parent can precede the onset of the symptoms.

While among adults, women with conversion reactions outnumber men, in children the discrepancy is not as large.

Dissociative Reactions. Somnambulism, amnesia, and fugue states have attracted less attention than conversion reaction among children. The main characteristic of this group of disorders is a sudden massive dissociation of consciousness that has a propelling force of its own. Janet (1876) viewed this phenomenon as a failure of the synthesizing function of the personality.

Treatment. Symptom removal, preferably without hypnosis and sodium amytal injection, is the first step in the treatment of these children, since the presence of the symptoms may expose the child to various medical and laboratory procedures and reinforce the sick role upon which the child has embarked. Environmental manipulation may be all that is needed to lessen the intensity of the child's conflict, or it may be the only practical help that can be offered under the circumstances. Psychotherapy may prevent the development of personality defects and cure not only the child's symptoms but the neurotic substructure of his style of interaction with his environment.

Hypochondriacal Neurosis

Kanner (1972) defined *hypochondriasis* as a "chronic complaint habit." in young children, complaints such as headache, stomachache, and so on are learned maneuvers for manipulation of the environment. Children notice very early in their lives that there are certain privileges associated with the sick role, such as being able to stay home and watch TV instead of going to school, being excused from doing customary chores, or having a deserved punishment suspended because of illness. Overprotective and oversolicitous parents may inadvertently encourage the child to pay an inordinate amount of attention to his bodily sensations and functions. Inadequate and overanxious mothers lavish such attention on their children's sickness that they teach the child a quick way of obtaining indulgence from them. In families in which ill health is equated with some form of religious punishment, children may express their guilt feelings by feeling ill. Hypochondriacal parents expect, or at least are not surprised, to find their children complaining about vague feelings of ill health and dysfunction of various organs. In some children, anxieties and psychic conflicts are actually felt as somatic distress, and their complaints and preoccupations are indications of their mental suffering. As with most other childhood neuroses, the parents style of coping with stress provides their children with models to imitate, and parental identification with the child's symptomatology may maintain a pattern of behavior in the child. In these children, bouts of anxiety and depression may underlie a period of somatic complaints.

Treatment. In treatment of children with hypochondriacal symptoms, a thorough medical checkup is necessary to reassure the family. However, such reassurances must be followed with a discussion of possible sources of stress as well as the pattern of intrafamilial communication. The overwhelming majority of hypochondriacal children are responsive to such intervention, although in a small group, hypochondriasis may become a lifelong habit.

Elective Mutism

Elective mutism is a condition in which the child limits his verbal transactions to few or all members of his own family and stubbornly refuses to talk to other people. The situation is usually brought to light when the child enters school and fails to communicate with his teachers and peers. Some children whisper; others remain totally mute. While in the beginning they may attract attention to themselves by their unusual silence, they are soon isolated and ostracized by other children and are a source of continuous frustration to their teachers. Even when they are intelligent and hardworking, their nonparticipation in those activities that require speech retards their academic progress.

Etiology. Although the condition has attracted clinicians' attention for over half a century, there is as yet no unified theory as to its etiology. Psychoanalysts view elective mutism as a defense against oral–aggressive impulses, though it is not clear why such control is required only when the child is in an unfamiliar situation. Behaviorists believe that mutism has come to acquire a fear-reducing function in a chronically anxious and timid child and is maintained by environmental reactions to it.

The background history of some children reveals a traumatic experience associated with the child's verbalization attempts during the early period of language development. Children who do talk to their therapists do not like to discuss their reasons for mutism or are unable to shed any light on the condition. When mutism is directed at a particular family member, the child has usually made a conscious decision not to talk in order to punish the person or to express his feelings of alienation from him. In some abusive families, children soon learn that to be silent is to be safe and may thus come to equate silence with safety everywhere. In still other cases, the child has been schooled in the necessity for remaining silent and noncommunicative with people outside the family. However, all these factors lead to complete mutism in only a very small group of children. Therefore one must assume that the child's particular style or personality characteristics play an important part in the development of the disorder.

The most commonly implicated factors are a combination of constitutional factors, such as initial withdrawal from novel situations and a tendency toward slow adaptation; speech difficulties or traumatic experiences associated with language development, and feelings of insecurity and fear leading to withdrawal as the most effective defense strategy.

Adams and Glasner (1954) view elective mutism as the child's reaction to a hostile environment. However, it seems that the child considers any new environment hostile, and his lack of participation and his noncompliance are a sign of his rejective attitude, which soon creates a hostile environment around him.

In reporting a series of 24 children who refused to talk in school, Wright (1968) found the majority to be strong-willed and oppositional. These findings are in contrast to the timidity commented upon by other authors. It is likely that a strong-willed child would be reluctant to give up the behavior that has served to set him apart in an unfamiliar environment. Furthermore, for such a child the coercive measures that are resorted to in order to involve him in verbal transactions may instead serve to maintain the motivation for mutism.

Treatment. There are almost as many therapeutic strategies reported in the literature as there are authors. Some have advocated removal from the home and placement in residential treatment centers. Others believe that the child should be engaged in long-term nonverbal therapy, with the hope that he may begin talking with others while preserving his nonspeaking stand against the therapist. Behavior modification and desensitization have been recommended in the classroom or in the therapeutic situation. The results of various therapeutic endeavors are mixed. In a follow-up study of four children who had been placed in an inpatient unit, Elson *et al.* (1964) found one child who still refused to speak to the teacher, two who had improved and performed well academically, and one whose adjustment was marginal. In the treatment of three cases with behavior modification techniques carried out by the teachers, Halpern and his co-workers

(1971) reported good results. In these cases, the plan for treatment was discussed and agreed upon by teachers and parents. The children were told in the class that they would be expected to say a preselected word before they could leave the classroom. The child's refusal to say the word would result in his staying with the teacher after all the other children had left the school. In subsequent sessions, the word was replaced by a sentence, and thus the mutism was slowly overcome.

CASE HISTORY

Rachel, an 8-year-old girl, was referred by the school because she had refused to talk since her entrance to school. She did her work and was considered a well-behaved child. However, she did not have any friends and had recently become victimized by several of her classmates, who had decided to make her talk by pulling her hair or destroying her property. The mother reported that Rachel was a talkative child at home. She would carry on long telephone conversations with a few of her mother's friends. Once she had answered the phone and talked until the caller identified herself as the assistant principal of the school, at which point Rachel refused to talk and passed the receiver to her mother. The mother further described Rachel as a "spoiled child," for which she took the responsibility, saying that Rachel was the youngest of her children and her only daughter. Birth history and developmental milestones were all within the normal limit. Rachel had been sent to kindergarten at the age of 5. However, she refused to stay without her mother and was discharged. She did not mind entering school the next year, but the mother was soon informed that Rachel was not talking in school, and the teachers would not be convinced that Rachel actually talked at home. The parents tried to persuade Rachel to speak in school and finally decided to record Rachel's conversation to convince her teachers. Rachel spoke animatedly for the recording session, but when the parents tried to ask her opinion about school, she turned the recorder off. The parents were not overly alarmed by Rachel's mutism at school, and her teachers decided to tolerate her behavior, even though at times they had to guess what she wanted or accept a single written word as an expression of her desires.

Rachel refused to talk or gesture to the examiner but readily agreed to draw pictures and do puzzles. When she was informed that she would have to return a week later, she seemed surprised but did not say anything. During the next five sessions, Rachel remained silent but was eager to play games. Once she chose a game that the examiner did not know how to play. Rachel tried playing the game to show the therapist, and having failed to convey her message, she became angry, banged the table, and finally called the therapist "stupid." She did not talk for the remainder of the session and refused to engage in any other activity. At the next session, when the therapist greeted her, she began to talk, though in a whisper. As the therapy proceeded, Rachel began complaining about her classmates, who did not leave her in peace. The therapist asked if she could yell for help when these children approached her; she said she did not think that she could do so but agreed that she would try. The teacher was informed of this possibility and remained within the vicinity of the class during the recess. That day only one of Rachel's customary tormentors was in school, but as she appeared from the far side of the corridor, Rachel called "Help," which brought the teacher to the scene. Rachel then began to speak to the teacher and a few children. However, she reverted to whispering whenever the teacher seemed in a hurry or did not stay long enough with her. Follow-up contact two years later brought the information that Rachel had decided to take singing lessons and would like to prepare for a singing career.

In this case, elective mutism seemed to be related to the earlier separation anxiety and lack of security of an overprotected child in a new environment. The tolerance exhibited by the parents and the school had maintained her behavior, resulting in the isolation and victimization of the child. At the time of referral, it seemed as if Rachel was searching for a face-saving way to break her silence. Her subsequent decision to become a singer may have been due to her awareness that audience expectations could help her perform verbally in public.

12

Childhood Psychoses

Before the turn of the century, the psychiatric literature on childhood psychoses in the United States was meager and essentially anecdotal in nature. Of the five writers mentioned by Leo Kanner in the years before 1900, two are French (Moreau de Tours, 1888; Manheimer, 1899), one German (Emminghaus, 1887), and two English (Irland, 1898; Maudsley, 1867). With the introduction of Kraepelin's nosological system, psychiatrists began to show an active interest in classifying various clinical pictures. Soon afterward De Sanctis (1906) in Italy described children with psychotic symptomatology who were not feeble-minded and in whom, according to him, dementia praecox was manifested at an earlier age than Kraepelin had suggested. In 1908 Heller reported six cases of progressive dementia in children in whom onset of the disease during the third or fourth year of life had caused rapid regression in behavior, loss of speech, and withdrawal of interest from the environment. Heller had assumed that these were cases of early dementia praecox and as such belonged to the category of functional psychosis. However, later developments showed Heller's disease to be due to acute and diffuse degeneration of the cerebral cortex.

Bleuler (1911) did not report any cases of schizophrenia among children, but commented that in some adult patients deviant behavior had been present since childhood. Other psychiatrists working with children soon began to apply Bleuler's criteria to the cases of abnormal behavior in children, and the term *childhood schizophrenia* was introduced into psychiatric literature.

There is relative agreement among various child psychiatrists about what constitutes severe psychotic behavior in childhood. However, its classification and the relationship between childhood and adult schizophrenia remain matters of controversy. Bender (1947) considers childhood schizophrenia a "deep-seated biological process, activated by a physiological crisis such as birth, which interferes with the maturation of the child in every area of functioning." In her view, the disorder persists throughout the individual's lifetime, but the clinical manifestations of the disease are different at various stages. Thus the clinical picture may resemble mental retardation (pseudodefective), neurosis (pseudoneurotic), or psychopathy (pseudopsychopathic).

Kanner, in 1943, reported cases of deviant behavior in young children that he called "autistic disturbances of affective contact." Later on, this cluster of symptoms was called the *syndrome of early infantile autism*. In 1949 Mahler described another variety of "developmental psychosis" as "symbiotic psychosis." Rank's (1949) designation of the "atypical child" was an effort to unify the various clinical pictures under one umbrella. According to Rank, the most consistent findings in these children were "ego fragmentation" and uneven or deviant development. While Bender's definition is considered too inclusive by some workers, the only active controversy is that of the existence of the distinctive syndrome of early infantile autism. Meanwhile, the term "autistic" has been used as analogous to *childhood schizophrenia* or even *childhood psychosis*.

In 1960 a group of British child psychiatrists attempted to provide a set of criteria for the diagnosis of the schizophrenic syndrome in children (Creak, 1961). The nine points of the British Working Party are as follows:

- Impaired relationship with people. This includes symbiotic relationship as well as autistic aloofness.
- Confusion of personal identity and unawareness of self, leading to such abnormal behavior as self-mutilation.
- Abnormal preoccupation with certain objects without regard to their functions.
- Resistance to change in the environment.
- Diminished or heightened sensitivity to sensory stimuli, such as sound or pain.
- Excessive and acute anxiety reaction in response to minor change.
- Disturbance of language and speech, which includes delayed acquisition of speech, loss of speech, peculiar use of language, echolalia, and reversal of personal pronouns.
- Disorders of motility. Hyper- or hypoactivity—strange postures or mannerisms (rocking, hand flapping, etc.).
- Scattered performance on tests of intelligence, with areas of normal to superior functionings interspersed with areas of backwardness or serious retardation.

The criteria of the British Working Party do not include such characteristics of adult schizophrenia as disturbed affect, ambivalence, or thinking disorder, even though schizophrenia in prepuberty manifests clusters of symptoms similar, if not identical, to adult schizophrenia.

There are very few prevalence studies of childhood psychoses. A survey of all children between the ages of 8 and 10 in Middlesex, England (Lotter, 1966), reported a rate of 2.1 per 10,000 of early infantile autism and 2.4 per 10,000 with "autistic" features, thus a rate of 4.5 per 10,000 children with psychoses of childhood. Treffert (1970) made a survey of all children under 12 years of age in Wisconsin who had received a diagnosis of childhood schizophrenia during the five years between 1962 and 1967. After removing duplicate reports, he found a total of 439 cases with the diagnosis of childhood psychoses (early infantile autism, psychoses complicated by demonstrable organicity, and psychoses of later onset with some autistic features). Based on the estimated population of children between the ages of 3 and 12 in the area, the prevalence rate of psychosis was 3.3 per 10,000 children. The prevalence rate for classical early infantile autism was only 0.7 per 10,000 cases. The incidence of newly reported cases in the area for all childhood psychoses was about 50 cases per year. This is one-tenth of the reported prevalence rate for adult schizophrenia. In Aberdeen, Scotland, Rutter (1967) found 4 cases of childhood psychosis among 9,000 children. The London County Council has records of 2 cases per 10,000 children. In all these studies, the ratio is 3.5–4 boys for each girl. No differences were found between urban and rural areas in the prevalence of childhood psychoses.

Clinical Pictures

Onset and Precipitating Factors. The onset of the disturbed behavior may be difficult to pinpoint because of the parents' lack of observational skill, their high tolerance for deviation, or insidious onset. Some authors believe that in some children abnormal development begins at birth; others report a period of normal development with slow acute deterioration of previously acquired skills. Kanner stated that in early infantile autism, there is no period of normal development, while Eisenberg (1957) described some cases in which the onset of illness was in the second year of life. Bender and Freedman (1952) and Fish (1960) have reported cases in which infants showed uneven development from their first few weeks of life. In some cases, parents become concerned when their infants fail to make differentiated social responses to them. Others report the infant's lack of anticipatory postures when parents try to pick them up. Some infants are reported to be unusually sensitive to noise, lights, or textures. Others are described as hypoactive and easy babies. Failure to develop speech is sometimes the presenting complaint of the parents. At times, acquired speech may be lost. In older children, failure to separate from the mother, lack of interest in the environment, sustained sleep disturbance, loss of acquired bowel control, a variety of phobias or unusual ideations, and excessive hyperactivity may bring the child to the attention of the psychiatrist.

In 100 cases of childhood psychoses, Creak (1968) reported normal development in 42%, retarded development during first year in 29%, and inconsistent, uneven development in 29%.

In the same group, the age of onset was reported as:

From birth 13%
First year 7%
Second year 18%
Third year 43%
Fourth year 10%
Fifth year 5%
After fifth year 4%

More than half of the sample was considered deviant by the parents from the early weeks of life, while in 31% the child's behavior regressed, and in 18% no further development took place. Precipitating factors in Treffert's Wisconsin sample were, in order of frequency, physical illness, birth of a sibling, and emotional trauma (death in the family, moving, abuse, and so on).

Early Infantile Autism

The syndrome first described by Kanner in 1943 was viewed by the author as the "earliest possible manifestation of childhood schizophrenia in the broadest sense of this term." (Kanner 1949). However, many investigators including Kanner have considered the clinical picture of autism of such a distinct nature as to warrant the designation of a separate entity. Characteristics of the syndrome are related by Kanner in several publications following the original description. These are as follows:

Age of onset. Signs of behavioral deviation are noticeable during the first two years of life. Parents comment on the infant's lack of social smile, his failure to assume anticipatory posture when being picked up, and his apparent nonresponsiveness to familiar people.

Aloneness or self-isolation. These babies impress their caretakers as being the happiest when they are left by themselves. They do not show any consistent desire to relate to people, avoid looking at them, and have aversive reaction to physical contact initiated by others.

Language development is delayed. Some children remain mute and others do not use their speech for communicative purposes. Peculiarities of speech include immediate and delayed echolalia, reversal of personal pronouns, and irrelevant utterances.

Excessive. Adverse emotional reaction is displayed by patients following changes in their surrounding. Kanner considers this desire to maintain sameness as one of the two fundamental symptoms of the condition, the other being lack of affective contact.

Unusual hyper- or hyposensitivity of patients to sensory stimulation may appear in the form of unresponsiveness to sounds to the extent that some are considered deaf. Others seek uncommon stimuli, and yet others do not respond to pinpricks.

Bizarre mannerisms, obsessive rituals, and stereotyped movements are prevalent. At times children engage in self-injurious behaviors such as head banging, or they rock their bodies, flap their hands, and walk on their toes.

Although a formal assessment of their IQs may not always be possible and their functioning is impaired, the children impress the observer as being intelligent and show exceptional abilities in auditory and visual memories and mechanical talents in manipulation of objects.

Patients are predominantly boys (4 boys to each girl). Their families are remarkable for their low rate of major psychiatric disorders and their high level of social and intellectual attainment. However, the parents are usually aloof and emotionally cold.

Follow-up studies reveal that the overwhelming majority of patients remain emotionally and socially defective regardless of the treatment. Those who do not speak by the age of five have poorer prognosis. Even those who have managed to make a better adjustment remain handicapped in interpersonal relationship, and their social judgment is impaired. More than three-quarters of patients are in need of life-long care in institutions. As adults they appear mentally retarded and psychotic. A significant number develop seizures during adolescence and this in spite of the fact that they do not have more frequent histories of prenatal and perinatal difficulties and do not exhibit signs of neurological involvement during childhood.

Studies of similar groups of patients have produced conflicting results regarding the families of autistic children. While the higher socioeconomic and educational status of the parents has not been universally reported, the majority of the reports indicate a low or unelevated rate of schizophrenia in the family. (Rimland, 1964; Rutter 1967; Ritvo, 1971).

About the children themselves, the majority of investigators have confirmed the serious nature of this disability and its poor prognosis. The nature of cognitive and language deficits of the patients has attracted much attention during the recent years. (Rutter, 1971; Bartak *et al.*, 1975). Because so many of these patients score on retarded range on various social, developmental, and intellectual tests, and remain retarded throughout their lives, Rutter (1971) has questioned the accuracy of the notion that the autistic child is endowed with average intellectual potential. According to him mental retardation and autism can and do coexist.

Symbiotic Psychosis. Margaret Mahler (1952) described a group of young children, aged 3 and 4, in whom states of extreme anxiety, usually in response to separation from the mother, could take a psychotic proportion. The child withdraws from normal interaction with the environment, is unusually attached to the mother, feels lost and confused without her, and may experience delusional bodily sensations and introjected objects. According to Mahler, in these children the process of separation and individuation has not been accomplished, and the child has failed to establish an individual identity. Mahler considers "symbiotic psychosis" a variety of schizophrenia in childhood and the opposite pole of early infantile autism. Bender (1947) stated: "Every schizophrenic child reacts to the psychosis in a way determined by his own total personality including the infantile experiences and the level of maturation of the personality." Thus she does not consider early infantile autism or symbiotic psychosis independent clinical syndromes. She described a variety of disorders in physiological and psychological aspects of personality. Thus children can manifest disturbances in:

- Vasovegetative functionings: for example, cold extremities, flushing, and perspiring.
- Growth disturbances: precocious or delayed puberty in boys and girls.
- Disorders of motor activities: hyper- or hypoactivity, awkwardness and peculiar gait, toe walking, grimacing.
- Postural reflex responses such as whirling beyond the normal age (6–7 years).
- Disorders of thought and language.
- Disorders of body image and problems of identity; introjected objects.

- Difficulties and preoccupation with sexual and/or aggressive activities.
- Extreme anxiety and unusual sensations or inappropriate affects.
- Disturbances in interpersonal relationships, particularly with family members.

Bender (1947) considers excessive anxiety to be the cornerstone of the clinical picture of schizophrenia and has gone so far as to state, "The presence of severe anxiety in a child, unaccounted for by a reality situation, is in itself suggestive of schizophrenia."

Bartak *et al.* (1975) consider infantile autism a distinct syndrome characterized by a specific cognitive defect—namely, language impairment—and severe failure in the development of social relationships, as well as ritualistic and compulsive phenomena. The language disability, according to the authors, is characterized by its severity, its extent across different language modalities, the presence of deviant language features, and the relative nonuse of speech for social communication.

In attempting to arrive at a consensus, one can divide the clinical picture of childhood psychoses into three categories: early, middle, and preadolescent and adolescent onset.

Early-Onset Psychoses. In these children, the onset of the deviation is within the first two years of life. The presenting complaint is usually delayed language development, lack of response, or extreme hyperactivity and irritability. Parents may give a history of normal or near-normal development for the first few months of life. It is not unusual to get a history of an infant who had been babbling, has even said a few words, and then has become mute. Sleep problems are quite frequent. Sometimes these children have manifested extreme irritability ever since birth and their mothers find it difficult to form an idea of what the baby's typical reactions are. In some patients, motor development may be precocious or on time. In others, the course of motor development is deviant: they walk before attempting to sit or lose a function after having acquired it. They may show interest in some objects and insist on having their food out of a particular container. Some children become very upset when slight changes are made in their environment. Others take major changes with minimal reaction.

CASE HISTORY

Vincent, a 2½-year-old black boy, was referred by the pediatric clinic of a general hospital. The mother stated that Vincent did not talk and had sleep problems. He ran around aimlessly, became "wild," twirled until dizzy, and banged his head. He had said, "Mommy," "Daddy," and "Get down" between the ages of 12 and 14 months but stopped talking at 18 months. He liked records but did not want to listen to them playing; rather he carried them around looking through the hole. He made his wishes known by grabbing his parents' fingers and pulling at them. He understood "no" only when his parents shouted at him; otherwise he did not seem to understand what was said to him. He responded to his own name once in a while by turning his head in the direction of the person calling him. He hardly ever looked at anybody.

During clinical examination, Vincent ran around the room, walked on tiptoes, and played with his fingers. He did not make any eye contact, disregarded blocks, and used dolls to hit himself on the head. At one point, he began to scream and took off his shoes. He allowed his mother to put them back on and smiled faintly. He did not imitate the examiner when she waved good-bye to him. The diagnostic impression was that of childhood schizophrenia with autistic features. This case history is typical of very young psychotic patients.

Middle-Onset Psychosis. In these children, the early development has been normal. The use of language is age-appropriate. However, the content of speech is bizarre. The child may show a high anxiety level in new situations, withdraw from any interaction with peers, or act superficially and aggressively toward them. There is a preoccupation with injury, violence, and death, and the contents of fantasy breaks through in the child's goal-directed speech. Hyperactivity or anergia and lack of interest in the environment may be the presenting complaints of the parents. Either attention span is short or any attempt at concentration is frustrated by the intrusion of irrelevant fantasy materials. The boundary between reality and fantasy is fluid, and at times the child becomes confused when he is confronted with reality. In highly articulate children, one becomes easily aware of the looseness of association and incongruity of perception. At times, the parents are aware that the child's speech does not "make sense" because the ideas are disconnected.

The three case histories that follow examplify different types of middle-onset psychosis. In the first case, a child with disordered development was brought to the psychiatrist when her parents complained that her speech did not "make sense." In the second, a psychotic picture appeared in a child with a normal development after his exposure to a series of frightening experiences. And in the third, psychotic symptoms developed in a child exposed to a psychotic mother.

Case History

Iris was a product of a full-term, uneventful pregnancy. The labor lasted eight hours and a Caesarian section was finally performed. Iris was a "blue baby," had an Apgar Index of 1 at birth, and required oxygen administration for 40 minutes. Her development was normal, though she did not talk until she was three and then began talking in sentences. She had learned to read before she talked. A hyperactive child, Iris nevertheless watched TV for a few hours each day and could imitate various TV personalities. Her mother complained that she could not understand Iris's talk because "she jumps from one subject to another." She had nightmares in which she would see the "whole world burning" and "all the buildings coming down because of an earthquake." During the interview, when she was 5 years old, Iris showed fluctuating inappropriate affects. She called the examiner Henry Fonda and then Carol Burnett, sang commericals, and said she would like to be candy so people could eat her or to be a tiger so she could eat people. The clinical impression was closely akin to hebephrenic schizophrenia. Neurological examination showed neither focal nor nonfocal findings, and her EEG was normal.

CASE HISTORY

Tony, age 6, was brought to the hospital following two sleepless nights during which he became unaccountably agitated, tried to jump out of the window, and begged his parents not to let him "go crazy." The father reported that the previous week Tony had come to his store with patches of burned hair and said that several teenagers had locked him in an abandoned building and tried to set him on fire. A police investigation failed to verify Tony's story. Following this episode, the school had called to ask about Tony since he had not been in school for a few days. When the mother asked Tony about his whereabouts during the school hours, Tony had become very upset and reported that the same teenagers were stopping him from going to school and forcing him to steal and to take "dope." Again the parents failed to find these teenagers and told Tony that they considered these stories his excuse for having played hooky. It was on the weekend following these episodes that Tony became agitated.

On admission to the hospital, Tony was found to be a highly articulate and extremely anxious and suspicious child. He protested that he would not be "safe" in the hospital, became agitated, and tried to run away. His associations were loose; he could not concentrate and felt that he was "going crazy." He was placed on tranquilizers, and within 48 hours he became less fearful and more organized in his thinking. He was then able to give a better description of the said teenagers, and the parents were able to verify a significant part of his stories. A check with the school and the kindergarten that he had attended revealed that Tony had been considered a bright, outgoing, and pleasant child with no indications of a behavior problem. The parents gave a history of normal development and excused their failure to pursue Tony's stories more vigorously as being due to the fact that Tony would make up excuses for all his infractions of parental rules. Tony was discharged after three weeks, with no subsequent lapses during the three-year follow-up.

CASE HISTORY

John, a 5½-year-old boy, was brought to the pediatric clinic because he had begun to soil himself after three years of complete bowel control. A physi-

cal examination failed to reveal any organic cause for John's problem. However, the pediatrician noticed that John talked incessantly and made little
sense. A psychiatric consultation was requested. John's mother greeted the
psychiatrist by stating, "John better not be crazy, or I will beat the craziness
out of him." She then gave the name of all the state hospitals in which she had
been hospitalized, stressing her belief that now she was quite healthy because
"I know that I am a saint and I know that John is King of Arabia." John's father reported that his wife had been hospitalized on numerous occasions
because she had become violent and agitated. He felt that John must be very
worried about his mother's unpredictable behavior and stated that he had
found John locked in the closet several times upon returning home from work.
He thought John would be all right if he stopped talking like his mother and
just went to school like all other children. John was a well-developed, well-
coordinated boy. He asked the examiner to tell his parents only that he was
doing good schoolwork. He then began to relate a story about seeing skeletons
on the window, being the king of Arabia, and wanting to kill his mother "so
she can come back as a nice person." He said he felt sick lots of times because
he had "high blood pressure" and could get a "heart attack" in his stomach

When admission to the hospital was advised, John's mother rejected the
advice. His father and John himself accepted it. During the first week of hospitalization, the mother disappeared and John's father suspected that she had
been hospitalized in another state. John did not seem upset by the news and
mentioned that his mother must have gone to Seattle since she had told him
that she would take him there. In the hospital, John stopped soiling himself
except for several occasions following fights with older children. He remained
aloof from his peers but played well with younger children. He became less
anxious and worked diligently in school. His thinking remained confused
whenever he talked about his life at home, but he stopped talking about his
aches and pains. He did not think that he was king of Arabia any longer.
While one could not rule out the possibility of childhood schizophrenia in this
child, it was quite clear that John had been frightened on numerous occasions
by his psychotic mother and had shared her delusional ideas. The chronic
state of anxiety in this child had been a reaction to exposure to a psychotic
mother.

Anthony (1969) described parapsychotic disturbances as those
conditions in which "delusions, hallucinations, and other psychotic
symptoms are imposed by the psychotic parent on one or other of the
children." He went on to describe the home environment in which
children of psychotic parents are exposed to conflicting messages, disturbing affect, and irrational motivations. In such an "environment of
irrationality," children, particularly the younger ones, are confused
and frightened and are unable to withstand the onslaught of various
crises without being overwhelmed and manifesting signs of distress.

Preadolescent and Adolescent Onset. Between the ages of 9 and 12,
childhood schizophrenia may be manifested by a neurotic picture of
obsessive–compulsive symptomatology, truancy from school, deterioration of work habits, withdrawal from social contacts, and vague

complaints about the external world. Some children manifest a variety of mannerisms, tics or, phobias.

CASE HISTORY

Peter, an 11-year-old boy, started to be truant from school sometime in September. He insisted that he could not attend his school because "everything has changed." More specifically he said, "They now have rules that you can't walk in the corridors." However, he admitted that he had never wanted to attend school during previous years. At his own request, he was transferred to another school, only to refuse to attend after a few days. He then began to spend the days in front of the TV without really watching it. He declared that he did not have any friends and did not want to associate with anybody. Soon he became obsessed with the idea of going to a private school and finally visited a child psychiatric clinic on his own initiative to ask to be sent to a private school.

The psychiatrist who interviewed Peter found him to be depressed, anergic, and withdrawn, with feelings of estrangement from his family and friends and concerns about the impending doom that was to overcome him. He expressed doubts about his own identity and the reality around him. He agreed to return for another appointment the next day but he did not come back until a month later, at which point he told the psychiatrist that he was planning to kill himself since no private school had been found for him. Upon admission to the hospital, Peter became even more depressed, with only one topic of conversation: he wanted to go to a private school. He was unable to describe his idea of a private school, could not explain in what way he hoped to be happier there, and finally stated that he was restless and would like to move on from one place to another every few days. There was a heavy background of psychiatric disorders in Peter's family, with his mother and one brother having had psychiatric hospitalizations in the past. Peter's depression did not change significantly during his hospital stay, but he began to show some interest in his surroundings. The clinical impression was of simple schizophrenia.

In the later years of adolescence, schizophrenia takes the classic forms of adult schizophrenia, with inappropriate affect, loose association, hallucinations, illusions, and feelings of loss of identity. In those cases in which the onset is insidious and can be traced to earlier years, the prognosis is poorer than when the psychotic picture develops abruptly out of a background of normal development.

Affective Psychosis. A review of the literature fails to reveal in children the presence of manic–depressive illness as encountered in adults. The youngest patients with the classic picture of manic–depressive psychosis are reported to be in their early adolescence. Some authors have considered examples of depressive moods, sleep disorder, night terrors, and vegetative disturbances occurring in children with a family history of manic–depressive psychosis, to be early indications of depressive illness (Annell, 1969). Others state that prolonged shifts in emotional states without appropriate basis in reality could be considered an early manifestation of affective illness (Feinstein, 1973). While it is reasonable to assume that affective illness, with its strong genetic basis, may be expressed in various forms during an individual's life, the testing of this assumption must await further clarification in terms of our ability to find the etiological factors involved in bipolar psychosis.

Epidemiology

Family History. In describing the characteristics of a group of children with early infantile autism, Kanner (1956) reported relatively few psychiatric disorders in the families and siblings of these children. Rimland (1964), in reviewing the literature on early infantile autism, supported Kanner's original contention. However, Bender's (1947) study found a high rate of psychiatric disorders in the families of childhood schizophrenics, including cases that could be diagnosed as early infantile autism.

There are also different findings regarding the social class backgrounds of children with early infantile autism. Kanner and Rimland found high educational and social status among the parents and a relative lack of representation from black and other minority groups. But Bender found that the socioeconomic status of parents with schizophrenic children did not differ from that of parents of children with different symptomatology.

No significant difference related to the social class were found by McDermott *et al.* (1967) in a group of children who had been diagnosed as psychotic in the University of Michigan's children's psychiatric hospital. However, they did note a significantly higher incidence of withdrawal and autism in the children of the professional executive group than among the psychotic children of skilled and semiskilled laborers. They hypothesized that differences in the clinical pictures of schizophrenia in childhood may reflect the varying styles of child-rearing practices among the social groups. In a study of the families of 148 patients at the UCLA Neuropsychiatric Institute, Ritvo *et al.* (1971) found no significant difference in the social class indices of children with psychosis relating to the child's symptomatology. In reviewing the literature on childhood schizophrenia, Miller (1974) found no conclusive evidence to support the contention of those researchers who maintain that epidemiological data support the existence of the distinct entity of early infantile autism.

Another interesting phenomenon in the epidemiology of childhood psychoses is the sex ratio. Boys outnumber girls in ratio of 4 to 1 in early-onset psychosis, while the number of girls with psychosis gradually rises with age and approximates the incidence in boys during adolescence.

Prenatal History. There are some reports that complications of pregnancy and a history of previous fetal loss by the mother are more frequent in childhood schizophrenics than in nonschizophrenic children with or without psychiatric problems (Knobloch and Pasamanick, 1962; Gittelman and Birch, 1967). Low birth weight and prematurity have not been specifically associated with childhood schizophrenia. However, various investigators have reported a high incidence of clinical signs that are ordinarily associated with central nervous system damage. Goldfarb (1961) divided childhood schizophrenics into "organic" and "nonorganic" groups and found the organic group to be "inferior in motor coordination, perceptual discrimination, body imagery, muscle tone balance, posture, and righting behavior." EEG findings have not settled the issue, although a higher incidence of EEG abnormality has been reported for hospitalized schizophrenic children (Kennard, 1959). The nature of these abnormalities is nonspecific.

Mental retardation, which has been reported in about two-thirds of schizophrenic children (Pollack *et al.*, 1966), has also been considered a sign of central nervous system damage or what Bender has called "diffuse encephalopathy in childhood schizophrenia."

Of special interest is the high incidence of autism in children with congenital rubella (Chess, 1971; Desmond *et al.*, 1970). In these children, the existence of central nervous system damage is unequivocally established, and a diagnosis of autism is made in accordance with the nine-point guide of the British Working Party (Creak, 1961) or Kanner's criteria.

Follow-up studies of some children with early childhood schizophrenia and autism have shown that a high percentage of them develop seizures in early adolescence, strengthening the assumption of the existence of central nervous system damage in these children.

Biological Abnormalities. Biochemical studies in childhood schizophrenia have duplicated similar investigations in adult schizophrenics, even though the criteria for diagnosis are even more controversial for children than for adult populations. The earlier search for a blood toxin, an inborn error of metabolism, and a decrease or increase in vitamins or trace elements, has so far yielded very little useful information.

A new impetus in biochemical studies has been provided by the advent of psychopharmacological agents that can mimic or suppress psychotic symptomatology. Recent investigations have been focused on the activities of biogenic amines in the brain and their derivatives in blood, spinal fluid, and urine. Because the levels of such neurotransmitters as dopamine and serotonin have been found to fluctuate in adult schizophrenics, and because psychotropic agents such as phenothiazines and amphetamine are known to alter the rate of the activities of the neurotransmitters, new hypotheses have been proposed to account for the production of psychosis based on biochemical abnormalities.

The group of psychotic children most freqnently studied for evidence of such abnormalities are the very young children with autistic features. So far, the results of investigations of the activities of the biogenic amines have been contradictory. However, the proponents of the biochemical hypotheses point out that present methods do not allow for the accurate testing of their formulations. For example, many investigators have tried to assess the concentration of monoamine-oxidase (MAO) in the blood platelets, reasoning that the activities of MAO in the platelets reflect the MAO behavior in the brain. However, although it is known that the brain MAO is directly involved in the metabolism of dopamine, it cannot be assumed that the MAO of the platelets is similar in structure or function to the enzyme in the central nervous system. Other researchers have noted that even if it is proved that such a relationship exists, it cannot be concluded with certainty that biochemical abnormalities are the causative factors in schizophrenia rather than the result of the psychotic state.

Psychological Test Results. Although some authors have stressed the fact that in early childhood psychosis the child is "endowed with good cognitive potentialities" or has islets of normal or superior functioning, follow-up studies have revealed that a large percentage of these children had deteriorated intellectually. Furthermore, Rutter (1971) and Gittelman and Birch (1967) have reported a high correlation between the IQ taken during the initial referral and the subsequent IQ, except for children with evidence of neurological damage, in whom the subsequent IQ was lower than the IQ at the time of referral. The functioning of the children on various subtests of the intelligence tests indicates lower scores on tasks requiring abstract thought and sequential logic. Verbal tasks may be particularly difficult for children with disturbances of language. Some children do not have any language, or their score on the test is dependent on their performance on the nonverbal part of the IQ test. On projective tests, some schizophrenic children show evidence of poor reality testing, illogical thought, and bizarre associations.

Some psychotic children exhibit evidence of special capacities, such as unusual sensory acuity, an extraordinary ability to remember or calculate dates, early reading skill, and mechanical, mathematical, and musical abilities. The nature of this unusually advanced and, for the most part, isolated functioning is another puzzling feature of childhood schizophrenia. The complex processes involved in each particular ability do not lend themselves to easy explanations, such as rote memory or a low threshold for certain kinds of sensory data. In each instance, the child has to pay selective attention to one or a variety of sensory data, to be able to discriminate between relevant and irrelevant cues, and to store and retrieve them from his memory. The deviant feature common to all these abilities is that, for the most part, they are not produced in response to request; rather, they are spontaneously exhibited and are not incorporated into the child's overall adaptive functioning.

Etiology

The genetic studies of schizophrenic adults, and particularly the studies of monozygotic and dizygotic twins, have essentially demonstrated that schizophrenia is an abnormality that occurs in families and the closer the relationship, the greater the possibility of its occurrence in particular family members (Mattysse and Kidd, 1976). However, most large-scale studies have been done among adult schizophrenics, although clinically it has been shown that families of schizophrenic children have numerous members who either are schizophrenic or have a variety of other psychiatric disorders. Kallman (1950) reported the prevalance of schizophrenia in full sibs as 14–15%, in parents as 9–10%, and in monozygotic twins as 46–86%. These studies have been interpreted as indicating that the organism is genetically deviant, though neither the nature of this deviancy nor the mode of genetic transmission is clear.

Earlier in this chapter, it was noted that in a group of children with schizophrenia, possibilities of injuries or presumptive structural damage to the central nervous system can often be obtained from the prenatal or paranatal histories and clinical examinations (DeMyer, 1975). Bender and Fish have conceptualized the primary deviation in schizophrenia as a defect in the organization and integration of the central nervous system. This defect is clinically manifested in disharmonious development, with lags, retardation, regression, or precocity in various developmental sequences. However, Fish (1971) found it necessary to use infantile "anhedonia, anergy, and apathy" as auxiliary concepts along with anxiety to explain the psychological manifestations of childhood schizophrenia.

Evidence for the view that childhood schizophrenia is the result of disharmonious family relationships has come from retrospective histories of the patients or observations of interactions between the family members. Some authors, such as Szurek (1973), have considered childhood schizophrenia to be the result of compromise solutions and defense strategies used by the child to cope with the conflicting relationships and interactions within the family. In this view, the child is biologically normal, but the experiences of his early years are deviant. Kanner, on the other hand, postulated a biologically damaged child within a psychologically unresponsive and cold milieu as the prototype of early infantile autism.

Studies used to prove the environmental causality theory of childhood schizophrenia have been criticized on the grounds of methodology, lack of corroborating scientific data, contradictory data, and the fact that the data are open to other interpretational possibilities.

Concerning methodology, the retrospective data used in these studies are collected during the time that an individual is designated as a patient. The data cannot, therefore, be treated as objective evidence because they are subject to distortion and retroactive interpretations by parents and patients alike. Furthermore, the designations used—such as "dominant mother" and "passive father"—are value judgments based on particular sociocultural premises that have been invoked to explain many behavioral deviations and do not provide the degree of specificity required of a sound etiological theory.

There is also a lack of corroborating scientific data. Attitude questionnaires and other objectively designed instruments have failed to reveal any significant difference between the mothers of schizophrenics and normal, or other psychiatrically ill, children. Schopler and Loftin (1969) have demonstrated that parents of schizophrenic children show more impaired thinking on tests when they are evaluated in association with their schizophrenic child than in relation to their nonschizophrenic children. Observations of the parents' pattern of response with their schizophrenic and nonschizophrenic children have failed to sustain the hypothesis that parental attitudes and behavior are significantly different toward their schizophrenic child as compared to their nondisturbed children (Waxler and Mishler, 1971).

Even if one accepts the validity of the reconstructed history or observed data regarding disturbed family interactions, they do not validate the etiological assumption of environmentally induced schizophrenia. Considering the genetic data on schizophrenia, it is not unexpected to find other family members who are also behaviorally deviant, with illness manifested by various degrees of chronicity and overt symptomatology. However, it is by now a truism that parental reactions may be totally or partially shaped by the child's pattern of responsiveness. Thus it is as reasonable to assume that parental distancing would develop in response to a child who does not take an "anticipatory posture" or "looks through" the parents as to consider "the autistic withdrawal of affect" a reaction to parental attitudes. Parents of schizophrenic children go through various stages in their attempts to socialize their children. At the time of psychiatric observation, their attitudes may reflect how they have learned best to manage the child. For example, they may have come to an intuitive understanding that any intense expression of emotions causes disorganization in their sick children and therefore practice a nonemotional, matter-of-fact strategy of interaction because it is the least trying one. Or they may believe that the intensity of their reactions will create a desirable response in their anergic, withdrawn children and are therefore in a chronic state of histrionic activity. Akerley (1975), borrowing Anthony's concept of the "invulnerable child of psychotic parents," applies the same criteria to what she calls the "invulnerable parents of psychotic children." She thus considers the objective attitudes, distancing stance, and detailed information collected by these parents about their sick children's symptomatology, and their responses to various intervention programs, the unique style of these parents' reaction to an experience that, although felt on a personal level, is not allowed to become overwhelming and incapacitating. She further suggests that such invulnerability is more likely to develop in those parents who have already raised normal children and are therefore more secure about their own adequacy as parents.

While no one theory or set of assumptions has been found to explain the pathogenesis of childhood schizophrenia, it is safe to assume that as in normal development, organismic and environmental variables are in continuous interaction. Healthy or abnormal elements in the environment are processed through a healthy or abnormal organism, and the end result reflects the interplay between the organism and the experiences that he selectively avoids or is exposed to. Just as the knowledge of chromosomal abnormality in Down's syndrome or enzyme deficiency in phenylketonuria has not explained the how and the why of mental retardation, advances in etiological information may not make it easier to account for the disturbing picture of childhood schizophrenia. And it may be possible to cure or prevent schizophrenia long before it becomes possible to understand it.

Differential Diagnosis

In the differential diagnosis of childhood psychosis, the most important consideration is the presence or absence of specific organic pathology. Acute and chronic brain syndromes due to toxicity, infection, trauma, and space-occupying lesions can present clinical pictures resembling early- or late-onset psychosis. Autistic-like behavior and even pictures indistinguishable from early infantile autism have been reported in children with congenital rubella, retrolental fibroplasia, and other brain syndromes.

In older children, temporal lobe epilepsy can present with behavioral abnormalities resembling psychosis. In these children, restlessness, inability to concentrate, shallow affect, hallucinations, reliving past emotionally charged episodes, outbursts unaccounted for by external stimuli, and confusions of thought may give the impression of childhood schizophrenia. The birth history may or may not reveal the possibility of brain damage. An EEG, if positive, could be extremely helpful. Hallucinations in children do not have the same morbid connotation that they have in adults. However, the content of hallucinations and whether they are evoked or are experienced as forced phenomena can give some clue as to their origins.

Children with a communicative disorder, such as dysphasia, may show extreme anxiety and disorganized violent outbursts and give confusing accounts of their subjective experience when under stress. In these children, particularly when aphasia has gone unnoticed, the clinical picture can be clarified only after the acute stress has subsided and one begins to realize that the child has difficulty in finding appropriate words and that his speech is characterized by frequent paraphasic statements and approximations of meaning (Cohen *et al.*, 1976; Piggot and Simson, 1975). In their desire to communicate the nature and intensity of their distress, these children answer queries about their feelings and motivations by choosing words from the statements made by their families without having a precise understanding of their meanings.

Treatment

Every weapon in the psychiatric armory has been used in the treatment of childhood psychosis. Electric shock, LSD, hormones, and various chemical agents have been experimented with. While each group of researchers has found some ameliorative effects in some children, none has claimed any long-lasting beneficial results. Over the years, psychoeducational approaches to the treatment of childhood psychosis have included strategies based on etiological theories, concepts of the basic defects, and eclectic combinations of all the available modalities.

Those authors who have considered the schizophrenias to be environmentally induced have advocated the removal of the child from his home environment as the first step in treatment. Others have maintained that the parents should be treated along with their children, and some have recommended that the parents be educated to act as co-therapists. The most important task in the treatment of early psychosis is to combat withdrawal and nonresponsiveness and at the same time to provide highly structured, predictable surroundings to which the child might adjust and respond. In such a situation, the presence of caring, competent, and compassionate adults is necessary to maximize the child's low ability to relate and to help in socializing. Within such a framework, the opportunities for teaching, stimulating, and practicing all forms of human communication are available to the child. Speech and language development is stressed—both the comprehension of others and the expression of one's needs. Children's special abilities are channeled toward social goals, and their lags and defects are taken into consideration in devising programs that could motivate them to engage in and draw pleasure from new activities. Stereotyped movements are either discouraged or incorporated into useful organized activities.

The use of sedating or tranquilizing agents is justified if it can be shown that they curtail disruptive hyperactivity and reduce panic reactions. No medication has been found to be of much help in lengthening a short attention span or in inducing enthusiasm in apathetic children. Barbiturates do not seem to be helpful in the sleep problems of these children. In fact, in some cases they have caused agitation and increased disorganization. Diphenhydramine (benadryl) has a mild sedating effect and a relatively large margin of safety (Campbell, 1973).

While in some cases family circumstances such as child abuse and parental rejection necessitate the removal of the preschool psychotic child from the home, in the majority of cases the child's attendance in a day care nursery school program is sufficient for therapeutic purposes. Speech therapy, perceptual–motor training, and experiences in group activity, as well as cognitive training, have to be provided on an intensive and continuous basis. Individual psychotherapy with the child is another opportunity for providing human interaction, in which the therapist patiently tries to understand the child's stage of development and help him exercise his potentials, explore his environment, and establish his own identity.

The treatment of childhood psychosis is a multifaceted enterprise in which professionals from a variety of backgrounds are needed. The role of the psychiatrist on such a team is that of a diagnostician who is able to use all the available data in order to devise a therapeutic plan for each child. By *diagnosis* we do not mean providing a label for insurance forms, but rather a profile of the child's weaknesses and strengths, an understanding of his style of reaction and response to the environment, and an analysis of the noxious as well as growth-promoting factors in his family interactions. The therapeutic plan should include efforts to help the child and the family by all available means. The psychiatrist's continuous involvement is necessary to assure the overall integration of the treatment plan as well as to reassess the child's progress in view of the changes within the child and his needs in every stage of development.

In treatment of children with late-onset psychosis, major tranquilizers have proved to be quite beneficial in reducing hyperactivity, anxiety, and aggressiveness. For these children, the removal or reduction of the amount of stress at home and at school is the first therapeutic task. Placement in special classes in school, remedial help, and habilitative activities are necessary. Individual psychotherapy with these children should be reality-oriented. Some children spend an inordinate amount of time daydreaming and are at the mercy of their violent fantasies. While such fantasies are dynamically interesting, their verbal expression by the child and even the interpretive efforts of the therapist do not help the child to organize his thinking or to be rid of the overwhelming affect associated with them.

Autoaggressive behaviors, particularly in severely psychotic children, have proved extremely difficult to control. Chemotherapy, aversive conditioning, and repeated interruption of the activity with the aim of distracting the child from self-injury have all been tried. Operant conditioning has been used in an attempt to teach psychotic children self-care and simple communicative skill—with some encouraging results. However, the response to all these programs has shown their limited usefulness. Churchill (1969) summarized the effort of his group at behavior modification with severely psychotic children as follows: there is a low ability to respond even when the child is highly motivated; there is a certain inability to respond to a combination of stimuli, which may be caused by specific learning defects; and some attachment behavior toward some adults appears. The children were considered less psychotic by the staff when they were successful in performing tasks set by the therapist because they showed less withdrawal and fewer rituals. However, when the tasks became difficult, the rituals returned and the child's overall functioning became more disorganized.

Prognosis

Follow-up studies in different countries and by various authors have been in fairly good agreement as to the outcome of childhood psychosis. Of children with early-onset psychosis, those with signs of organicity have the poorest prognosis. These children do not seem to progress easily and at times lose some of their acquired skills and deteriorate. Their IQs show slow but progressive decrement and, finally, they become unmanageable except within the confines of an institution. About one-third to one-half of early-onset psychotics are part of this group.

Children who have some communicative language by the age of 5 have shown better prognosis, although even these children do not necessarily grow up without various degrees of maladjustment. In fact, only about one-sixth to less than one-third in various samples have been found to be fairly well-adjusted individuals. The remainder of the group are in need of lifelong psychiatric support, be it in the form of repeated hospitalizations or marginal outpatient adjustment. Bender has described some cases in which the individuals became inmates of correctional institutions because of their criminal acts. The outcome of childhood psychosis has not proved to be dependent on any particular therapeutic procedure. In a follow-up study of 63 psychotic children, Rutter *et al.* (1967) found four variables that seemed to be associated with the outcome: IQ, speech, schooling, and the severity of the illness. Children with higher IQs seemed to fare better in their ultimate social adjustment. While in some children with better-than-average IQs speech is delayed, it is generally observed that speech development and the amount of schooling that a child receives are closely associated with IQ. Either severely psychotic children are untestable or their illness has permeated all those functions that are measured by IQ tests.

While it is reasonable to assume that psychotic children coming from more disturbed and unstable families would contribute a large proportion to ranks of the maladapted individuals, no study has specifically tested this assumption, particularly since children coming from such families have a higher chance of being institutionalized in early life. In patients who have made marginal adjustments in adulthood, the psychiatric diagnosis of adult schizophrenia has been repeatedly made. However, the relationship between childhood and adult schizophrenia is far from being clarified.

13

Mental Retardation

Mental retardation is the current terminology of the nomenclature of the American Psychiatric Association (DMS II) and has replaced the previous designations of *mental deficiency*, *feeblemindedness*, and *mental subnormality*.

In their most recent manual on terminology and classification in mental retardation (Grossman, 1973), the American Association on Mental Deficiency gives the following definition: "Mental Retardation refers to significantly subaverage general intellectual functioning existing concurrently with deficits in adaptive behavior and manifested during developmental period." As can be noted, the above definition describes behavior and does not include any reference to etiology, pathogenicity, or the prognosis of the condition. Furthermore, in the new definition, as in all the previous ones, the scores on psychological tests of intelligence play a central role in the determination of mental retardation. The average intellectual functioning is the score obtained by 50% of a random population on IQ tests (usually the Stanford–Binet or the Wechsler Intelligence Scale for Children). The "subaverage" is defined as more than two standard deviations from the average norm. The standard deviation is 15 points on the WISC and 16 on the Stanford–Binet. "Adaptive behavior" includes level of communicative skill, competency in self-care, social interaction, play activities, and, later on, the rate and speed of academic learning and ability to make age-appropriate judgments as to safety standards and goal-directed behavior. The normative measures of "adaptive behavior," such as the Vineland Maturity Scale, are devised for younger children and therefore are applicable only when the retardate's mental age does not exceed 3–4 years. The level of competence and the deficiencies of "adaptive behavior" in an older child are impressionistically determined by the diagnostician. "Developmental period" is the period covering the span from birth to 18 years of age.

Classification. Based on IQ scores, mental retardation is classified into four categories:

	IQ Score on Stanford–Binet	IQ Score on WISC
Mild	52–67	55–69
Moderate	36–51	40–54
Severe	20–35	25–39
Profound	below 19	below 24

Children whose measured intelligence falls between 1 and 2 standard deviations (70–85 on WISC or 68–84 on Stanford–Binet) were formerly called *borderline retardates.* This designation has now been replaced by *borderline intelligence.*

Although there is no direct correspondence between the obtained IQ score and the underlying pathology causing the deficient intellectual functioning, in practice, the majority of children with mild and even moderate retardation do not exhibit identifiable organic pathology, while severe and profoundly retarded individuals are more likely to show signs of damage to the central nervous system. The heterogeneity of the retarded population necessitates a careful appraisal of each individual retarded patient, since conclusions and statements about mentally retarded children are generalized principles that may not apply to a particular child.

Epidemiology. It is estimated that about 3% of the population of the United States falls within the category of mental retardation. About 1% are diagnosed as retarded before school years. These are children whose retarded development is of such a degree that their developmental deviation is clear. The remainder of the group is identified during the first few years of school attendance. Mercer (1976) reported that in a Southern California community with a 130,000 mixed population of Hispanic and English background, the children who were identified and labeled as retardates during their school attendance showed low academic performance, poor adjustment, few social interactions, and low competence in English. However, some children, when tested, received the same low IQ score but had not been identified by the school. The members of this latter group were more easily manageable in the classroom, were liked by their peers, and could communicate in English. Therefore, the social designation and meaning of retardation, although overlapping with the clinical description of mental deficiency, is not identical with it.

ETIOLOGY

The most widely accepted definition of intelligence is the ability of an individual to find solutions for new problems by the process of reasoning based on his previous experiences. Successful problem solving depends on factors such as interest in the task, motivation for performance, accurate analysis of the task, availability of previous relevant experiences and strategies for problem solving, and, finally, the capacity to generalize and synthesize information.

Intelligent behavior can thus be viewed as the end product of organismic and environmental factors. The relative importance of each factor can be surmised only through the investigation of all relevant data for each individual. Our knowledge regarding the activities of the higher nervous system responsible for cognitive functioning is at an elementary stage. Nor have we managed to define all aspects of the environment that enhance or hinder the development of such functions. While it is logical to assume that genetic factors play a part in the makeup of the biochemical and structural aspects of the central nervous system, the statistical data based on those aspects of cognitive functioning that are assessed by IQ tests cannot be the sole criteria for the heritability of intelligence. Genetic factors responsible for the clinical manifestation of mental retardation must be clearly differentiated from the statistical data, which show that the majority of children with mild and moderate retardation come from the low socioeconomic and certain minority groups. In this class, the highest incidence of poor prenatal care, malnutrition, and ill health is combined with a myriad of other disadvantages associated with poverty that affect the integrity of the central nervous system and the quality and the quantity of the relevant experiential background of the child.

The overwhelming majority of children with moderate and mild mental retardation (70–80%) come from disadvantaged, multiproblem families. Although some may exhibit indications of general dysfunction of the central nervous system, the contribution of organic factors to the causation of mental subnormality in this group remains hypothetical. On the other hand, in a smaller but still significant number of patients, particularly those with severe and profound retardation, associative clinical findings are of such a nature that causative links may be surmised.

It must be stressed at the outset that the presence of medically identifiable causative factors does not negate the importance of the environmental contribution to the inadequate functioning of these children. On the contrary, treatment, education, and management strategies employed with mentally retarded children are all based on the assumption that environmental manipulation is an effective method of enhancing the functioning of mentally retarded individuals.

The causative factors associated with mental retardation are classified as follows:

- Genetic factors: These include the chromosomal defects as well as the defective genes reflected in various disorders of metabolism.
- Prenatal factors: These may be of a general nature, such as maternal malnutrition and toxemia of pregnancy, or the more specific illnesses due to viral infections.
- Intrapartum and neonatal factors: Difficulties due to the birth process or the immaturity of the fetus.
- Postnatal factors leading to damage to the central nervous system of the infant.

Chromosomal Abnormalities

Genetic aberrations due to chromosomal abnormalities may affect the sex or the somatic chromosomes. In general, abnormalities in sex chromosomes—such as Klinefelter's syndrome, with xxy or variations with xxxy or xxyy, or female gonadal dysgenesis (Turner's syndrome) with xo and numerous other combinations—are not invariably associated with mental retardation. Some children are reported to have normal to superior intelligence, while others have been noted to show inadequate intellectual ability.

Aberrations of autosomal chromosomes, on the other hand, are known to be associated with lower intellectual functioning. The most common and the best-known example of this group is Down's syndrome (mongolism).

Down's Syndrome. Down's syndrome was first described by the British physician Langdon Down in 1866. The report was based on the physical characteristics associated with mental subnormality. These children were called *mongoloid* because with their slanted eyes and flat nose, they resembled members of Mongolian tribes. The particular karyotype associated with Down's syndrome was first reported by Lejeune in 1959. The majority of patients with Down's syndrome have an extra chromosome in all their cells. This is called *trisomy 21*: instead of two chromosomes in Group 21, they have three chromosomes, resulting in a total of 47 instead of 46 chromosomes. Another group shows the trisomic picture in a variable proportion of the cells and is called *trisomy 21 with mosaicism*. At times, chromosome 21 is fused with another chromosome. This is called *translocation*. In this group, the total number of chromosomes is 46 or 45, and mosaicism may or may not be present. This kind of karyotype is usually inherited, so that translocation and mosaicism can be found in the karyotype of the parents.

The incidence of Down's syndrome in the United States is one in every 700 births. In mothers above age 35, the incidence increases to approximately 1 out of every 100 births. The risk for Down's syndrome in children is 1 out of every 3 births when parental translocation is present. Mental retardation of moderate to severe degree is one of the most important findings. Because of such distinguishing clinical characteristics as low nose bridge, slanting eyes, epicanthal folds, small head, protruding tongue, and general muscular hypotonia, the diagnosis can be made on clinical grounds alone. Special configurations of the palm and the sole and the chromosomal studies are used to verify the diagnosis. Patients with Down's syndrome comprise the most easily identifiable group of the mentally retarded and represent about 10% of the retarded population in residential care.

Other autosomal aberrations associated with mental retardation are less prevalent than Down's syndrome. Trisomy 13 is characterized by the presence of minor motor seizure and apneic spells. Trisomy 18 occurs more in females than in males and is believed to be associated with radiation to the gonads prior to conception. In *cri du chat*, severe retardation is accompanied by the characteristic cry during infancy, and the chromosomal picture reveals defects in the 5th chromosome.

Genetic Defects

Enzyme deficiency and metabolic disorders are usually caused by recessive inheritance. Parents are unaffected since each is heterozyotic for the defective gene, and only when the infant inherits the defective gene from both parents does the condition become clincally observable. The most well known example of this group is phenylketonuria.

Phenylketonuria (PKU). The disorder was first described by Fölling in 1934 as an example of inherited enzyme deficiency. The basic defect is absence or inactivity of the liver enzyme called phenylalanine hydroxylase, which is responsible for converting phenylalanine to tyrosine. In the absence of the enzyme, the level of phenylalanine in both blood and cerebrospinal fluid is elevated (10–25 times normal value), phenylalanine is excreted in urine (30–50 times normal value), and such abnormal metabolites as phenylpyruvic acid are found in the urine. Furthermore, the metabolism of other amines, such as tryptophan, tyrosine-melanine, epinephrine, norepinephrine, and serotonin, is disturbed. Deficiency in melanine in young children is responsible for the blue eyes and blond hair characteristically associated with phenylketonuria. While previously the disease was diagnosed on the basis of a urine test, recently the more reliable assay of phenylalanine in the blood is used as a screening test (Guthrie inhibition assay). Mandatory screening for newborn infants has been legislated in many states in this country.

PKU occurs in approximately one in every 10,000–15,000 live births. However, once a child with PKU is born to a family, the risk for having another child with PKU is one in every four successive pregnancies. The mass screening test has revealed that a larger proportion of the population are carriers of the recessive gene for phenylketonuria than had previously been thought. However, the disease can become clinically manifest only when two such individuals mate.

Infants with phenylketonuria may exhibit such clinical signs as eczema, vomiting, and a characteristic urine odor. Later on, untreated children manifest such symptoms as mental retardation of varying degrees, hyperactive and unpredictable behavior, and seizures and are commonly blue-eyed with blond hair. Infants who are placed on a special dietary regimen that excludes phenylalanine may show below-average to above-average intelligence, depending on the age at which the diagnosis was made and the success of dietary control. As a general rule, children who are diagnosed prior to 3 months of age and are maintained on good dietary control are more likely to have normal intelligence. Although the diet is not without danger of producing protein deficiency, at the present time it is the only effective treatment modality available. Genetic counseling of the parents is the logical preventive measure when a child with PKU is born or the couple are identified as carriers for PKU.

The list of disorders due to enzyme deficiency associated with mental retardation is a long one, and new entities are added to the list as new discoveries are made. Some children who in the past did not survive the first few months of life are now maintained on special diets that exclude the need for the absent enzyme. Galactosemia and maple syrup disease are other examples of this category (Crandall, 1977).

Prenatal Factors

Maternal health during pregnancy, general state of nutrition, and freedom from severe emotional stress are considered important for the overall development of the fetus. However, systematic research in this area is still sadly lacking, and only clinical impressions, unsupported by well-designed studies, can be reported. It has been known that chronic maternal illness such as hypertension, uncontrolled diabetes, and anemia, and the ingestion of drugs such as alcohol and narcotics will expose the unborn infant to noxious substances that may result in damage to the central nervous system. However, the causative role of such deleterious factors in mental retardation cannot be ascertained. On the other hand, the role of maternal viral infections in producing various fetal damage including mental retardation has been clinically verified. The type of viral infection, the severity of the illness, and the gestational age of the fetus are important variables as to the degree of damage done to the fetus as the result of maternal infection. A large number of infectious diseases of the mother have been tentatively associated with damage to the fetus. However, the two conditions in which high risk for mental retardation has been definitely established are maternal rubella and cytomegalic inclusion disease.

Maternal Rubella (German Measles). Maternal infection with rubella, particularly during the first trimester, has been shown to be associated with various congenital anomalies among children. The clinical manifestations of congenital rubella include low birth weight; eye lesions, such as cataracts, glaucoma, and blindness; deafness; cardiac defects; brain lesions associated with mental retardation; hydrocephalus; microcephaly; and meningoencephalitis.

Cytomegalic Inclusion Disease. This disorder remains dormant in the mother but gives rise to a variety of clinical symptoms in children. Some infants are stillborn. Others show jaundice, hepatosplenomegaly microcephaly, and radiographic findings of intracerebral calcification. Mental retardation may be associated with cerebral calcification and microcephaly or hydrocephalus. The presence of the virus in throat swabbings and urine, as well as the recovery of inclusion-bearing cells in the urine, affirms the diagnosis.

A variety of other viral and nonviral infections have been shown to present a risk to the unborn infant. Untreated syphilis, toxoplasmosis, and the arthropod-borne encephalitides have all been noted to infect the fetus and cause damage to the central nervous system.

Intrapartum and Neonatal Factors

When the birth process is prolonged, or bleeding due to placenta praevia or rupture of the umbilical cord deprives the infant of the normal supply of oxygen, the resultant damage to the central nervous system may lead to mental retardation. Uncommon fetal positions such as breech or transverse presentations, uterine anomalies, and deformities of the birth canal may all result in a prolonged period of anoxia, birth injury, and fetal distress. Such conditions are associated with various degrees of brain damage and may contribute to lower intellectual ability.

Immediately following birth, the newborn may be noted to suffer from anoxia, which will be reflected in a low Apgar score, or it will be observed to have developmental abnormalities of the brain or skull, such as hydrocephalus, porencephaly, and microcephaly. Mental retardation associated with such developmental abnormalities is usually of the severe type and is occasionally incompatible with life. Rh blood incompatibility causing jaundice and subsequent damage to the central nervous system is treatable with exchange transfusion. If untreated, mental retardation, cerebral palsy, hearing defect, and kernicterus may follow a hyperbilirubinemia of more than 20 mg/100 cc.

Postnatal Factors

Postnatal causes of brain damage that produce lower intellectual ability in children may be easily recognizable. Damage due to infection, trauma, poison, and endocrine and metabolic disorders are easy to diagnose, but unspecified factors such as general nutritional deficiency, sociocultural deprivation, and psychiatric disorders are also found in association with mental subnormality. Infection of the meninges due to hemophilus influenza, pneumococcus, meningococcus, or tuberculosis may leave irreversible damage causing severe to moderate mental retardation and other symptoms of neurological involvement. Disorders of metabolism of fat carbohydrates and amino acids are all diagnosed after birth. Some disorders such as Tay-Sachs disease, Gaucher's disease, and Neimann-Pick disease are not clinically demonstrable during early infancy and cause intellectual deterioration only after the neurons in the brain are destroyed by the storage of various lipid end products.

A major endocrine disease associated with mental retardation is hypothyroidism. The disease results from defective thyroid hormone. Clinical signs include lethargy, dry skin, coarse facial features, anemia, stunted growth, and weight gain. Diagnosis is verified by laboratory studies and signs of growth retardation in the skeletal system found in X rays of the wrist. If the diagnosis is made during the first few months of life and thyroid hormone replacement is prescribed, mental retardation can be prevented.

Chronic poisoning with lead may cause severe mental retardation because of cellular damage in the central nervous system. Poisoning with neurotropic agents is usually accidental, but it can lead to devastating consequences. Serious injuries to the brain also cause tissue destruction that may be extensive enough to cause mental retardation. Skull fracture and acute or chronic subdural hematoma may be the consequence of accidental traumas or may be associated with the battered-child syndrome. Destructive lesions due to neoplasm of the brain are fortunately uncommon during childhood years. However, abnormalities of the skull such as premature closure of the sutures (craniosynostosis) or obstructive hydrocephalus may cause pressure and atrophy of the cortex, resulting in mental retardation.

Psychiatric disorders of childhood may cause mental retardation or may be superimposed on or coexistent with lower intellectual functioning. Of children diagnosed as autistic or schizophrenic, a large percentage present defective intellectual ability on tests of intelligence. Some of these children show cognitive deficiencies only on the verbal portion of the IQ tests; others do poorly on tests of perceptual organization. Some researchers, such as Rutter (1971), believe the retardation to be independent of the autism; others, such as Kanner, view the uneven performance on IQ tests as a characteristic of early infantile autism.

The sociocultural factors associated with mental retardation have been the subject of numerous studies. Children of the lower socioeconomic class are disproportionately represented among the mentally retarded population. At the same time, the incidence of reproductive casualties such as prematurity, low birth weight, and paranatal complications is higher among members of this group. Furthermore, chronic ill health, poor nutrition, overcrowding, substandard housing, and finally poor schooling plagues these children during their postnatal period. The unenviable status of the "disadvantaged child" represents exposure to such deleterious factors as physical and emotional ill health in the parents, unavailability of caretakers because of alcohol and drug abuse, and over- or understimulation and general chaos resulting from the cumulative effects of deprivation. The known facts do not allow any conclusion to be drawn as to the relative importance of the various interrelated factors in the causation of mental retardation.

Pathological Findings

The mentally retarded population is not a homogeneous group, and pathological findings, as well as the psychological characteristics of each group of retarded individuals, may not be applicable to the entire population of retardates. Neurological examination in retarded children suffering from identifiable damage to the brain may reveal localized signs of pathology, while in the majority of these children only nonfocal generalized signs can be discerned. The EEG, except when seizure disorders are present, is not helpful in the diagnosis of mental retardation. Even in a condition such as PKU, in which about 80% of the patients show abnormal EEG, the abnormalities are nonspecific. Microscopic examination of the brain tissue may reveal a generalized decrease in the neural cells in the cortex and disorganization of the cortical structures. Or depending on the nature of the underlying disease, it may show a variety in disease-related pathology, for example, storage of the gangliosides in the cells in cerebromacular degeneration.

Psychopathological findings in mental retardation include various degrees of intellectual deficiency as measured by IQ tests. The severity of the retardation does not show a one-to-one correspondence with the causative factors of intellectual disability. However, in general, children with severe or profound retardation show evidence of organic damage to the central nervous system.

Some theorists believe that mentally retarded children are fundamentally different from their normal peers; others consider retardation to be a lag in cognitive development. The idea of qualitative similarity is stressed by Inhelder (1968), who has stated that severely retarded individuals do not progress beyond the sensorimotor stage in Piaget's theory (2 years), while the moderately retarded can be expected to achieve the stage of intuitive thoughts (5–6 years). The educable or mildly retarded individuals are arrested in the stage of concrete operation (11–12 years of age). Luria (1963), in reference to retarded children with clear indications of brain damage, stated that "The mentally retarded child is fundamentally different from his normal peers by the range of ideas he can comprehend and by the character of his perception of reality." Zigler (1973) considers the essential difference between mildly and moderately retarded children and their normal peers to be in the rate of cognitive development and the final stage achieved by the former. He has asserted that the lower-than-expected performance of the retarded child matched in mental age with normal children on various cognitive and learning tasks can be explained on the basis of motivational factors and failure orientation in the retarded group.

No one theory or combination of theories has been adequate in delineating the nature of cognitive impairment in mental retardation. Furthermore, very little attempt has been made to find a link between the psychological and the biological aspects of mental retardation. Only recently have some researchers tried to study the medical subgroups of mental retardation and attempted to correlate specific aspects of behavior with the known biological findings. O'Connor and

Hermelin (1961) compared mongoloid and nonmongoloid retardates of the same mental age on several cognitive tasks and concluded that mongoloids are poorer on tactile discrimination than nonmongoloids. Their skin conductance also proved inferior to other retardates and normals. However, these studies are still too sporadic and the number of subjects too small to prove any significant difference. Most researchers in the field of mental retardation have devised various tests that compare the functioning of retarded children with their normal peers of the same mental age. This invariably results in the comparison of younger normal children with older retardates. The possible effects of this difference in chronological age—be it enhancing or inhibiting in character—cannot be delineated. This factor is particularly important when the effects of environmental factors and expectation are considered. For example, if one is to assume with Zigler that the history of repeated failure plays a part in the test performance of the mentally retarded children, it is reasonable to assume that the older child has more cumulative experiences of failure than the younger one.

Cognitive Functioning

Studies of the cognitive functioning of the mentally retarded have for the most part used moderately to mildly retarded individuals as subjects. These investigations can be divided into several categories.

Language Behavior. The majority of investigators in the field of mental retardation have reported some deficits in the verbal production of mental retardates. These deficits have included a higher percentage of immature speech with misarticulation, a higher percentage of delayed language acquisition, and, in the profoundly retarded, a complete absence of speech. However, Wood (1960) found that in a large group of children with language delay, only 20% were mentally retarded. Furthermore, the incidence of hearing loss of various degrees among the retarded is much higher than in the general population (4–5% for public school students as opposed to 20–40% for institutionalized retardates). Therefore, the poor verbal production of retardates may be partially due to factors other than low cognitive functioning.

In the speech of mentally retarded children, sentences are shorter, vocabulary is more limited and repetitious, and syntax is inferior to what one expects of a normal child of the same age. Retarded children use fewer pronouns, verbs, and prepositions than their normal peers. Some theorists believe that inferior speech production is not the only defect in the linguistic behavior of retardates; rather, another important function of speech, which is the effective direction and control of behavior, is also impaired. Furthermore, according to Luria (1963), "The mental (semantic) associations of the mentally retarded child are much more spontaneous and primitive and develop on the basis of a vocabulary system which is much less stable." Milgram (1973) cautioned against equating language with cognitive functioning. Although language as a channel of communication can impart information and furnish ready symbols for abstraction, he believes that the ability of a child to decode and encode verbal communication and his level of intellectual functionings are two distinct areas. Even in the normal child, there is a lag between the child's ability to process nonverbal information and his ability to use language, although this is expected to disappear with age. This lag is even more pronounced in the retarded child. Therefore, language training alone is not sufficient since the basic deficit is in the cognitive area, and cognitive training should be provided along with language enrichment.

Learning. Laboratory studies have failed to show a slower rate of learning among moderately or mildly retardates than among normal children. However, when the tasks become complicated, there is a decrement in the performance of the retardates. Ross and Ross (1973) found that the IQ score is unrelated to simple conditioning, while in differential conditioning the performance of retardates is inferior to their mental-age–matched group. Ross and Ross believe that for classical conditioning to be used as a diagnostic test in the mentally retarded, parameters other than simple unconditioned stimuli and responses should be taken into consideration. For example, to make differentiation possible, the interval between two effective stimuli must be longer for retardates than is necessary for normal children. This may reflect the longer time for information processing needed by a retarded child.

Attention. Zeaman and House (1963) postulated that the retarded child attends to the wrong stimuli and that the "breadth of retardate's attention" is limited in that the retardate cannot use the redundant aspects of the stimuli in solving problems; that is, he cannot use incongruent elements in order to rule out certain classification. Zigler *et al.* (1968) believe that retarded individuals, having in the past failed in tasks too difficult for them, have come to rely on external cues and that the irrelevant nature of those external cues accounts, in part, for their poor performance. Routh (1973) postulated that retardates are unable to disengage their attention from irrelevant stimuli even when they are aware of their irrelevance. Other studies have shown that retarded noninstitutionalized children are inferior to their mental-age–matched normal peers in the number of relevant stimuli with which they can deal.

Memory. Studies by Spitz (1963) and others have shown that the immediate memory span of the retardate is shorter than that of normal children of the same age. While a nonretarded person can process 7 ± 2 bits of information over a short period of time, in mild retardates this capacity is only 4 ± 1 bits of information. According to Spitz, while the grouping of stimuli facilitates the task of memorizing for normal individuals (for example, seven-digit telephone numbers are grouped into three and four digits), retardates do not find it easier to memorize such a grouping. The nature of memory impairment in retardates is a subject of much speculation. Their short-term learning and extinction rate do not differ from those of normal children, but their long-term retention is inferior to that of their normal peers. Some researchers believe that retardates are deficient in the use of rehearsal strategy and that therefore what has been learned over a short span does not become a part of memory storage. Others postulate that this group has a rigid preference for old information, which they maintain in place of allowing the new material to be registered.

Thinking and Reasoning. Various tests have been devised to measure the effectiveness of cognitive strategies for problem solving. In tasks ranging from logical classification to problems relating to maintaining a spatial relationship after rotation, it has been shown that mental retardates' performance is lower than that of a mental-age–matched group. This has been taken to mean that mental age does not accurately represent the developmental status of the mentally retarded and that there are generalized deficits in the reasoning and the cognitive functioning of the mentally retarded children.

Motivation. Zigler (1973) believes that the performance of the mentally retarded cannot be judged without a consideration of the life history of the retarded individual. He stated that one of the characteristics of the problem-solving strategy of the mentally retarded is his outer-directedness. Because of lifelong experience with failure, he has come to mistrust his own judgment and is engaged in seeking helpful cues from the environment. This factor accounts for what is considered his attention to irrelevant stimuli and his distractability, as well as for the greater suggestibility of the mentally retarded. He further pointed out that the retarded individual's ability to work for an inordinately long time on boring and monotonous tasks is a function of the individual's preferring to avoid failure and his pleasure in cognitive mastery. Zigler's view regarding the effects of motivational and personality factors on the performance of the mentally retarded has shed some light on the contradictory findings among the various institutionalized and noninstitutionalized groups and the problems related to their social and vocational adjustment.

Personality Development and Behavioral Disorders. The mentally retarded child is not impervious to those factors that influence the personality development of intellectually normal children. Adverse environmental and attitudinal factors may indeed have a more deleterious effect on a retarded child, who is, to a greater degree and for a longer period of time, dependent on his caretakers and also less capable of analyzing and synthesizing his experiences. The temperamental quality of the retarded child in interaction with his environment can create the same range of personality types as in the general population.

Even severely retarded children can develop some capacity for normal interpersonal interactions within the limits of their cognitive ability. However, the mentally retarded child faces more hazards in achieving emotional growth because of factors related to his slow rate of development, difficulties associated with possible central nervous system damage, and parental rejection or overprotection. Furthermore, the retarded child does not have the same opportunities for socialization as his normal peers. His tolerance for anxiety and frustration is lower than would be expected of his chronological age, and because of his frequent failure, his self-evaluation is unfavorable. These factors, if not taken into consideration is rearing a mentally retarded child, may result in various behavioral disorders. As the child grows older, his school experience can be rewarding or frustrating. Later on, not only peer relations but relationships with authorities and co-workers are new sources of emotional conflict or emotional support.

Various studies have shown a higher incidence of psychiatric disorders among the mentally retarded, although most of these studies have been carried out among institutionalized retardates and do not represent the risk of emotional disorder in the retarded population. In a sample of 100 consecutive admissions to the Mental Retardation Training Program of the Langley Porter Neuropsychiatric Institute, Philips and Williams (1975) found only 13 children who did not suffer from emotional disorder; 38 children were diagnosed as psychotic and 49 had various symptoms of neurotic or behavioral problems. In the nonpsychotic group, disturbed social relationships, aggressive behavior, and school problems comprised the majority of presenting complaints. The nature of the behavioral difficulties did not differ from those found among the nonretarded population referred to the clinic. The psychotic group were younger at the time of first referral, and their symptomatology included disorganized behavior, self-abusive and uncontrolled temper tantrums, and varying degrees of disturbed communication.

In a group of 616 children from the ages of 7 days to 8 years evaluated at the Mental Retardation Clinic of the Nebraska Psychiatric Institute, Menolascino (1969) reported that 191 were psychiatrically disturbed. Of this group, 151 children showed both mental retardation and emotional disorder. Furthermore, it was noted that among children in whom the cause of mental retardation was unknown and uncertain, emotional disturbances were more prevalent. Psychiatric symptoms manifested by the severely retarded group included a high frequency of primitive disorganized behavior, while the moderately retarded showed hyperactive, impulsive behavior. The mildly retarded children were characterized by neurotic symptomatology and depression.

Psychosis in severely retarded children may be caused by the underlying pathology of the central nervous system. Functional psychoses such as schizophrenia have been reported to develop in children with Down's syndrome. However, because the peculiarities of cognitive functioning in the mentally retarded and the overwhelming reliance on thinking disorder for the diagnosis of schizophrenia, the differential diagnosis between organic and functional psychosis may be quite difficult.

Diagnostic Evaluation

As is the case with all psychiatric evaluation of children, the clinician's direct observation and assessment of the child must be supplemented by information obtained from the family, the school, the pediatrician, and all other appropriate sources. Detailed questioning of the parents or other caretakers is necessary if one is to evaluate the child's level of competence and the degree and nature of impairment in his adaptive behavior. A behavioral profile of the child must include information regarding his interpersonal relationships; the extent of his contact outside his immediate family; possible factors responsible for his isolation or acceptance by other children and adults; the degree to which the parents can rely on him to perform age-appropriate tasks relating to his personal care and safety; and the explicit and implicit rejection, hostility, acceptance, and protection that he is receiving from his siblings (Szymanski, 1977).

The data regarding parents' attitudes toward the mentally retarded child may come from inferences made by an astute clinician or may be directly expressed by each parent. The emotional atmosphere of the home may be surmised by the manner in which parental accounts of the child's behavior or reports of their own child-rearing practices are or are not in accord with each other. Some parents are eager to focus attention on the shortcomings and the temperamental or personality characteristics of their spouses as the alleged cause of the child's behavioral difficulties. Others are ready to take the blame on themselves and thereby disqualify themselves as appropriate caretakers for the child. An assessment must be made as to whether the emotional outpourings of the parents are reactions to the interview situation and without serious consequences for the child's daily life or are disguised messages of rejection of the child stated at the outset to alert the psychiatrist that the family is seeking an expert opinion in order to bow out of its responsibilities toward a deviant member.

The history of mental retardation or other developmental disabilities in close relatives and sibs must be investigated as to the possible genetic or familial causes of retardation and the need for further studies and counseling for the affected members. Inquiries into prenatal, paranatal, and postnatal hazards are important as the physician attempts to establish a probable etiology and to alleviate the family's apprehension about the risk of retardation in future generations. The child's developmental history may give valuable clues as to the nature of deleterious influences on development, rates of acquisition of various skills, and regressions.

Physical examination includes a search for the various stigmata associated with some forms of mental retardation, such as low-set ears, hypertelorism, and epicanthal folds. The measurement of the various indices of physical growth, such as head circumference, height, and weight, are necessary, as is a neurological examination and assessment of the sensory systems. Pathological findings in other systems may or may not be directly related to mental retardation; however, any sign of ill health must be noted, since the evaluation of retarded status and treatment of the child as a person are indivisible.

Specific laboratory investigation in mental retardation is somewhat more extensive than in other psychiatric disorders of childhood. Apart from conditions that may necessiate surgical or medical treatment, such as hypothyroidism or chronic subdural hematoma, the identifiable organic causes of mental retardation, even when not treatable, may require genetic counseling. Chromosomal studies, screening tests for aminoaciduria, skull X ray, and EEG are among the laboratory tests most commonly obtained when clinical indications point toward particular etiologies. Audiological studies are of particular value when deviation in language development is not accounted for by general retardation in cognitive functioning.

Psychological Testing. Because measured intelligence on standardized tests comprises such an important part of the diagnosis of mental retardation, the child psychiatrist must be familiar with the basic procedures by which the level of intellectual functioning is determined and the validity and reliability of the test scores.

During the first two years of life, the tests used are scales of development. They provide the examiner with a systematic observation of the developmental status and the presence or absence of physical and sensory handicaps, which may or may not retard the subsequent development of the child. When the infant's developmental quotient (DQ) is sufficiently below the expected level for his age, a three- to six-month follow-up and reassessment are necessary in order to ensure that developmental deviations do not go unnoticed and appropriate corrective measures are not postponed.

The intelligence quotient, as measured by standardized tests, has certain implications in terms of the child's overall functioning that must be understood by the child psychiatrist and conveyed to parents. Furthermore, the psychologist assessing the "measured intelligence" also observes and evaluates some aspects of the child's adaptive behavior, emotional state, and personality characteristics, and it is the task of the child psychiatrist to integrate data obtained from all other sources and devise a treatment strategy based on such information. For example, while a child with an IQ of 51–70 is expected to be able to reach a certain level of competence compatible with independent life in society, lack of a supportive family, lack of educational and vocational opportunities within the community, and certain behavioral problems may lead to the early institutionalization of such a patient. On the other hand, a severely retarded child may be cared for by parents when their expectation of the child's optimum functioning is not significantly different from the child's capability. Such assessment and interpretation cannot be based on IQ alone, although the test scores provide a valuable predictor of the child's optimum level of achievement (Zigler and Balla, 1977).

Clinical Interview. Psychiatric observation of a mentally retarded child must provide information and impressions about the patient's relatedness to the examiner, his level of competence in play, his breadth of interest and curiosity regarding his surroundings, and his predominant mood and activity level. The child's willingness to imitate the examiner's activities upon request, his approach to problem solving, the appropriateness of his requests for help, and the ease with which he can be persuaded to change activities or the amount of perseverance that he exhibits are important characteristics that are of crucial relevance to his adjustment. Verbal interaction with a retarded child may be limited by the child's underdeveloped speech or his reluctance to engage in conversation. The examiner's speech must of necessity be kept simple, concrete, and within the child's level of comprehension. Information regarding the child's interpersonal conflicts, his self-evaluation, and his fantasy life can be obtained through the child's graphic production and comments solicited from him about his wishes, hopes, and expectations of the future. Impulsivity, timidness, easy discouragement, low frustration tolerance, unusual fears, or primitive and disorganized behavior are all observable phenomena when the child psychiatrist allows enough time for clinical evaluation; if need be, the child can be observed over an extended period of time.

Treatment

The medical treatment of mental retardation can be best described in terms of the concepts of preventive medicine, that is, primary, secondary, and tertiary prevention.

Primary Prevention. Primary prevention includes those measures that will reduce or eliminate the causative factors. These include such broad public health policies as the provision of maternal and infant care and the eradication of diseases that can cause pre- or postnatal damage to the central nervous system. The identification of genetic disorders and proper genetic counseling are also effective methods of combating mental retardation. Continuous public education is necessary in order to maximize the use of health care facilities and to implement newly acquired knowledge in every area of preventive medicine. Supplementary care and early enrichment programs minimize the impact of parental limitations as primary caretakers and the deleterious consequences of the low socioeconomic status of the parents on their children.

Second and Tertiary Prevention. The early identification and appropriate treatment of such remediable conditions as PKU and hypothyroidism will limit or eliminate the risk for low intellectual functioning in later life. Prompt therapeutic intervention in a variety of diseases of early childhood, such as lead poisoning or posttraumatic subdural hematoma, decreases the likelihood of a chronic damaging influence on the brain. The early diagnosis and correction of sensory defects maximize the child's opportunities for receiving appropriate amounts of environmental stimuli and thus prevent retardation due to experiential deficiencies.

When mental retardation is suspected, the task of the treating physician is to devise a management strategy that includes the elimination of factors that impede the child's chances of utilizing his capacities, as well as providing guidance as to the type of educational facilities that may best serve the child in his quest for mastery over his environment.

It has been frequently noted that emotional and behavioral disorders impair the individual's capacity for optimum functioning. Mentally retarded children are no exception to this general rule, and, in fact, because of their limited resources, they are less able to afford the heavy toll extracted by such added burdens. While all appropriate modalities of psychiatric treatment may be employed to help a retarded child, those methods that are heavily dependent on verbalization and abstract conceptualization do not provide the main strategy for treatment. Play therapy and an opportunity for group interaction and socialization help the child to reveal his internalized conflicts and give him an opportunity to receive clarification and sympathetic understanding from the therapist. Behavioral modification methods may be extremely effective in changing the child's maladaptive behavior and teaching him alternative means of response. Chemotherapy, when appropriately used, may help in curtailing the child's level of anxiety and in combating his depressed mood or hyperactive and impulsive behavior.

The family of the mentally retarded child is in need of special consideration, since it is the family that provide for or fail to support the special needs of a retarded child. The informing interview with the parents may not answer all parental concerns and questions regarding the diagnosis and its implications. Most parents are so distraught when their own fears, apprehension, and insights are confirmed by the opinion of the expert that they cannot be expected to remain goal-oriented and to focus their attention on the detailed explanations of the child psychiatrist during the first interview. They must be given time and repeated opportunities to express their feelings of distress, guilt, despair, and rejection in response to the diagnosis before they can formulate their questions regarding the child's future. Parental questions regarding etiology and the implications for future pregnancies must be answered on the basis of current medical information and knowledge, and recommendations should be given for a further medical workup based on the factors that have been identified as possible causes.

The designation of the level and severity of retardation on the basis of "measured intelligence" does not provide the necessary information for the parents, who need to plan for the child's future. The diagnosis must be explained on the basis of the optimal level of education and self-sufficiency that the child is expected to achieve. Factors that may impede or enhance the child's use of his intellectual abilities must be reviewed. Children with mild retardation may be expected to learn to read and write and do simple computation. This obviously excludes any possibility of their obtaining a high school diploma and limits their future employment opportunities. Moderately retarded children are even less capable of learning academic skills. Furthermore, their limited judgment requires that their routine jobs be under close supervision. Severely retarded children can be expected at best to achieve independence in regard to their own personal care and are in need of lifelong support and care. Profoundly retarded individuals are totally dependent on their caretakers and may be inmates of institutions for life.

Parental questions and concerns, as well as the child's behavioral and emotional status, undergo various changes because of factors within the child, the family, and the community. Younger normal siblings soon outstrip the retarded child in competence and social awareness, and their attitudes toward the retarded member of the family may become rejective and hostile or accepting and protective. They may need assurances and understanding along with their parents. The service of a family counselor may be needed on a long-term basis to provide guidance and support for all members of a family with a retarded child.

A crisis situation may arise when the family is no longer able to provide care for the child, when the child's behavior becomes dangerous to his own safety or the safety of others, or when he becomes unacceptable to the community because of his behavior. Decisions regarding long-term or short-term institutionalization may have to be made based on the support system available to the family, as well as on the supportability of the child's behavior in the community. In making such decisions, families are in need of information about and an evaluation of the consequences of institutionalization, as well as clarification of their own feelings toward the child. The retardate himself, even when not emotionally disturbed, may need counseling and guidance about his own personal concerns and desires at various points during his life. The child psychiatrist must advise the family regarding all these eventualities where counseling services are not available in the community or must provide them with information regarding such services for the retardate.

Education. The history of educational attempts in the rehabilitation of retarded children begins with Itard, who in the beginning of the 19th century dedicated five years of intense effort to educating the "wild boy of Aveyron." Edward Seguin, a student of Itard's, later came to the United States and pioneered educational programs for the retarded. Maria Montessori in Italy considered mental deficiency an educational problem and developed methods to strengthen children's sensory and motor abilities. Present educational programs for retarded children are based on these earlier insights and on principles borrowed from learning theory, psychiatry, and education.

Special education for the retarded has undergone numerous changes during the 20th century. Special classes within the public school system have replaced the larger institutions that were entrusted with the education of retardates. Preschool programs are designed to provide enriched experiences for children between 3 and 6 years of age. Classes in the elementary school typically enroll children from 6 to 13. In these classes, the retarded child is expected to learn basic academic skills, while secondary school programs have the ultimate goal of leading adolescents into vocational placement. Services such as speech therapy and language training are offered as part of preschool and elementary school education.

While with better facilities for treatment, education, and rehabilitation the majority of retarded children can remain in their own homes or be placed in foster homes, there remains a group of profoundly retarded patients and those with severe behavioral problems who are in need of long-term institutional care. The goal of the treatment and education in these institutions is to help the retardate achieve the highest possible degree of self-sufficiency and independence.

14

Learning Disabilities

The literature on learning disorders contains a variety of definitions and terminologies. Some writers, such as Silver and Hagin (1964), have described reading retardation as a reading level one year or more below the expected grade placement of a child with average intelligence. Rabinovitch (1959), on the other hand, defined reading retardation as a reading level two or more years below the child's mental age as obtained by performance scores on the IQ test. This reliance on the performance score on the IQ test indicates the author's belief that the verbal scores on IQ tests are significantly affected by the child's school achievement, and specifically his proficiency in reading. The incidence of reading retardation among school-age children also varies in different reports. Most authors believe that about 10% of school-children are retarded in reading.

Reading Retardation

Backwardness in reading is the end product of a number of different processes. Learning to read is a highly complex task, which, like all other learning, is dependent upon organismic and environmental factors. Among the important environmental factors are such things as the availability of the relevant stimuli under optimal conditions, for example, appropriate teaching techniques, effective teachers, and opportunities for individual interaction between teacher and pupils. Overcrowded classrooms with high noise levels and continuous disruptions are not conducive to learning even when the child is highly motivated to learn. On the organismic level, freedom from anxiety and other unpleasant feelings, such as hunger, ill health, depression, and anger, is a prerequisite for a child's attention to the learning task.

The term *reading readiness* refers to a variety of physiological and psychological states, the nature of which is not clearly defined. The age at which instruction in reading should begin is a matter of controversy. Some authors, such as Bender (1957), state that teaching at an early age, before 5 years, could be detrimental to the child's later progress, while others consider the age for reading readiness to be influenced by such factors as social class and the previous verbal stimulation at home. Children of the lower socioeconomic class may show less evidence of reading readiness as compared to their age mates of middle-class background because of their impoverished experiential history or their lack of a scholastic-oriented value system.

Reading requires the visual discrimination and recognition of the letter symbols and the translation of the visual configurations of the words into phonemes that are meaningful auditory stimuli for the individual. Furthermore, this information has to be stored and retrieved audiovisually for reading to be mastered. Visual analysis, visual memory, and visual synthesis are necessary parts of the reading process. Similar phenomena are involved in the reproduction of the phonemes: besides the individual sound of each letter, the temporal sequence of the sounds and the rules of the blending of sounds must be associated with visual configurations and stored in the memory. In addition, sight and sound pairing should produce words that are meaningful in the context of the child's language milieu. Any disturbance in one or several areas in this chain could result in reading retardation or reading disability.

Since achievement in school is the highly valued cultural task of a child in all industrialized societies, psychological reactions to underachievement are an important part of the clinical picture of reading retardation. At times, children are referred to child psychiatrists with behavioral problems ranging from school phobia to fighting and disruptive behavior. Clinical evaluation reveals a child with a severe reading disability who has resorted to avoidance, denial, and defiance in reaction to his own functional backwardness in school.

Children with reading retardation are by no means a homogeneous group. Reading retardation has been divided into several groups, although, as will be noted later, there is considerable overlap between various groups, and cases of pure clinical forms are uncommon.

Psychological Factors. Lack of motivation to learn may be due to devaluation of learning by parents or other significant adults in the child's immediate environment. In subcultures in which the obligatory nature of schooling is actively resented, parents may convey their lack of interest in or outright hostility toward the educational system to their children, and the children in turn may view school learning as contrary to their parents' wishes.

For some children, fear of failure and an obsessional desire for perfection may act as an emotional block against learning. Various anxieties and worries can also weigh heavily upon a child and divert his attention from the task of learning. Emotional conflicts related to the child's identification, or rivalry, with a sib or parent could result in a neurotic avoidance of learning to read. In these children, reading has acquired a personalized neurotic meaning and is looked upon as an activity with deep emotional significance. Some writers in the psychoanalytic field consider neurotic conflicts to be the cause of reading disability in as many as 20% of children with reading retardation; other workers have found little evidence to support such a view. De Hirsh (1974) stated that "neurosis in children with neurogenic learning disabilities may be part of the biologic dysfunction." According to this view, the neurotic conflict surrounding learning to read may stem from the child's denial of his inability to master a task and his subsequent rationalization and devaluation of reading. In psychotic children, reading disability may be the result of the child's withdrawal from his environment, his preoccupation with internal stimuli, his inability to focus and maintain his attention on any external happenings, or his inability to organize and pattern his perceptions. In those children in whom psychosis is associated with various signs of organic deficits, these deficits could, in and of themselves, account for the inability to learn to read.

Unless it can be shown clearly and logically that psychological factors have resulted in reading retardation and that the process by which reading has been thus affected can be delineated, reading retardation must always be considered an independent symptom in a clinical picture and must be diligently investigated. Recently researchers have become interested in those psychological variables that influence the child's strategies in intentional learning, such as selective attention, memory development, and expanding awareness of one's own cognitive processes (Mackworth, 1973; Torgensen, 1977).

Environmental Factors. A significant number of children attending schools in the slums of large cities are educationally backward. This backwardness is manifested particularly in their low level of achievement in reading when they are compared with students from suburban schools. Aside from the high incidence of undiagnosed neurological defects, chronic subclinical malnutrition, and other consequences of ill health, these children are experientially ill-equipped for the variety of demands that school entrance places upon them. Even when children speak the standard language of society, their language production and facility to manipulate verbal symbols is less advanced than those of their middle-class peers. Furthermore, in some children, chaotic and highly unstable home environments have resulted in what could be called *protective inattention*. In some families, the sense of despair and helplessness in the parents produces the feeling that school learning will not help their situation, and the parents give the child no active encouragement to perform academically. Other parents view the school establishment as another symbol of oppression by the majority and do not provide the necessary guidelines for conforming with the demands that school attendance places upon their children. In some ethnic groups, the emphasis in child rearing is more on social relations than on task performance. For these children, the impersonal atmosphere of large classrooms and the paucity of interaction with teachers act as a hindrance to effective learning.

The techniques of instruction in reading reflect the dominant belief of educators at any given time and place. In large classrooms, only those children who can benefit from a particular technique are receiving adequate and relevant instruction; the child who is weak in the prevalent perceptual modality will remain confused and illiterate. Orton (1937) estimated that children who were at that time predominantly taught by the sight-reading method showed three times as many reading problems as those who were taught by phonetic techniques.

Neurological Factors. Pre- or postnatal insult to the brain causes a generalized, nonspecific dysfunction that is clinically manifested by hyper- or hypoactivity, impulsivity, attentional disturbance, and a high vulnerability to anxiety. On psychological tests, these children may demonstrate disturbances in visual and/or auditory memory, lag in the acquisition of concepts, difficulty in differentiating figures from the background, distorted body image, problems with spatial orientation, and confusion in directionality. Reading retardation in these children is due to combinations of these factors. Short attention span and hyperactivity limit the amount of instruction available to the child, while perceptual problems destroy the quality of the stimuli, and the high anxiety level caused by the child's uneasy interaction with the environment produces further disorganization.

These children usually have a history of difficult birth or complicated pregnancy. Clinically some evidence of brain dysfunction, such as poor motor coordination, asymmetric reflexes, uncertain dominance, and other nonfocal neurological signs, can be elicited. The electroencephalogram may be abnormal in a large proportion of these children. On the Bender–Gestalt test, these children frequently draw primitive "fluid" forms, dots are replaced by loops, the squared figures are "rounded," the horizontal forms are "verticalized," and open figures are closed. Five types of distortion by these children on the Bender test have been described: angulation, rotation, primitivation, separation, and slant. These anomalies are particularly seen in the younger age groups. During adolescence, most of these signs have disappeared or have been compensated for, and reading retardation and the psychological reactions to it dominate the picture. These children may be truant from school, may engage in group delinquency, and may drop out of the educational system completely. Their attitude, hardened by years of failure, is that of underlying depression and helplessness, with a facade of noncaring and hostility toward any societal goal. Even those children who have received appropriate help during the early years and have been raised in supportive and accepting families will remain partially handicapped, in that reading is a slow, laborious process, more dependent on sounding individual words than on the more efficient visual scanning method.

Reading Disability

The Research Group on Developmental Dyslexia of the World Federation of Neurology has defined this condition as "A disorder manifested by difficulty in learning to read despite conventional instruction, adequate intelligence, and sociocultural opportunity. It is dependent upon fundamental cognitive disabilities which are frequently of constitutional origin."

The term *dyslexia* was first used in reference to those patients who lose their ability to read as the result of a specific injury to the brain in the parietal or occipital region. In these patients, dyslexia is associated with a variety of other conceptual deficits, such as impaired spatial orientation and difficulty in sorting colors and naming objects. The patient may be able to read and understand silently, with only oral reading being impaired.

In developmental dyslexia, on the other hand, the reading skill is not learned and there is no dissociation between reading, writing, and spelling. Form perception may be impaired even for nonsymbolic and nonlinguistic visual stimuli. The child may have difficulty in learning math and musical notations or other scientific formulas. On nonverbal tests for visual perception, the performance of the child in areas such as recognition of similarities and differences in pictures and abstract designs or recognition of incomplete pictures may be below what is expected of his general intellectual level. These children either fail to recognize the significance of the visual configuration of the letters (word blindness), or they do not retain the overall visual gestalt of a series of letters in a meaningful sequence that comprises a word (deficit of visual memory). Therefore they fail to learn to read by the visual scanning that is characteristic of the mature reader. Spelling and writing, which are the reproductions of the visual memory of the words, also manifest this fundamental impairment.

Developmental dyslexia has been reported from all Western countries. Critchley (1970) believes that dyslexics are more easily identifiable in English-speaking countries because of the particular character of the English language. Among Japanese children, dyslexia is more distinguishable in Kana script, which is phonetic script, than in the ideographic symbols of the Kanji script, which is of Chinese origin. The instruction technique of sight reading leads to earlier recognition of dyslexia than the synthetic methods, whether phonic or syllabic.

The incidence of specific reading disability or developmental dyslexia is not known. Boys show a higher proportion of dyslexia than girls, and there are indications that among the families of dyslexic children, there is a higher incidence of language disorders and reading disabilities. Mixed dominance is a relatively frequent finding among dyslexics. Refractive errors do not cause dyslexia; rather, faulty eye movements and difficulty in binocular coordination may be the outcome of the reading difficulty. In those children who show choreiform movements of the small muscles of the tongue, face, neck, and eye, the reading difficulty is a part of minimal brain dysfunction. Disorders of articulation are not associated with reading disability, although the child may exhibit other disorders of language development (developmental aphasia) (Thompson, 1973; Witelson, 1977).

Clinical picture. Although dyslexia can occur in children of any level of intellectual functioning, the dyslexic child is frequently of above-average intelligence. Mistakes in oral reading include:

- Incorrect pronunciation of vowels, such as *big* for *bag* or *cat* for *cut*.
- Incorrect pronunciation of consonants, such as *sad* for *sat*.
- Interpolation of inappropriate phonemes, such as *trick* for *tick*.
- A tendency to guess wildly at the phonic structure of an unfamiliar word.
- An inability to differentiate between the auditory properties of letters or words, such as *bat* for *but* or *blud* for *blood*.
- A confusion of words with minor differences in configuration, such as *quiet* and *quite*.
- Reversal of letters or whole words, such as *big* for *dig* or *saw* for *was*.

- Confusion and reversal of concepts, such as *stop* for *go* and *up* for *down*.

The performance of the dyslexic child shows variability from one occasion to the next. When reading a subject of interest to him, the child may achieve a higher score for accuracy than when he is performing on a test. His performance tends to deteriorate as he becomes fatigued or his attention is distracted. In writing, these children show poor handwriting, produce malformed letters, and omit or add letters to words. Capital letters are found in the middle of a word, letters are malaligned or rotated, and the serial order of the letters is confused, as in *nto* for *not*. Reading is a laborious and slow process, and writing is the outcome of successions of guesswork and mistakes, so that these children are not able to read their own writing. Their spelling mistakes are not consistent, and a child may make different mistakes in writing the same word at different times. Some children are able to do calculation in their heads but cannot perform the same process on paper. Their comprehension of reading materials may be below age level because of their poor memory for the serial order of the spoken words or their inability to differentiate various sounds.

In extreme cases of dyslexia, the child is painfully aware of his inabilities and tries to compensate for them by various means. Some children try to uncover some rules of pronunciation or spelling and generalize these rules in order to assure some degree of accuracy in their performance. Others find themselves overwhelmed with their handicap and engage in protective withdrawal. In all cases, the child is depressed and has low self-esteem. This is particularly true in those children whose high intelligence leads to critical self-evaluation and comparison with their peers. When the child's problem has not been recognized, his teachers and his parents become frustrated by his lack of motivation, and his inability is taken as unwillingness to perform. This negative environmental attitude is accepted by the child and further lowers his self-regard, with resultant feelings of unworthiness and hopelessness. At times, the obvious psychological and emotional problems of the dyslexic child are made the focus of attention, and years of psychotherapy are embarked upon in order to remove the "reading block," only to the detriment of the child's early diagnosis and appropriate corrective measures.

Etiology. The cause and the basic defect in developmental dyslexia are unknown. Various authors have described the deficits and disturbances encountered in the functioning of dyslexic children, and efforts have been made to hypothesize about the nature of the central nervous system dysfunction in dyslexia. Orton (1937) postulated a developmental lag in the areas of the brain responsible for the acquisition and maintenance of reading and writing skills and their association as the cause of the dyslexic syndrome. The concept of developmental lag indicates the author's belief or expectation that the deficits will disappear as the individual matures; however, it must be noted that such disappearance is not the rule and that some functional deficits are not compensated for. The circumstances leading to the lag in development and their persistence into adulthood are not clear. According to Cruickshank (1977), "Learning disability, specifically defined, is a manifestation of a perceptual processing deficit." These deficits are of a varied nature and may include one or more sensory modalities. They may reflect inadequacies in such areas as recognition of subtle differences between the auditory and visual features of written symbols, retention or recall of these discriminating features, and difficulty in the sequential ordering of sounds and orthographic forms.

Among the basic deficiencies of functioning found in dyslexic children, the following are most prevalent:

- Inability to use forms and sounds as symbols with meaning.
- Language deficits such as imprecise articulation and primitive syntax.
- Difficulty in translating perceptions into symbols; for example, a child knows which of the two persons in front of him is taller but cannot translate this perception into units of measurement.
- Problems with body image.
- Problems with directionality and three-dimensional spatial relationships.
- Poor visual memory for forms.
- Poor auditory discrimination and auditory sequencing.

It must be emphasized that not all children who show poor directionality or some backwardness in visual–motor skill present a dyslexic picture. In the diagnosis of reading disability, it is necessary to map each individual child's cognitive and perceptual weaknesses and strengths. In the present state of knowledge, such a map is needed in order to provide a rational strategy for treatment.

Treatment. In recent years, a variety of programs have been devised to identify those children who might develop reading difficulties in later years and to provide practices that are believed to correct faulty habits and perceptual deficiencies. Difficulties in left and right orientation and motor problems have been particularly stressed. Some researchers have reported a high degree of success with early preventive measures. Early enrichment programs in language development and concept formation could theoretically help eliminate some deficits in the background of those children who have not achieved reading readiness by the time they enter school. In children with minimal brain dysfunction, high activity level and disturbances of attention can be alleviated or minimized by medication, and chemotherapy can supplement other special programs for helping these children. Children who suffer from psychiatric conditions that interfere with their learning need appropriate psychiatric treatment along with remedial schedules.

In primary dyslexia, as well as in those children in whom dyslexia could be said to result from neurologic damage, the program of instruction must consist of two basic strategies. First, the child's preferred sensory pathway must be strengthened. And second, the necessary practice must be provided to link the weak pathway with the stronger ones by the simultaneous use of several pathways (such as auditory, visual, and tactile). In such a program, the child is taught to differentiate between auditory stimuli and to blend the sounds of the individual letters in order to obtain a phoneme. This strategy uses the child's auditory memory in order to compensate for his poor visual memory, so that the child first begins to read by sounding out each word. Even though such a child will be a slow reader, he will still acquire enough skill to decode the written language. For some children, flash cards may help to make each letter, and then each word, stand alone without interference from other visual symbols for better registration in visual memory. Tactile manipulation of letters and numbers can strengthen poor auditory and/or visual memory. If the information is received via several pathways—pictures, gestures, and presentation of objects—the visual memory of a word and later on of each sentence is reinforced. All techniques for getting the child to attend to stimuli, be they visual or auditory, are helpful in learning. Supportive psychotherapy is needed to overcome the child's reluctance to engage in an activity in which he has failed on numerous previous occasions and to maintain his motivation in the face of the slowness of the learning process.

The prognosis in all types of learning disabilities depends upon the time of the diagnosis, the thoroughness with which all the pertinent factors have been identified, and finally, the appropriateness of the remedial program, In general, children who have been identified in the early years of their schooling respond more favorably to programs of intervention. Sometimes, after years of persistent effort and slow learning the dyslexic child seems abruptly to gain an insight into the whole process and becomes a proficient reader within a short period of time.

15

Disorders of Language Development

Speech Lag

Children with average intelligence and without any auditory defects are expected to have a small vocabulary of 15–20 meaningful words by 18–20 months of age. By 2 years, most normal children can and do communicate their needs and wants. Speech development occurs earlier in girls than in boys, although boys show a greater rate of progress later on and catch up with the girls. Physical maturation influences language development by providing the child with a variety of experiences that stimulate his desire and ability to talk. Furthermore, fine motor coordination of the muscles of articulation is a prerequisite for speech development. The emotional atmosphere of the home and the amount of verbal interaction between the parents and the child and the child and his sibs are all instrumental in the child's rate of language acquisition and ability to communicate. The impersonal exposure to the language emanating from communications media such as television and radio has not proved to be a helpful model for language enrichment, although television sets and/or radios are found in the majority of American homes. The failure to acquire speech by 2–2½ years of age calls for an investigation into etiology and the initiation of a treatment program for the child.

Mental Retardation. The most common cause of speech delay is mental retardation. Although the degree of language defect is not directly proportional to the intellectual retardation, language and cognitive functioning are interrelated. In these children, motor development may be only slightly retarded, but the acquisition of language is considerably later than in the normal child. Furthermore, speech is limited in vocabulary and simple in syntactic structure and may show various articulatory defects. Echolalia, a tendency to perseverate, and an inability to comprehend or use abstract concepts are other characteristics of the language of mentally retarded children. If the retardation is of a very severe degree, language may not develop at all. Some mentally retarded children may suffer from hearing defects unrelated to their mental retardation; others are neglected or overprotected by their parents and have to be motivated and encouraged to use language.

Hearing Impairment. Language development depends on the intactness of the hearing apparatus. Impairments of the conductive system, as well as damage to parts of the central nervous system involved in the perception of auditory stimuli, can impede the acquisition of speech. Congenital abnormality of the external ear, traumatic perforation of the tympanic membranes, or early otitis media can result in conductive hearing loss. These children present with delayed speech, speech defects, or lack of volume control of the voice. They are often considered retarded, since they do not seem to understand what is being said to them, until hearing tests uncover their difficulties. The earlier the possibility of hearing impairment is suspected and recognized, the more favorable the outcome of medical intervention, particularly if the process is a reversible one.

Damage or congenital anomalies of the inner ear and the acoustic nerve give rise to sensorineural deafness. Maternal rubella during the first trimester, meningitis, and damage to the acoustic nerve resulting from fracture of the base of the skull are among the more frequent causes of sensorineural deafness. Early diagnosis of such a child is necessary so that he may obtain amplification of sound through the use of a hearing aid and be trained in the use of visual cues (lip reading) in communication.

When hearing loss is profound and prostheses do not restore a significant degree of sound recognition, speech training is usually ineffective. Sign language can be learned by the child and the family to provide an opportunity for communication.

Damage to the areas of the brain involved in auditory perception and associative function may result in an inability to perceive and differentiate aural stimuli (central deafness). Infection, traumas, or structural malformation may be the cause.

Infantile Autism. In infantile autism, language acquisition is significantly delayed, and a good proportion of those who do not develop language by 5 years of age remain mute. Some children begin speech at the usual time and then lose this function. Furthermore, even when speech is developed, language remains impaired and deviant in various aspects. The child's speech may consist of a succession of words, some meaningful, others repetitious phrases that he has heard in different contexts and that have little communicative value. These children are usually withdrawn, more involved with inanimate objects than with people, and show other peculiarity of behavior and affect (Bartak *et al.*, 1975; Simon, 1975).

Developmental Lag. Sometimes in an otherwise normal child the onset of speech is delayed until 3–3½ years. The rate of progress is slow and the speech is unclearly articulated. The family history reveals speech lag or other language disturbances. Such a child may be quite happy and free of emotional conflicts during the preschool period. However, when speech remains incomprehensible into the school years, the difficulty in making himself understood may be very upsetting to the child. Although peer relationships during the first few years of school are not heavily dependent on verbal interactions, the child may become timid and shy in his relationship with adults. In some instances, reading disability is associated with language lag, and this presents a new source of stress in the child's adaptation. The prognosis in children with speech lag is good. Most children will have normal speech by 8–9 years of age. Corrective speech therapy can help these children overcome their speech defects earlier, and the family is reassured when it is reminded that other members who were late talkers in childhood now have normal language.

Defects of Articulation

Defective articulation can be caused by structural defects of the organs of articulation, such as the lips, jaws, tongue, and hard or soft palate. The faulty use of normal organs of speech is called *functional misarticulation*. Symptomatic misarticulation is found in hearing defect, mental retardation, and aphasia.

Dysarthria. The most frequent cause of dysarthria is congenital failure of fusion of the upper lip. The condition is correctable by plastic surgery, and the speech does not show any defects after repair of the cleft lip. Tongue tie, formerly frequently diagnosed, is not very common. This malfunction is due to a short frenum, which limits the movement of the tip of the tongue. Dysarthria in cases of a cleft or other abnormality of the palate is characterized by nasal escape during pronunciation of certain vowel sounds, such as "a" and "e."

Neurological disorders such as cerebral palsy can affect speech production by involving the muscles of articulation. Incoordination of these muscles gives rise to various defects in articulation and hampers the smooth production of speech.

Functional Misarticulation. Infants produce vowel sounds first, and as they grow older they master the consonant sounds. The first group of consonant sounds are labial sounds, such as "b," "p," "m." Three-year-old children can produce these consonant sounds without any distortion. The dental and guttural sounds, such as "t," "d," "n," "k," "g," and "ng," are accurately reproduced by about 4 years of age. The labiodental sounds, "f," and "v," and the complicated sounds such as "l," "r," "j," and "ch," "s," "z," "sh," are mastered by the beginning of school. "Baby talk" is the characteristic phonetic distortion of young children. These distortions are due to factors such as lack of perfect auditory discrimination, slow fine motor coordination of the articulatory muscles, and stages of dentition. At times, overindulgent parents encourage baby talk beyond the point in maturation by which the child is capable of accurate articulation. In those children who continue to have defective articulation beyond the normal stage of development, various researchers have found differences in competence with regard to auditory and visual discrimination, speed of motor performance, and fine motor coordination.

Substitution, distortion, and omission of sounds are the most frequent disorders of articulation. A lisp is the most common type of articulatory defect, and since the sound of "s" occurs frequently in the English language, the mispronunciation of this sound is very noticeable. Other frequently distorted sounds are "z," "zh," "j," and "ch." Another type of distortion is the substitution of the sound "w" for "h" and "r." Omissions such as *cool* for *school* and *pay* for *play* and insertions such as *warsh* for *wash* create a language that becomes difficult to comprehend. In longitudinal studies of articulation in children, it has been found that the number of articulatory defects decrease up to the fourth grade. From then on, while the number of omissions and substitutions decreases, the number of indistinct sounds increases or remains unchanged.

In the treatment of articulatory defects, the first step is an expert assessment of the degree of deviation and identification and localization of the defective sounds. Auditory training for discrimination of sounds along with strengthening of the correct sound in isolation and later on in words and sentences is a process by which defective articulation can be corrected. Some children retain their habitually mispronounced words of the earlier years while learning the correct pronunciation of more sophisticated words. The child must become aware of his defective articulation; however, this awareness should be imparted in such a way that he does not become extremely self-conscious or resentful toward the speech therapist.

Stuttering

Stuttering is a disturbance in the rhythm of speech. There is spasmodic blocking or repetition of sounds and words. The spasm may be clonic, causing explosive utterance of the same sound, or it may be a tonic spasm of the muscles of speech, such as of the tongue, lips, and larynx. At times, the tension in the muscles involved in speech production is visible to the observer. Karlin (1950) believes that stuttering occurs in 1–2% of the population. The ratio between boys and girls is 4 to 1. No differences have been found between the socioeconomic backgrounds or intelligence of stutterers and nonstutterers. Some familial tendency has been noted.

Theories regarding the pathogenesis of stuttering are numerous. some authors consider stuttering an expression of personality problems or a neurosis (Coriat, 1928). Others state that emotional problems are caused by stuttering rather than inducing the condition. Shames (1968) considers stuttering a learned behavior. According to this view, parental behavior causes the normal repetitions and hesitations of 2- to 3-year-old children to become a fixed pattern of stuttering. Orton (1937) believed that stuttering is a neurologically based disturbance of language function resulting from the disturbances of cerebral dominance. More recent experimental studies (Beech and Fransella, 1968) have disclosed the interrelationships among various factors in the maintenance of stuttering. None of the present theories of stuttering have been able to account for all the known clinical facts regarding this condition.

The onset of stuttering is during the preschool years. Symptoms include simple repetition, hesitation, and mild anxiety. While the normal preschooler may repeat words or phrases, the prestutterer often repeats sounds. Spasms of the muscles (tonic and clonic) soon appear. The child becomes aware of his speech problem, and as he grows older, the fear of stuttering directs much of his behavior. He may become shy, avoid participating in class discussions, and refrain from asking questions. During adolescence, marked anxiety causes disturbances in interpersonal relationships and feelings of isolation and alienation. Speaking causes great fear, particularly since the pattern of stuttering is unpredictable and can change from one occasion to the next. Sounds such as "b," "d," and "g" tend to cause more stuttering than "p," "t," and "k."

While in normal speech sound is produced only during expiration, the stutterer at times tries to speak while inspiring. The subsequent spasm may thus involve the muscles of chest, neck, and abdomen, resulting in considerable psychological strain in the listener as well as in the stutterer. The compensatory mechanism developed by the stutterer further distorts communication. Some stutterers come to rely on some words as starters, since they are confident that they will not stutter on these words and therefore such utterances will give them time to prepare the next phrase. Words such as *now, well, so,* and *see* are used for this purpose. Other stutterers insert meaningless words into their speech in order to maintain the flow of speech (embolophrasia). Invisible stuttering refers to the feeling of apprehension that besets the stutterer while thinking about what he wants to say. Singing, whispering, and reading aloud in solitude or learning a foreign language may diminish the stuttering. The reason for these beneficial effects is not at all clear. In singing, the vowels play a more important part than the consonant sounds; therefore there is less possibility of stuttering. Whispering eliminates the laryngeal component of speech production, and therefore there is less chance of stuttering.

Prognosis and Treatment. In a large-scale study of 8,000 public school children, Johnson and co-workers (1948) found that 42% of the stutterers outgrew their dysfluency without any intervention. No test has been developed to differentiate between this group and the majority who continue to stutter.

During the preschool years, treatment consists of lessening environmental stresses through guidance and counseling of the parents. Direct remedial work with the child is indicated during the school years. Treatment consists of methods of muscle relaxation, coordinated breathing and talking, control in the pace of speech, and prolongation of vowel sounds (Ryan, 1974). Placing a ticking miniature metronome in the ear has been reported to minimize or eliminate stuttering. Adolescents and young adults may exhibit secondary emotional problems because of the difficulty in communication. Speech therapy is the cornerstone of treatment, although the patient may need support and encouragement to reestablish peer relationships and overcome the feeling of low self-esteem.

The stutterer may obtain some degree of secondary gain, such as greater attention from the listener and sympathetic treatment by some people with whom he comes into contact. The therapist must make sure that these secondary gains do not become powerful motivations for maintaining stuttering and must provide rewarding replacements for them.

Aphasia

While issues in the genesis of language are far from settled, it is universally accepted that language development is dependent upon intact sensory organs, coordinated motor apparatus for sound production, and a brain capable of integrating sensory data and executing the necessary motor behavior. Disorders of language can be conceptualized as impairments of this complex and interdependent system. Various degrees of sensory impairment and defects in the sound-making apparatus can be directly tested, but the impairment of the integrative part of the system (aphasia, or central language disorder) can only be inferred. Head (1926) classified language disturbances resulting from damage to various areas of the brain into four categories:

- Verbal aphasia characterized by defective word formation.
- Syntactical aphasia.
- Nominal aphasia (difficulty in the use of nouns).
- Semantic aphasia (lack of comprehension of the meaning of spoken or written words.)

Other neurologists have divided aphasia into expressive (Broca's) and receptive (Wernicke's) aphasia. In all these instances, the impairment of language function can be traced to the time of the pathological insult or injury to the brain. The comparison of language functioning before and after the event provides convincing evidence of the relationship between the lost function and the damage to the brain. In children, this form of acquired aphasia due to acute or subacute brain pathology is of a transitory nature, and the younger the child the better is the prognosis for full recovery.

Developmental or Congenital Dysphasia

In some children who show adequate motor and intellectual de-velopment and no sign of overt neurological disorder, language development is slow and shows deficits resembling those found in acquired aphasia. Some authorities oppose the use of the term *aphasia* for this dysfunction and have proposed the term *developmental dysphasia* to differentiate impairment in the acquisition of symbols from post-traumatic loss of language function (Eisenson, 1968). *Word deafness*, *congenital verbal–auditory agnosia*, and *congenital verbal imperception* are among the terms used to define this condition. The etiology of the defect is a matter of speculation. The underlying pathology is believed to be in the auditory cortex, most likely in the dominant hemisphere.

While some degree of hearing loss may be present, the results of audiometric studies are inconsistent. A majority of researchers consider developmental dysphasia primarily a problem of receptive language with subsequent deviations in expressive speech (Ingram 1969). The child with dysphasia reveals difficulties in discriminating among language sounds and the sequencing of incoming sounds and words. His ability to recall words and sounds is impaired, resulting in unpredictable word loss, unstable syntactic structure, and inconsistent grammar. The clarity of speech is further compromised by the compensatory mechanisms adopted by the child suffering from discorders of communicative skills. The findings of neurological examinations of the child are within normal limits. Language is limited and late in appearance. Comprehension of language is below that expected of the child's chronological age. The child is unable to find words to express his thoughts and makes statements to that effect. Naming objects is more difficult than pointing to objects named by the examiner. Semantic confusion is revealed by the observation that words associated in meaning and function are substituted for each other (*chair* for *table*, *sky* for *blue*). The syntactic structure of sentences is of primitive quality. Parts of speech other than noun and verb are frequently missing or underutilized. A combination of auditory inaccuracy and approximations of word meanings results in jargon or meaningless words. Visual cues may help the aphasic to find the appropriate word or to recognize an object that is named. However, aphasic children may have difficulty in learning to read as a part of their defective ability with symbols. The intellectual functioning of aphasic children is impaired because of these cognitive deficiencies. The aphasic child, however, has adequate intellectual ability in nonverbal areas. Emotional problems are related to the consequences of difficulty in communication (de Ajuriaguerra *et al.*, 1976). The child may be withdrawn and shy, irritable, or aggressive and may give a clinical picture resembling psychotic disorganization or neurotic behavior.

Aphasia in children is often diagnosed by exclusion since no reliable test is available. Hardy (1960) considers the study of pattern perception and foreground–background recognition in both the visual and the auditory spheres helpful in the diagnosis of aphasic children. He also believes that failure in auditory and visual tracking, or the inability to integrate a succession of sensory stimuli over a span of time, is the most important aspect of aphasia in childhood. In children with above-average intelligence, language functioning eventually approaches an adequate level of communication. In the treatment of aphasic children, speech therapy and educational placement at an early age are of utmost importance. Appropriate school placement fosters easy socialization and prevents maladjustment. Speech therapy is directed toward the use of those sensory and motor pathways that are unimpaired while helping the child to establish new patterns of sensory integration.

16

Organic Brain Syndromes

Epilepsy is a periodic, recurrent state of impaired consciousness associated with abnormal brain activities that may be clinically manifested by localized or generalized seizures, disturbances of the vegetative system, and alteration in sensation, perception, thinking, and emotional state.

Epilepsy is always a symptom of underlying brain dysfunction, though the exact nature of the brain pathology may not be easily identifiable. Metabolic disorders such as hypoglycemia, anoxia, electrolite imbalance, uremia, pyridoxine deficiency, and chronic or acute infections involving the central nervous system may cause convulsions. Intracranial pathology such as space-occupying lesions, malformations of the cerebral vascular system, or cerebrovascular accidents is associated with convulsions, particularly when convulsions first appear after the third decade of life. A history of head trauma and birth injuries associated with pre- or postnatal complications has been obtained in a substantial majority of patients with idiopathic epilepsy. Some authors have reported the existence of an inheritable tendency toward epilepsy. While all authorities in the field consider epilepsy to be symptomatic of brain pathology, the lack of an identifiable cause in the majority of patients has led to the introduction of the term *idiopathic epilepsy* to describe those cases in which epilepsy appears as a clinical disorder in an otherwise healthy individual with or without a history of presumptive birth injury. In our discussion of epilepsy, only the idiopathic epilepsy is under consideration.

The estimated incidence of epilepsy in the United States is between 3 and 4 per 1000 population. Of all epilepsies, 35–50% begin in childhood, with a peak incidence during the first four years of life. The incidence in families of epileptic patients is five times greater than for the general population. One study has shown 85% concordance for epilepsy in monozygotic twins (Cooper, 1965).

Clinical Pictures

Epilepsy is classified into two general categories. The first is called generalized (centrencephalic) seizures and includes grand mal and petit mal varieties of epilepsy. The second category is focal seizures, such as Jacksonian seizures and temporal lobe epilepsy.

Seizures. Grand mal seizure, in its classic form, usually begins with a brief aura and a cry followed by loss of consciousness. The patient falls, all the muscles are in an extreme tonic phase, and the body is fully extended. This phase is followed by alternating clonic movements of the extensor and flexor muscles. Relaxation of sphincters results in the loss of urine, feces, or semen. The seizure terminates with noisy breathing. The patient regains partial consciousness but is usually confused or may go to sleep for a few minutes to a few hours. After each attack, the patient has amnesia for the episode. Biting of the tongue or injury to the head during the clonic phase is added to the injury due to the fall, and the patient may complain of various aches and pains after he has regained consciousness.

Petit mal is a brief (20–30 seconds) lapse or absence of consciousness with or without myoclonic or atonic seizures. Myoclonic movements may take the form of jerks of a group of muscles (salaam seizures). Atonic seizures may cause momentary loss of upright position. Because the lapses are of such short duration, patients either may be unaware of them or may at times try to conceal them. Parents and teachers may notice frequent staring or a faraway, dreamy look on the child's face. At times, the short period of confusion that follows each lapse may be the only thing that attracts the parents' attention. When these transient lapses are frequent, the patient spends most of his waking time in a confused state.

Focal seizures of the Jacksonian type are usually caused by localized and identifiable pathology. They are characterized by the twitching of a specific group of muscles, always in the same area. When the seizures are of a sensory character, they are felt as parasthesia, a tingling sensation in one part of the body. Occasionally these localized seizures become generalized, and a seizure that begins as a Jacksonian type will progress toward a grand mal convulsion with loss of consciousness.

Temporal lobe seizures, which originated in the anterior and midtemporal lobe of the brain, are usually accompanied by disturbances of affect and thinking processes, at times some motor phenomena, and occasionally grand mal seizures. Thalamic and hypothalamic seizures are most frequently seen in children. In these seizures, disturbances of the autonomic system are particularly prevalent. These visceral disturbances (abdominal seizures) are difficult to diagnose (Aird, 1968).

Psychic seizures (temporal lobe) are behavioral phenomena that may occur without any motor components and without loss of consciousness, or they may precede a grand mal seizure or be mixed with petit mal seizures. Temporal lobe seizures comprise about 20% of all seizure disorders. Although the diagnosis of temporal lobe seizures is particularly difficult in early childhood, their peak incidence is during the second decade of life. Awareness of these seizures is especially important for psychiatrists since they are manifested clinically by perceptual changes; disturbances in consciousness, mood, and thinking processes; and complex, stereotyped automatisms (Pond, 1969; Ounsted, 1966).

Behavioral Disturbances. In the perceptual changes that occur during the attack, objects may be seen as smaller or larger than their usual size. They may recede or move forward in the field of vision. Hallucinations may be experienced in all sensory modalities. They may take the form of a forced reliving of emotionally charged memory strips and therefore are not alien to the personality of the patient and can at times evoke appropriate moods. In uncinate fits, patients experience unusual and unpleasant odors. *Déjà vu*, as well as a feeling of unfamiliarity with the surroundings, has also been reported. Paroxysmal, unexplainable changes in mood and affect, such as feelings of extreme well-being, despair, terror, or anxiety unrelated to external stimuli, may be experienced.

Thinking disorders are manifested as forced thinking in which a sentence, a word, or a complex thought intrudes upon the patient's consciousness. This is another form of psychical seizure. Patients may or may not remember the content of such thoughts, although they are aware that the experience is identical to their previous attacks (Flor-Henry, 1969; Herrington, 1969).

Automatisms are complex acts that are accompanied by impaired consciousness and consequently are followed by complete amnesia. These acts are stereotyped, may appear purposeful, and may be compatible with the dynamics of the individual personality. However, their self-limited, periodic character, their execution without the patient's awareness, and the subsequent amnesia provide important diagnostic clues as to their organic nature.

Twilight states are characterized by a clouded consciousness that follows seizures or are themselves the manifestation of abnormal brain activities. These patients are disoriented, suspicious, agitated, and delusional and may wander around aimlessly. Various combinations of these abnormalities may be noted during one episode, or a patient may manifest different symptoms during various attacks.

Sometimes children with a history of behavior problems, such as hyperkinetic syndrome, eventually develop the clinical picture of epilepsy. On the other hand, behavioral disturbances such as paroxysmal rage, hyperactivity, and severe temper tantrums that are disproportionate to external stimuli are reported in children with abnormal EEG activities in the temporal lobe area.

Assessment

When the presenting complaints of a patient include periodic, recurrent phenomena such as abnormal motor movements or impairment of consciousness, a general medical workup is necessary to rule out such things as hypoglycemia and tetany. A careful history of drug intake should be obtained. Hysteria and malingering should be particularly kept in mind. A skull X ray can give clues about possible abnormalities of the cranium and cyst formations within the brain.

EEG. An electroencephalogram, a brain scan, and, if necessary, a lumbar puncture can further clarify the diagnosis. The electroencephalogram is still the single most important test for diagnosing epilepsy. However, it should be pointed out that while the presence of an abnormal EEG verifies the diagnosis of seizure disorders, a single normal EEG in between the attacks does not rule out this diagnosis. Even in grand mal seizure, only 20% of the patients show an abnormal EEG during the interseizure period. In focal seizures, an abnormal EEG record is even less common, and the focus of abnormal activities may actually disappear during a psychic seizure.

Special procedures are used to stimulate and intensify the abnormal activities during the recording of the EEG. Physiological maneuvers such as sleep can produce abnormal EEG recording during the interseizure period of the grand mal in 80% of patients. The abnormalities of the petit mal are more likely to be seen in waking records. Hyperventilation activates all abnormalities, particularly the petit mal variety. Flickering lights is another maneuver that will intensify the abnormal activities. When particular stimuli are found to precipitate seizures in some patients, these stimuli can be used to produce a diagnostic record. In some patients activation with drugs, such as a subconvulsive dose of Metrazol, is attempted during EEG recording. Special leads are sometimes necessary to record the focus of an abnormality. It should be noted that even with the best efforts, an abnormal EEG record can be found in only 80% of patients with seizure disorders.

During a grand mal seizure, the EEG shows high-voltage, fast activities in all leads, which will then end on the isoelectric line with no activities for a few seconds. During the petit mal attack, about three to four waves and spikes per second are found in all leads. Hyperventilation usually results in evoking a burst of seizure activities.

In focal seizures, focal spikes over a particular lead may slowly spread to involve other areas of the brain. In some patients, 14 and 6 positive spikes per second have dominated the EEG record in one or more leads. Episodes of destructive rage had been reported previously in these patients. but these findings have not been substantiated.

As can be noted from the above description, the abnormal activities of the brain in epilepsy are of a specific nature and do not resemble the generalized slow activities and rhythmic abnormalities of the EEG that are found in a sizable portion of children with behavior disorder. The mechanism through which these abnormal activities lead to the clinical manifestations of epilepsy is as yet unknown.

Psychiatric Problems

Epilepsy is a chronic illness that incapacitates the child from early life and influences his adaptation. In some children, seizures are only one manifestation of generalized damage to the central nervous system. In these children, intellectual backwardness, learning disabilities, and other behavioral disturbances associated with chronic brain syndrome combine to handicap the child. Poor medical control of the seizures may cause further injury to the brain, while high doses of an anticonvulsant result in toxicity, sleepiness, and feelings of ill health. Fear of an unannounced seizure, with the dangers implicit in loss of consciousness, may keep the child from participating in a variety of activities, or conversely, the need to deny the disability or defiance against such a fate may prompt the child to be careless and forget or refuse to follow the medical regimen. Older children may be concerned about their illness and its meaning for their future in terms of their ability to find a mate, produce normal children, or engage in productive activities. The social stigma associated with epilepsy may cause worries about acceptance by peers and society in general (Shaffer, 1973; Voeller and Rothenberg, 1973).

Children with petit mal epilepsy may go undiagnosed for a long time and may be accused of a lack of motivation to concentrate and learn. Their confusion is considered a sign of strangeness, and their inability to stop "daydreaming" an indication of defiance of authority. They may be hyperactive, have poor concentration, and be generally unpredictable. Some children use a variety of maneuvers to conceal short lapses in their awareness and earn a reputation for lying and confabulation. The frequently interrupted awareness of self and environment makes it impossible for these children to comprehend what goes on around them; the consistent relationship between causes and effects escapes their attention. These children may be perplexed, suspicious, and nontrusting because they are unable to form an uninterrupted impression of people. In cases of mixed seizures, the child may present with a puzzling picture of sudden rage, unwarranted happiness, or terror that is impervious to environmental responses and vanishes as suddenly as it appears.

The incidence of behavior problems in children with epilepsy is higher than for nonepileptic children. In children with psychomotor epilepsy, behavioral problems are fairly common.

In a study of children with behavior disorders and EEG abnormalities indicative of temporal lobe focus, Nuffield (1961) concluded that these children are somewhat more aggressive and less anxious than the nonepileptic group with behavior disorders. In 100 children with behavior disorders, Aird and Yamamato (1966) found that 49 showed abnormalities on the EEG; in 40 of these, some form of focal abnormality could be seen, with the majority showing abnormal focus in the temporal lobe area. The authors concluded by stating:

> Children who have behavior disorders which are inappropriate in character for the individual and which are disproportionate in degree to the environmental factors involved, and who have an abnormal EEG with a temporal focus, represent dysfunction of the temporal lobes and/or underlying limbic systems. However, the relationship between temporal abnormality as indicated by EEG and behavior disorders of childhood would appear to be a secondary predisposing one.

In some epileptic children, the prodrome of an attack lasts from a few hours to a few days, during which the child is irritable, hypersensitive, restless, and impulsive. Parents usually talk about the child's behavior building up toward a seizure. Unusual nocturnal phenomena such as sleepwalking and night terrors in the presence of temporal lobe abnormality have been reported in some studies. In the literature of the early part of this century, the concept of an "epileptic personality" is repeatedly discussed. Such a personality is said to be rigid and hypersensitive, with an unstable mood, a perseverative tendency, and egocentricity. The role of adverse environmental experiences in the creation of such a personality type is neglected. The concept of an epileptic personality has been disregarded, since research studies have failed to prove the existence of an independent personality type in epileptics.

Psychosis and Epilepsy. The presence of psychotic states with schizophrenic-like symptomatology, particularly in adults with psychomotor epilepsy, has been the subject of numerous investigations. Flor-Henry (1969) found such episodes to be particularly prevalent among patients with focal abnormalities in the dominant hemisphere. In younger patients, episodes of labile affect and lack of impulse control with hysterical features could mimic a psychotic episode. Disturbances in perception and sensation may evoke extreme panic in children who do not know what is happening to them, and during such attacks, the child may be mistakenly diagnosed as suffering from psychosis.

Differential Diagnosis. It should be noted at the outset that most authorities in the field of epilepsy consider emotional stress an important triggering factor in inducing an epileptic fit. Therefore the presence of conflicts and various psychodynamic factors in the child's inter- and intrapersonal milieu should not be construed to rule out epilepsy. Some patients are able to activate their own seizures through various maneuvers and may do so for secondary gain. They cast the responsibility for their behavior onto their epilepsy and simulate a fit when it is necessary for their purposes. Conversion hysteria and malingering are particularly troublesome in view of the fact that one normal EEG does not rule out epilepsy.

In younger children the possibility of petit mal seizure, and in older ones the question of temporal lobe epilepsy, should always be kept in mind when episodic, recurrent, and unprovoked behavioral phenomena with impaired awareness and partial or total amnesia are present (Pond, 1961).

The following case reports are examples of epilepsy presented as psychiatric problems.

CASE HISTORY

Eric was a 9-year-old boy who was hospitalized in a pediatric unit following an overdose of Librium. Eric was living with his aunt, who reported that Eric had had a fight with his older brother the previous afternoon but did not seem very upset by it. He ate dinner that night and went to his room to sleep. The following morning, Eric's aunt found that her supply of Librium was missing from her handbag. When she went to awaken Eric, he was drowsy and finally stated that he might have taken the Librium since the aunt found the empty bottle of Librium in his room and questioned him about it. He was taken to the hospital and was admitted. Eric's behavior in the ward puzzled and alarmed the treating physician. Eric would change from a cheerful boy to a suspicious, hostile, threatening youngster. He would accuse doctors and nurses of wanting to kill him and then calm down and begin joking with them. It was also observed that at times Eric would stop in the middle of a sentence, look preoccupied for a few seconds, then finish his sentence or start from the beginning as if the pause were intentional.

Eric told the psychiatrist that he did not feel sad or unhappy, was not nervous or angry when he had the fight with his brother, and had never intended to kill himself. He simply did not know why he had taken all those Libriums. He reported only one experience that was disturbing to him. Some nights, while preparing for sleep, he would see his dead mother looking at him with an expression that frightened him. Eric had lost his mother five years before, and the frightening look on her face shortly before her death was the only vivid memory of her that he had.

Eric was of average intelligence; his birth and developmental history were normal. He was about a year below his grade in academic skills. His teachers described him as "elusive and unpredictable." He was the youngest child in his family and had been told that his mother had become pregnant with him against the advice of her doctor. He sought reassurance that he had not caused his mother's death.

Laboratory tests and neurological examination were within normal limits. Two EEG records revealed a mixture of petit mal and abnormal left temporal lobe foci. The brain scan was normal. He was placed on anticonvulsant medication, which resulted in the prompt disappearance of visual hallucinations and a decrease in the number of absences. His behavioral style of interaction improved to a lesser degree.

CASE HISTORY

Pierre, a 12-year-old boy, had a long history of hyperactivity, impulsivity, and poor peer relationships. He awoke one night in an agitated state, called for his mother, began to sing and whistle, talked about the devil having entered his body, and tried to run away from the house in obvious terror. He finally calmed down, asked to be fed, and demanded that both parents stay in his room. He went back to sleep. The next morning he accused his younger sister of trying to kill him in his sleep, became agitated again, and kicked his sister. He finally calmed down and agreed to go and see his therapist. He said he did not know what had happened the night before, could not remember having awakened, and explained his fight with his sister as a "regular argument." While talking about the devil and his ideas of being possessed, Pierre became agitated, uttered a loud cry, and had a grand mal seizure in the office. An EEG verified the diagnosis.

Prognosis and Treatment. Petit mal seizures are more frequent during early childhood and may disappear with maturation. However, the prognosis of epilepsy in terms of the long-term adjustment of the individual child is dependent upon medical control of the seizures, avoidance of toxicity due to anticonvulsant medications, parental attitudes toward the child and his illness, and the social and academic opportunities available to the child. Epilepsy need not unduly hamper a child's emotional and intellectual growth, provided that he is supported and encouraged and his seizures are reasonably under control.

The treatment of epilepsy in children is first and foremost a medical treatment. The drug regimen should be under the careful supervision of an expert physician who uses a drug, or a combination of drugs, to achieve a seizure-free state with a minimum slowdown in intellectual functioning. The psychiatrist's role in the management of epilepsy is important for identifying and treating indications of maladjustment, low self-esteem, and discouragement in view of a chronic illness. Overprotectiveness in the parents or carelessness and defiance in following the medical regimen in adolescents are detrimental to the normal development of an epileptic child and should be handled with understanding and firmness.

ORGANIC BRAIN SYNDROME

Behavioral deviations in association with various injuries to the brain have been long noted by clinicians among adult patients. However, even in adults, the nature of behavioral symptomatology is not of unfailing diagnostic significance in localizing the damage to the brain or in determining the extent of tissue destruction. Some clinicians maintain that the patient's premorbid personality is an important factor in the type of psychopathology that follows structural damage to the higher central nervous system. Others consider behavioral symptoms significant of the patient's attempts at a new adaptation to environmental problems.

The consequences of brain injury in children are more problematic: on the one hand, depending on the age of the child, some functions have not yet been acquired or are in various stages of development; and, on the other hand, because of the plasticity of the central nervous system, the loss of some functions may be compensated for by the establishment of new associative links and a different level of integration.

From a psychophysiological point of view, the function of the central nervous system may be divided into three broad categories. First is the *sensory or receptive function*, which, in ascending order of complexity, includes the perception and organization of primary sensation, recognition of objects and processes, and finally, the conceptualization and understanding of verbal and nonverbal symbols. Second is the *expressive function*, such as voluntary but purposeless contraction of muscles, performance of purposeful, complex movements, and production of meaningful symbols and speech. And third is the *affective or emotional aspect*, which is experienced and expressed along the same hierarchial line from vague awareness of pleasure and pain to more articulate, well-defined, and modulated feelings and emotional expression. Every environmental stimulus passes through the receptive channel, is influenced by the degree of integration in the higher cortical area, and is expressed through an individual's behavior. Maladaptive and deviant behavior may reflect dysfunction in the receptive, expressive, affective, or integrative activities of the central nervous system. Conversely, any impairment in one part of the system may be manifested in the form of deviant behavior.

The severity of behavioral pathology is not a direct consequence of the extent of structural damage, although diffuse destruction is more likely to produce significant global disturbance than localized impairment. Furthermore, the nature of environmental stimuli and the complexity of tasks requiring solutions are factors that influence the behavioral outcome. Sensory defects or motor disabilities may have a less disorganizing effect on the overall behavior of a patient than central language disorder, since in the latter, concept formation is impaired, verbal communication is defective, and socialization is delayed. Diffuse cortical damage may prevent cognitive development and result in mental retardation or may cause loss of cognitive abilities and dementia. The child's behavior may be so globally impaired and disorganized as to be designated psychotic, or deviations may be circumscribed and mild in nature and phenomenologically indistinguishable from disorders related to experiential defects.

The incidence and prevalence of behavior disorders associated with structural damage of the central nervous system in the total population are unknown. However, studies of children with neurological damage and of severely retarded youngsters have consistently revealed a higher rate of behavioral pathology. In the epidemiological survey on the Isle of Wight, Graham and Rutter (1968) found psychiatric disorders to be five times more frequent among children with neuroepileptic conditions than among the general population, although the rate was only three times higher than that of children with chronic physical illnesses unrelated to the central nervous system dysfunction. Furthermore, children with bilateral brain disorders were more likely to have associated psychiatric symptoms than those with unilateral brain damage. Unfavorable environmental factors, disturbed family relations, and educational difficulties were associated with psychiatric disorders, though their etiological contributions could not be assessed. Childhood psychosis and hyperkinetic syndrome were diagnosed with higher frequency among these children, even though the authors reemphasized that no constellation of symptoms or diagnostic category could be said to be invariably related to organic brain damage.

While infections, intoxication, head trauma, congenital malformations, neonatal anoxia, brain tumor, and a variety of metabolic disorders are all known to cause various degrees of structural damage to the brain, psychiatric disorders are not the inevitable concomitant of all these diseases. The relationship between the age at the time of injury and subsequent outcome is not clear. The neurological and psychiatric sequelae of meningitis and encephalitis are reported to be more serious when the disease occurs during the first two years of life, while localized cortical damage resulting in language impairment tends to be corrected when the patient is younger. The effects of tissue destruction in various areas of the brain on the psychiatric status of children have not been systematically investigated, although studies in adult patients indicate a higher probability of psychiatric disorders in injuries to the left temporal, left parietal, and both frontal areas.

Organic brain syndrome may be acute or chronic, progressive or stationary; it may be manifested at the time of injury or appear after a symptom-free interval. Some diseases are acquired, while others are the late manifestations of metabolic or genetic disorders.

Clinical Pictures

The behavioral symptoms accompanying acute brain syndrome are fluctuation or total impairment of state of awareness, ranging from confusion and drowsiness to stupor and coma; disorientation and misidentification of objects, people, and places; illusions, hallucinations, and delirium; and agitation and panic. Anxious agitation is more often noted in febrile illnesses, although some young patients may react with psychomotor retardation and apathy. Other children may be very irritable and show regressive behavior. Neurological findings may include convulsion, paralysis, or disturbances of sensory functions. Speech is incoherent, associations are loose, and terrifying dreams interrupt the patient's sleep. Abnormalities of a diffuse, nonspecific nature in the form of slow waves with high amplitude may be seen on the electroencephalogram, and lumbar puncture may reveal high pressure of the spinal fluid. Other laboratory findings are dependent on the nature of the causative agent. For example, in acute bacterial meningitis, the bacteria may be isolated from the spinal fluid, while in acute lead encephalopathy, the blood lead level is elevated. Although the mortality rate for acute organic brain syndrome has decreased substantially because of advances in medical diagnosis and treatment, permanent disabling sequelae in the form of cortical atrophy, hydrocephalus, mental retardation, motor or sensory deficits, convulsive disorder, and behavioral pathology are frequent.

Chronic brain syndrome is characterized by intellectual impairment, poor memory, difficulties in changing set perseveration, obsessive concern about details, limitation of ability to abstract, deficiencies of attention and concentration, and problems with impulse control and affective regulation, as well as hyper- or hypokinesis. More severe damage may be manifested as varying degrees of mental retardation and/or psychotic behavior.

Psychiatric disorders have been reported in association with nontreated phenylketonuria, Down's syndrome, head injuries, and congenital cerebral palsy and in children with chronic excessive blood lead level.

Lead Poisoning may be the causative factor in encephalopathy or may aggravate the preexisting problem, since mentally retarded or severely psychotic children may ingest nonnutritious, lead-containing materials. While the most common source of poisoning is eating lead-based paint and plaster, a number of other sources of lead, such as canned foods, printed papers, and respiratory absorption of dust, dirt, or auto emissions, have also been identified. When the amount of lead absorbed through respiration or ingestion is not excessive, excretion through bile, urine, and sweat is adequate. But when increased uptake continues, lead is depositied in soft tissues such as the brain, bone marrow, kidneys, and long bones, and blood lead level reaches values of 80 mg or higher per 100 ml in the whole blood, which is the definition of lead poisoning suggested by the Center for Disease Control. In the presence of clinical symptoms of encephalopathy, blood lead level of 50 mg/100 ml of whole blood is considered diagnostic of plumbism. Encephalopathy due to lead may appear suddenly with symptoms such as convulsion, delirium, partial or complete blindness, transient aphasia, and paralysis, or it may be ushered in by apathy, sluggishness, restlessness, parasthesia, hallucination, insomnia, and terrifying dreams. Toxic episodes are more frequent during the summer months and are more like to afflict children between 2 and 4 years of age. Even though the mortality rate has appreciably decreased since introduction of chelating agents such as calcium disodium versenate (EDTA), about 25% of the survivors of acute encephalopathy sustain severe permanent neurological damage. Some studies have revealed that chronic elevated blood lead levels (40 mg and above) and/or radiologic findings without clinical symptoms of acute toxicity are associated with intellectual deficits and behavioral deviations (de la Burdé and Choate, 1975).

Psychotic reactions associated with chronic brain syndrome may present a problem in differential diagnosis, particularly when focal neurological signs are absent and mental retardation beclouds the picture. Menolascino (1969) regards a period of early, near-normal psychosocial development, followed by global regression and personality disintegration, as signifying a functional psychosis superimposed on mental retardation. Psychotic reaction due to chronic brain syndrome, which is a recurrent feature of the clinical picture of mental retardation, may be more responsive to environmental manipulation and psychotropic medication.

Progressive brain syndrome is often due to degenerative diseases of the central nervous system. Some of these disorders are clearly genetic; others are of unknown etiology. In some disorders, such as Niemann-Pick disease, Tay-Sachs disease, and Gaucher's disease, enzyme deficiencies have been identified. In others, such as Schilder's disease, progressive demyelinization remains unexplainable. Although the clinical manifestations of each disease may begin differently and appear at different ages, the signs of various progressive brain disorders are similar. Patients slowly lose the acquired functions; periods of apathy or agitation are accompanied by disturbances of language comprehension and expression; and disorders of perception and sensory functions are added to disturbances of the neuromuscular system, such as convulsions and paralysis. Finally, decorticate rigidity and profound dementia set in and death follows.

The loss of skills, deterioration in intellectual functioning, and appearance of bizarre or aggressive behavior should alert the clinician to the possibility of progressive organic brain syndrome. While focal neurological signs may not be present in the early stage of the disease, repeated evaluations will soon reveal the nature of the disorder. Although at the present time no treatment is available for these conditions, accurate diagnosis is of preventive value through genetic counseling for the parents.

17

Hyperkinesis and Attentional Deficiencies

The term *minimal brain dysfunction* (MBD) defines a cluster of clinically observable behavioral deviations among children. Although such terms as *brain-injured, brain*-damaged, and *hyperkinetic impulse disorder* of the previous era have been dropped in favor of MBD, the change in terminology was not occasioned by the discovery of the etiology, extent, or type of the presumed lesion(s) in the brain. In fact, the clinical picture of MBD is not considered the direct consequence of damage to the central nervous system. Instead, it is hypothesized that structural and/or functional impairment in the organization of the central nervous system leads to a disturbed interaction with the developmental environment, which includes the social, interpersonal, and objective world surrounding each individual. The behavioral deviation is the expression of such faulty interactions. The term *hyperkinetic syndrome* has often been used interchangeably with *minimal brain dysfunction,* and brain damaged has been inferred despite the absence of any history of prenatal insult or any clinical evidence of central nervous system findings. In some of these children, careful observation shows that while a high activity level is indeed present, it is not in the abnormal range. Attention span, while briefer than average, is not defective. These children typically react to stress by an exaggeration of their normal tendency. This seems to be the basis of some clinicians' opinion that hyperactivity is the equivalent of anxiety or depression in children.

There have been reports that a high percentage of children raised in institutions or coming from deprived backgrounds demonstrate the hyperkinetic syndrome. Inadequate socialization may account for this outcome, since it is usually in school that the behavior is first designated a problem.

Clinical Pictures

Hyperkinesis. Overactivity and restlessness is the most consistent presenting symptom. Parents and teachers find the child involved in an inordinate amount of aimless motor activities. At times, while the amount of motor activity may not be excessive, the quality of the activity and its aimlessness, intensity, and unpredictability set the hyperkinetic child apart from his normal peers. The hyperactivity may fluctuate in different settings and under varied circumstances. In stressful situations, the child may exhibit an excessive amount of motor activity, while in the one-to-one situation of the clinical interview he may be capable of inhibiting his motor discharges.

Defects of Attention. Children with MBD show fleeting and superficial attention with a high degree of distractibility. They appear unable to screen out the irrelevant environmental stimuli and consequently do not learn as fast as their normal peers. Their attention span is below their chronological and mental age. At the same time, some activity may absorb the child's attention to the exclusion of all other stimuli. Parents and educators may mistakenly view this perseverative tendency as evidence that if the child wanted to do something he could be attentive, and they assume that his failure to do so is a sign of lack of motivation rather than a deficit in concentration ability.

Learning Deficits. Attentional abnormalities, independent of any perceptual deficits, have important consequences for learning. The educational curriculum is based on the characteristics of the average child with the average attention span. When a child does not attend to the educational tasks, he fails to acquire the fund of knowledge necessary for the more complex learning of the later years. The easy distractibility makes the selection of the significant common properties of sensory data extremely difficult, and consequently the acquisition of abstract attitudes and learning sets is delayed, so that a child with average intellectual potential may fail to perform the educational tasks required of his age group. In some children with MBD, disturbances of perceptual–motor integration provide a further obstacle to learning.

Impulsiveness and Emotional Lability. The child with MBD is unable to delay acting on his immediate intentions. He cannot regulate his own actions, and the consequences of his activities do not inhibit his subsequent behavior. He may engage in unacceptable aggressive and sexual behavior and may have unpredictable and unprovoked verbal outbursts. Rapid and unexplainable changes in mood and affect puzzle the parents and are frowned upon by peers. Other children try to avoid interaction with the child and consider him "strange" or "crazy." The child's disruptiveness and temper outbursts are sources of continuous irritation in every social situation. He alternatively becomes withdrawn and aggressive. He slowly comes to view himself as incompetent and worthless. Being unable to regulate his actions, he comes to believe that he is "bad" and undesirable. The resultant depression and anxiety cause further deterioration in attention span, and aggressive and hyperactive behavior become more indiscriminate.

Etiology. Given the complexity of the clinical picture of minimal brain dysfunction, it is clear that no single etiological factor can account for the disturbances of the behavioral pattern. Some investigators have found a higher incidence of psychopathology in the families of the children with MBD (Cantwell and Statterfield, 1972). Others have reported a higher incidence of MBD in sibs reared away from home. However, these findings cannot be construed as an indication of genetic etiology, since the effects of subclinical maternal malnutrition and abnormal intrauterine development on the central nervous system are not fully understood.

The prenatal history of children with MBD reveals a significantly high incidence of abnormal pregnancy and difficult birth, necessitating resuscitation. Neurological examination, in some cases, shows a variety of nonfocal neurological signs reflecting deficits in sensorimotor coordination. The child may be clumsy and show poor motor coordination, which can be seen when he is attempting to fasten his buttons or tie his shoelaces. Some children have difficulty in rapid alternate movements. Others may have mild nystagmus or fine tremors in the upper extremities when the arms are outstretched and the fingers widespread. In children with visual perceptual problems, there is confused laterality and difficulty with spatial orientation (Clements, 1966).

Electroencephalographic abnormalities of various kinds have been reported in about 40–50% of these children as compared to 10–15% of normal children of the same age group. Slowing of frequency, poor background rhythm, absence of age-appropriate well-organized alpha rhythm, and paroxysmal abnormalities have all been reported as EEG findings in children with the clinical picture of minimal brain dysfunction. The significance of the electroencephalographic findings is a matter of controversy. Some researchers have found a better response to stimulant drugs in children with slow activity in EEG and neurological signs.

Psychological Testing. In psychological testing, children with MBD may show circumscribed cognitive and perceptual deficiencies, presumably based upon the site and the extent of the brain dysfunction. Copying block designs on the Wechsler Intelligence Scale for Children is a difficult task. On the Draw-a-Person test, the child's production is inferior to that expected of his mental age because of perceptual–motor disturbance, difficulty with spatial organization, and finally, the child's poor evaluation of himself. On the Bender–Gestalt tests, figures are rotated, the spatial relationship is not accurately copied, and the figure–ground discrimination is poor.

Birch (1963) believes that synthesis of the sensory data received from various modalities, such as visual, haptic, and kinesthetic, is especially poor in children with brain damage and that the performance of these children on tests designed for investigating the level of intersensory integration is inferior to that of their normal peer group.

Clinical Course and Prognosis. As infants, these children may exhibit high sensitivity to various stimuli, such as noise and light. They may be hyper- or hypoactive for the first year of life, but as toddlers, they begin to show hyperactivity, destructiveness, aggressivity, and negativistic behavior. During their school years, low tolerance for frustration, disorganized working habits, poor judgment, lack of control, and noncooperation with teachers are sources of constant complaints by teachers and parents. Most observers have reported a decrease in hyperactivity during adolescence. However, the short attention span, a poor fund of knowledge, and impulsivity may continue to exert their deleterious effects on the scholastic and interpersonal areas of the adolescent's life.

In several anterospective studies of children with MBD, investigators have found a high percentage of psychopathology in adult life (Morris *et al.*, 1965; Menkes *et al.*, 1967; Mendelson *et al.*, 1971). Retrospective studies tend to corroborate these findings, in that the childhood histories of adult patients hospitalized for a variety of psychiatric disorders reveal possible MBD-like behavioral patterns in childhood (Hartcollis, 1968; Quitkin and Klein, 1969).

Treatment. The goal of the counseling of parents is to clarify the nature of the child's problems and to provide the parents with helpful suggestions regarding their handling of the child's behavior.

Most children with MBD are in need of special educational programs that take their slow rate of learning and their attentional deficits into consideration. Special activities and exercises to improve their coordination and enhance their power of intersensory organization are needed in order to allow the child the maximum development of his intellectual potentials and to facilitate his participation in social interactions with his peer group. Supportive and directive psychotherapy are necessary when a child has come to view himself as a worthless individual who is doomed to failure in every interaction with his surroundings.

In 1937 Bradley noticed the calming effect of amphetamine on some hyperactive children. This was considered a paradoxical effect, since in adults amphetamine is a stimulant to the central nervous system. The mechanism of action of dextroamphetamine (Dexedrine) and methylphenidate (Ritalin) is unknown. Some authors believe that one group of children with MBD suffer from underarousal of the central nervous system and that in this group the effect of stimulants is to increase the attention span, with a consequent decrease of motor activities. Others believe that some abnormalities in serotonin, norepinephrine, or dopamine metabolism in the brain may be present in those children who respond to dextroamphetamine and methylphenidate, since it is known that these medications alter the metabolism of the catecholamines and indolamines of the brain. Reports on the efficacy of the stimulant drugs are not always in agreement. Most researchers have reported beneficial results with stimulant drugs in one-half to two-thirds of the treated children with MBD. Other authors have found marked placebo effects. The duration of effectiveness and the extent of improvement are not unlimited.

The starting dose is 2.5–5 mg/day for dextroamphetamine and 5–10 mg/day for methylphenidate. The dosage is then increased until the desired effects are achieved or side effects appear. The total dosage can be given in the morning or divided; however, no medication should be given after 3–4 P.M. In some children, there is a "letdown" effect at the end of the day, and the medication may make sleeping easier. Temporary discontinuation on weekends and holidays assures that the child will not accommodate to the drugs (Grinspoon and Singer, 1973).

Sometimes a child who is unresponsive to dextroamphetamine may respond to methylphenidate and vice versa. The duration of the drug therapy cannot be predicted. The dosage range for Dexedrine is 5–40 mg and for Ritalin 5–80 mg daily. Possible side effects are increased activity, anorexia with resultant weight loss, headache, abdominal pain, irritability, depression, excessive crying, and aggravation of previous symptoms. Rare instances of urticaria, facial tics, and hallucinations have been reported. Temporary suppression of the rate of growth on higher dosage of stimulants has been noted (Safer *et al.*, 1975). After nearly 30 years of clinical usage, there is no evidence that the use of the stimulant in early childhood causes drug abuse in later life.

The tranquilizers chlorpromazine (Thorazine) and thioridazine (Mellaril) are helpful in some cases of children with MBD. Anticonvulsants have generally been ineffective and barbiturates are contraindicated.

18

Disorders of Habit

Stereotyped Movement and Self-Injurious Behavior

Stereotyped rhythmic movements usually involve one or more segments of the body and take such forms as head banging, rocking, and flapping of the hands. Epidemiologic studies have shown that a considerable percentage of normal children under 2 years of age engage in such behavior for short periods of time and that the incidence is higher among boys than among girls (DeLissovoy, 1961). However, in abnormal populations, such as retardates or psychotics, the stereotyped movements persist beyond the age of 2, take exaggerated forms, and may comprise a significant part of the child's activities. Furthermore, while in young normal children such behavior is limited to situations in which the infant is fatigued, understimulated, or left alone in the crib, in deviant groups the behavior for the most part appears regardless of the nature of environmental stimuli and seems to be the preferred activity for the patient. At times, these stereotyped movements become positively dangerous to the child—head banging results in repeated severe traumata to the skull, or pulling of the ears or the penis causes laceration and infection (Green, 1967).

Theories of etiology have been numerous and at times contradictory. Some authors consider stereotyped movements an indication of understimulation and point to the high incidence of such behaviors in blind children or institutionalized inmates as confirmatory proof. Others believe that excessive stimulation in the environment outstrips these children's capacity to organize and respond to the incoming stimuli and that the child's behavior is therefore a defense strategy. Behaviorists regard such stereotyped movements as having a high attention-getting value and as being modifiable through withholding social reinforcements. Studies in laboratory animals have shown that animals reared in isolation engage in stereotyped behavior and thus

have lent support to the theory of understimulation. Because neurologically damaged, mentally retarded, and disorganized psychotic children are particularly vulnerable to the development of such behavior,
it seems that the common factor in etiology may be the child's inability to receive, organize, and integrate environmental stimuli. The behavior may then be further maintained and strengthened by a variety
of social reinforcements (Baumeister and Rollings, 1976). What is
amply clear is that these activities are undesirable because of their potential danger to the child and because such stereotyped movements
utilize an enormous amount of the child's time and energy and make
normative experiences less probable (Chess, 1970).

Treatment. In management of these children, efforts should be
directed at providing the patient with appropriate activities to engage
his attention, withholding social reinforcements when the behavior is
exhibited, and finally, when the child's activities are clearly dangerous
to himself, restraining him from inflicting further damage. A variety
of devices and programs have been designed to attempt to manage the
most exaggerated and dangerous types of behavior. These include a
special helmet, restraints on the hands, and aversive electric shock
treatment. Sedation with tranquilizers may be helpful.

Tics

Tics are the involuntary, aimless, and repetitive movements of a
group of muscles. They usually originate in the head and neck and at
times generalize to include other parts of the body (Gilles de la
Tourette's disease). Lapouse and Monk (1958) reported the frequency
of tics to be 12% among children between 6 and 12 years of age, with
peak incidence after age 9. The course is benign and most children are
not seen by psychiatrists. While in psychiatric clinics more boys are
seen with tics, in epidemiologic studies boys outnumber girls by only
a slight margin. Although in one group of children with tics studies
by Pasamanick (1956), the incidence of complications of delivery was
higher than in the control group, no clear association between tics and
minimal brain dysfunction has been established.

Kanner (1972) considers tics a concomitant sign of anxiety, while
psychoanalysts, notably Mahler (1949), have emphasized the symbolic
significance of tics. She described five categories of tics: tics as a transient sign of tension; tics as a sign of reactive behavior disorder; psychoneurotic tics; organ neurosis; and character disorder (Gilles de la
Tourette's disease).

Learning theorists believe that for some children tics have a ten-
sion-reducing quality because they have been fortuitously associated

with anxiety reduction. Some authors have reported a family history of tics in such children. Others have reported case histories in which a friend or a neighbor is said to have exhibited the same kind of tics and has presumably functioned as a model for the child's imitation. Torup (1962) found a variety of tension symptoms associated with tics and thus lent credence to the generally held view that tics are seen in inhibited, overanxious children.

Prognosis. In a follow-up study of children with tics, Zausmer (1954) found that 25% of the children were free of symptoms one to five years after referral, 50% were greatly improved, and 25% had remained the same. The longer the period after original referral, the higher was the percentage of improvement. Girls showed a better prognosis than boys. Torup's follow-up four to six years after referral found that only 6% of the children had not improved (Torup, 1962).

Generalized Tics. Gilles de la Tourette's syndrome is a generalized tic, characterized by episodes of explosive, involuntary utterances in the form of inarticulate noises or articulated obscenities and concomitant involuntary movements of various muscles. In most cases, the tics begin from the head, with twitching and blinking. They progress to neck, shoulders, trunk, and finally the upper and lower extremities. Vocal tics may be added to the picture years after bodily tics, or they may be the first symptom. Coprolalia may be a combination of barking, coughing, grunting, and obscene language. On rare occasions, obscene gestures may accompany other movements. Anxiety and excitement may precipitate an attack, and parents report a build up of tension shortly prior to an episode, with relaxation following it. Attacks vary in frequency, with some children having numerous episodes per hour. Tics disappear with sleep.

The incidence of the syndrome is not known. Woodrow (1974) gave the figure of 4 per 100,000 as the incidence of Gilles de la Tourette's syndrome. Onset may be before the age of 10. The disease may be arrested spontaneously or may become progressively worse, though no mental deterioration has been reported. Various psychopathologies in patients or their families have been reported, although none seems to be unique to patients with this syndrome. EEG abnormalities of a diffuse and nonspecific nature are noted in about half of the published reports, but no organic etiology has been so far established. Recently some theorists have postulated a possible disorder of brain catecholamine as the etiological factor. Evidence for this hypothesis is still uncertain.

Treatment. Psychotherapy, alone or in conjunction with phenothiazine or Haloperidol, has helped these patients. In a follow-up study of 44 cases, Kelman (1965) found that of the 11 cases treated with psy-

chotherapy, two-thirds were improved, while phenothiazine or bu-
tyrophenone had been effective in 83% of the cases.

Hair Pulling

Hair pulling (trichotillomania) is a rather uncommon symptom
described in the literature in children as young as 17 months and as
old as 16 years of age. It may or may not be associated with thumb
sucking and nail biting. Some children only occasionally pull their
hair. Others may systematically indulge in the habit to the point of
baldness. In some, eyebrows and eyelashes are pulled. Others limit
their hair pulling to the scalp area. No particular psychopathology can
be said to differentiate these children (Manningo and Delgado, 1969).
In various case reports, they have been diagnosed as being obsessive–
compulsive neurotics, schizophrenics, borderline mental retardates,
and normal. Some authors believe that hair pulling is more prevalent
among girls. Others have reported equal distribution between the
sexes.

Conflicts between the child and the mother and other members of
the family are said to antedate the hair pulling by the child, though
there does not seem to be any convincing hypothesis about symptom
choice. Once the symptom is exhibited, it can be expected to provide a
nucleus for further conflict and a focus for intense attention. Some
authors have pointed out that while hair pulling in a young child may
be a form of bodily manipulation, particularly in children who are
understimulated, in adolescence symbolic meaning may have become
attached to the behavior and may obscure the original intent of the
child. In obsessive–compulsive children, hair pulling, like most other
symptoms of neurosis, is disturbing to the child, though he is not able
to stop the behavior. On the other hand, highly disturbed psychotic
adolescents may find the sensation desirable. The prognosis of the
symptom varies with the degree of the underlying disturbance. In
older children, the symptom is harder to eliminate.

Treatment. Treatment is dependent on identifying the circumstances—internal and external—that maintain the behavior. In some
very young children, environmental manipulation and provision for
more gratifying interaction is all that is needed to overcome the habit.
Other children require motivation and treatment of their conflicts and
fears. Behavior modification of various kinds may be helpful in treating the symptom while the underlying disorder of relationship and
communication is rectified.

19

Physically Handicapped Children

The psychiatric problems that arise in physically handicapped children can be divided into two major categories: those in which the physical defect is complicated by primary psychiatric disorders, and those in which the behavioral pathology is of a reactive nature. Examples of the first group are retardation, chronic brain syndrome, psychosis, and developmental delays. The same causative agent may produce different constellations of symptoms in a particular child, such as a combination of spastic diplegia, mental retardation, and brain damage, each with its own set of symptoms. In the reactive category, behavior problems may reflect stress on the child who cannot cope with the normative environmental demands because of his physical limitations, or they may appear as the consequence of inappropriate handling. An example of the latter is the failure of some parents to expect as much self-care activity as the child is capable of, thus creating unnecessary helplessness. Both primary and reactive psychiatric disorders may coexist in a particular child.

Primary Psychiatric Pathology

Mental Retardation. Retardation is defined as an impairment in adaptation as determined by the level of intellectual maturation, learning, and social behavior. The statement that a child is retarded at the time of assessment does not indicate the irreversibility of this status. In physically handicapped youngsters, the possibility of an alteration of retarded level may depend on the degree of exposure to optimal stimulation. Ideally, the developmental pattern should be compared with that of children with similar disabilities who have achieved a normal adaptive level. Unfortunately such normative data are not available for all types of handicaps. Formal test performance is only one element of judgment of intellectual level. It is important that the tests selected be appropriate in that they do not require the use of the defective function itself for task completion. For example, one should not employ tests that require listening to directions and giving verbal responses with a hearing-impaired child, visual scanning with a visually impaired youngster, or motor skill with a muscularly deficient patient. If specialized tests are used, they must be standardized with normal children or with those tests in common use with the physically intact group, so that valid comparisons can be made.

Brain Damage. The presence of one set of symptoms of central nervous system damage, such as neuromuscular defects, is not necessarily accompanied by all other possible sequelae. Behavioral manifestations of brain dysfunction, such as hypermotility or perseveration, may or may not coexist. On the other hand, if behavioral symptomatology of the types often associated with brain damage is present but no signs of neurological pathology are evident, the behavioral disorder in itself does not warrant a diagnosis of brain damage. However, the combined presence of neurological findings and certain, but not all, behavioral manifestations can together be considered sufficient for a diagnosis of behavior disorder due to cerebral pathology, or chronic brain syndrome. Such symptoms would include hypo- or hypermotility, constriction or lability of mood, unresponsiveness or hyperirritability, brevity of attention span or an inability to shift from an ongoing activity, hypo- or hyperdistractibility, difficulty in sequencing, central language disorder (aphasia), and perseveration. It is important to distinguish the pathological behavioral manifestations from both normal temperamental extremes and temporary lags due to individual developmental styles.

Since the internal structures of both eyes and ears develop in the embryo as outpouchings from the layers that form the brain, the factors that cause the defective development of these organs may simultaneously interfere with the normative formation of the brain structure. Consequently, in children with eighth-nerve deafness or a defect in the organ of Corti, or in those with blindness due to retinal insult or malformation, the possibility of central nervous system damage as a basis for behavioral aberration should be suspected and explored.

Developmental Delays. The sequences of affective, motor, and language development depend upon the interaction between the maturational processes in the child and stimuli of diverse modalities and characteristics from the environment. In a child with a physical defect that interferes with the reception and processing of stimuli in one or more areas, normal developmental sequences are delayed. Specific developmental milestones occur later than usual, or the order of their appearance may be different. For example, motor milestones are delayed in blind babies, who lack the experiences of seeing interesting objects and thus fail to pull to sitting or standing position at the usual age in order to see better. Only later do they make use of auditory cues for crawling or walking toward an object or a person of interest. However, such developmental lags are not permanent. The cumulative effect of the stimuli received through intact pathways and the compensation for impairment by the increasing use of cognition eventually accelerate development.

Psychosis and Infantile Autism. The criteria for schizophrenia, organic psychoses, and infantile autism in the physically handicapped do not differ in their essentials from those employed in diagnosing these disorders in physically intact youngsters. It is important, however, that a distinction be made between behaviors directly representing the physical incapacity or compensatory actions, and those behaviors that represent disorganization of thought, bizarre motility, or loss of interest in surroundings. Touching and clinging in a blind child may be an appropriate way of making affective contact; the smelling of food and objects in blind or some deaf youngsters is a typical mode of exploration of the environment through an intact sense. Certain behaviors, such as head weaving or eyeball pressing, are so typical of blind children that they are called *blindisms*. The difference between these behavioral peculiarities and those of psychosis or autism is the ease with which the child puts these mannerisms aside in favor of human interaction. Odd gaits or peculiar hand movements that are caused by muscular spasticity, atonicity, or athetosis are not to be confused with the bizarre motor patterns of these major psychiatric disorders.

Reactive Behavior Disorders

Most parents with physically handicapped children do not have easy access to guidelines for their management, particularly during infancy. Without knowing what the techniques are for compensatory stimulation or what their babies are capable of doing, the general tendency is for parents to overservice and to make insufficient demands for task accomplishment and/or impulse control. The child's reactions depend, in part, on his temperamental qualities. He may become passive and more helpless than necessary, or he may become a tyrant with tantrums whenever frustrated. He may give up easily or persist in his attempts, thus developing maladaptive techniques to dominate his environment. Social rules and safety regulations are hard to explain to sensorially deprived youngsters: with deaf children, the reliance is on demonstration; for the blind, verbal explanations plus haptic techniques are available. Because of these limitations, parents often rely to a great extent on unchanging rules. The same is likely to be the trend regarding children with motor disabilities, for whom the dangers of falling or otherwise hurting themselves are very real. Such children are at risk for such psychological reactions as a denial of the limiting effects of their handicap or rigidity of behavior. The resulting lack of flexibility in accommodating to changes in plans, accepting deviations from the rules of games, or responding to cues to guide social behaviors may become even more of a limiting factor than the handicap itself. When the child's distress is expressed intensely, as in tantrums or hostile and destructive acts, management problems and social unacceptability can become a major issue. In such cases, plans that are appropriate in terms of physical needs may be impossible to implement because of behavioral interference.

If the behavior disturbances are reactive to parental handling, a program introducing gradual modifications can be quite effective. When such children enter a school attuned to their needs, the combined effects of appropriate handling by the environment and the observation by the child of the activity and reactions of others with like defects create a salutary attitudinal change and help in learning more effective coping techniques. On the other hand, without intervention, inappropriate attitudes can become fixed and neurotic in nature; for example, the assumption of a helpless stance leads to ineffectual efforts, which reinforce the attitude of helplessness. A hostile approach to people evokes hostile counterresponses, thus reinforcing the child's assumption that he must protect himself by attacking first.

A crucial decision of psychological import is whether youngsters with physical defects are to be placed in normal or special classes. A general guiding principle is that children should be kept in the mainstream if this can be a constructive experience. The next choice may be to supplement instruction with special help, such as home tutoring or a resource teacher at school. Should such mainstreaming result in poor learning because the child's need for special teaching techniques and/or individualized attention exceeds what can be provided in a class of the usual size, a special class or school is required. One of the goals of special education is that such children should be returned to the mainstream of education if and when constructively possible. Such decisions should be made on an individual basis. The needs of many children are such that the permanent use of specialized teaching facilities is necessary, while for others periodic reassessments and changes in educational arrangements are more appropriate.

A handicapped youngster in a normal class may be very self-conscious about his deformity if it is visible. This is particularly true of a spastic gait and uncontrollable movements of the head, face, or upper extremities. These children must often realistically be excluded from sports and find themselves social outsiders. In preadolescence, the reactions of demoralization, self-denigration, depression, or denial may be found. In adolescence, the full force of the social stigma may be felt for the first time, resulting in deep depression and a danger of suicidal ideas or attempts. In fact, the youngster who had been well integrated into normal child society may be most vulnerable to such reactions because of his sudden exclusion from adolescent social activities. Adolescents often refuse to use prostheses that had previously been well accepted.

Assessment

The history taking follows the same format as with physically intact youngsters. There may, however, be more rigor in exploring familial defects, the possibility of maternal infections or exposure to environmental toxins during pregnancy, and the presence of difficulties during delivery. Neonatal status and childhood illnesses whose complications may include both physical and behavioral defect would also be areas for close scrutiny. The developmental history is to be considered with reference to type, severity, and the age at onset of physical defect or cluster of defects. Is the handicap of an improving, worsening, or fluctuating nature? If corrective measures have been employed, at what age were these started, how much improvement has been obtained, and for how long prior to assessment has the new status of competence been a part of the child's daily functioning? Observation techniques and conclusions must be related to the facts of the defect as ascertained in the history. These will be detailed below.

SENSORY IMPAIRMENTS

The major sensory impairments are those of vision and hearing. Defects of taste, smell, touch, and pain are either infrequent or of little importance in daily interactions. Hypersensitivities of these senses are more commonly noted as possible nuclei of problem behaviors.

Hearing Defects

The definition of deafness is given in measurements of decibel units of loss. Decibel loss and functional hearing are combined in the classification reported by Mindel and Vernon (1971). Since decibel units "are generalizations based on pure tone averages" and individuals vary greatly in capacities at different tones, the following classification does not function as a full guide for prosthetic correction:

- *Normal*: Up to 25-decibel (dB) loss. No significant difficulty.
- *Slight deafness*: 26–40 dB loss. The child may have difficulty hearing faint or distant speech.
- *Mild to moderate*: 41–55 dB loss. There is difficulty in understanding conversational speech in the distance range above 3–5 feet. However, fatigue and competing sound may create practical difficulty in hearing even within this range.
- *Moderately severe*: 56–70 dB loss. If the child is to hear conversation, sounds must be loud, distance small, and conversation directed exclusively to the child.
- *Severe*: 71–90 dB loss. Even shouted conversation most likely will not be heard.
- *Profound*: greater than 90-dB loss. The child perceives only vibrations and occasional loud sounds.

Speech sound consists of pitches between 300 and 4,000 cycles per second, and hearing loss may selectively occur in one range of pitch, with normal or better hearing in other ranges. High-frequency deafness is not unusual, although the reverse may be true, with normal hearing only in the high frequencies.

The acquisition of language by conventional means is not possible for children with severe or profound hearing loss, and if there is this degree of hearing loss prior to the age of 2, whatever language had been acquired will be lost. When hearing loss is slight or restoration through aids can bring the child's hearing to this level, speech can be normal. With mild or greater loss and with fullest correction, expressive language is below chronological and mental age.

Prevalence of Psychiatric Disorder. No general population survey of deaf children has been made that can provide precise data regarding the prevalence of psychiatric disorders in this group. Because deafness may exist alone or in the company of other handicaps, for maximum usefulness such data would need to be subdivided in terms of kind, number, and severity of other disabilities, since the nature of each additional handicap profoundly alters the stresses on and the limitations of the hearing-impaired child. Surveys of the adult deaf (Rainer and Altshuler, 1967) have indicated that schizophrenia rates are comparable to those in the general population and that depressions accompanied by guilt feelings are virtually nonexistent. The surveys have described many deaf adults as having personality characteristics that include egocentricity, rigidity, impulsivity, paucity of empathy, and failure to realize the effects of their behavior on others.

Some surveys of specific groups of deaf children have been done. While these cannot be safely generalized to all deaf children, they do provide important information. Bowe (1974) reported from a survey of 21,000 hearing-impaired students in the year 1968–1969: of those on whom appropriate information was available, 80.5 per 1,000, or 17,000 children were retarded as well as deaf. In a study of psychiatric casualty among children with congenital rubella (Chess *et al.*, 1971), of the 243 children in the study sample, 72.8% had a hearing defect. Of these hearing-impaired youngsters, 65 had only this single defect. Their psychiatric status was charted with reference to unspecified, moderate, or severe degree of hearing loss:

Psychiatric Diagnosis*	Degree of Hearing Loss		
	Unspecified (N = 4)	Moderate (N = 14)	Severe (N = 47)
No psychiatric disorder	1	7	31
Reactive behavior disorder	2	3	7
Chronic brain syndrome	1	1	1
Mental retardation	1	4	7
Autism (complete)	0	0	2
Autism (partial)	1	1	1

*Total is greater than 65 because of multiple diagnoses.

While half the children in this study whose hearing defect was accompanied by visual or neurological impairment were mentally retarded, only 1 of the 10 youngsters whose deafness was complicated by cardiac defect showed mental retardation. The complexity of distinguishing the behavior disorder due to deafness from the pathology conferred by additional handicaps was demonstrated when the children with two handicaps in addition to the deafness were categorized psychiatrically. Thus 11 children had combined hearing, visual, and neurological defects, and only 2 of these were without psychiatric disorder. Of the 17 preschoolers with a combination of hearing, visual, and cardiac pathology, 2 had no psychiatric disorder. And 27 of the sample had defects in all four areas: hearing, vision, cardiac, and neurological. Of these, 1 was without behavioral pathology, and 1 showed reactive behavior disorder, while the other 25 were all retarded.

When the same children were studied again at ages 8–9, 50% of those with profound hearing loss had five or more behavioral symptoms of moderate or severe degree, as against 32.4% for the entire rubella sample. A group whose hearing could not be estimated at all in audiologic examination because of behavioral interference contained 92% of the children with moderate or severe symptomatology; most were autistic (Chess, 1974a,b).

The difficulties of separating out the behavioral effects of deafness *per se* is illustrated by the 1971–1972 survey conducted by Gallaudet College, a major educational facility in the United States devoted to deaf pupils. Data were obtained on 42,513 students enrolled in 636 special education programs for the hearing-impaired in the United States. Of these students, 32% had one or more additional handicapping conditions. Hearing loss above 65 dB and the fact of the loss having been present from birth were both associated with a higher rate of additional handicap. The three most frequently reported additional handicaps were emotional or behavioral problems reported for 18.9%; mental retardation reported for 18.1%; and visual disorders reported for 16.3%. However, the survey report noted that the schools were given as a definition of additional handicap "any physical, mental, or behavioral disorder that significantly adds to the complexity of educating a hearing impaired child," and judgments were made individually by the participating programs. This survey can thus be used as a suggestive rather than as a rigorous statement as to the prevalence of psychiatric casualty among deaf students. It was also noted that deaf children whose additional handicaps were so severe as to exclude them from special education programs were consequently not included in the survey. In a study of 172 deaf children at the Children's Psychiatric Institute in London, Ontario (Goldberg *et al.*, 1975), 70% had an additional nervous system disorder, further documenting the difficulty of ascertaining psychiatric problems in deaf children and distinguishing those due to deafness as opposed to those ascribable to accompanying handicaps.

Qualitative statements on the behavioral characteristics of deaf children (Lesser and Easser, 1972) have identified motor restlessness, impulsivity, and a mixture of doubt and uncertainty coexisting with rigidity, obstinacy, and a tendency toward compulsive personality. On the other hand, Goldberg *et al.* (1975) came to the conclusion that deafness did not produce any specific psychiatric syndrome, although there was a tendency toward hyperkinesis and immaturity.

Intelligence. While the term *dumb* is used in reference to the absence of speech in deaf individuals, its connotations as meaning intellectual retardation are in keeping with widespread opinion. Psychologists for many years failed to use tests that did not require oral fluency or linguistic experience. As has been noted above, Bowe (1974) reported 8% of 21,000 hearing-impaired students to be retarded. Mindel and Vernon (1971) analyzed more than 50 studies in which the selection or modification of standardized tests eliminated the direct effects of deafness and inexperience in language development, and they concluded that these data confirm that the deaf have essentially the same distribution of intelligence as hearing individuals. In addition, these authors share the opinion of Furth (1971) that capacity for abstract thought does not differ in the deaf and in the hearing.

Academic Achievement. There is general agreement among educators of the deaf that academic achievement is below expectation for mental and chronological age. Schools for the deaf often have grade-level expectations below the national norms. Children who, because of oral and lip-reading proficiency, transfer to the mainstream of education are often behind their new grade, despite apparently adequate academic achievement within the special education program. They may then be able to catch up, but typically they have difficulty with those subjects in which discussion in class is an essential part of the learning process. Only a small percentage of deaf children manage to finish secondary school (Mindel and Vernon, 1971). Some studies have shown that children exposed to manual language from a young age are more proficient in reading and are equally capable in speech as compared with children restricted to oral training.

Work and Social Functioning. Vocational opportunities for the deaf are limited by the exclusion of work requiring oral skills, by educational inadequacy, and by the negative attitudes of prospective employers toward deaf employees in general. As reported by Mindel and Vernon (1971), 87% of deaf people are employed in manual labor as compared to less than 50% in the general population, and 17% of deaf people are white-collar workers as compared to 46% of the general population. Hearing people who have not been exposed to deaf individuals do not know how to communicate and are often uncomfortable in their presence. Avoidance is a frequent manner of coping with such embarrassments. Because of this and also because of the realistic communication difficulty, deaf adults tend to form social groups with each other. Almost all deaf adults use sign or manual language. Ninety-five percent of deaf people marry deaf partners (Rainer, *et al.*, 1963). Social organizations composed entirely of deaf members are common, as are those attended exclusively by the oral deaf, in which speech and lip reading are the language modality employed. Thus social separation is reinforced by attitudes of both the deaf and the hearing population.

Developmental Issues. The child born with a significant degree of hearing loss must develop his interpersonal awareness and relatedness and his comprehension of concepts of time, space, and danger through his intact senses, namely, the visual, olfactory, and haptic systems. Cause and effect, in terms of both physical reality and social conventions, are ordinarily conveyed to infants by the nurturing adults through combinations of imitation, approval and disapproval, permitting certain explorations, and removing the child from others and also, to an increasing degree as the child matures, through explanation. Language used with infants with intact hearing includes not only the spoken word but nonverbal communication of a rich degree through facial expressiveness, tonal quality of the voice, gesticulation, and different types of body contact of an affectional, approving, or disapproving nature. All of these, with the exception of speech, are available to the deaf infant. However, the experience of deaf babies depends upon their caretakers' knowledge and competence in utilizing such communication modalities.

Since the deaf child's early babbling is no different from that of the hearing infant, the fact of the deafness may not be suspected until there is a failure to imitate and practice sounds. When the possibility of deafness is finally suspected, its establishment as a fact is not easy. The audiologist projects sounds of various types and loudness into the testing room through speakers located at the child's right or left. Sound awareness is expressed by the infant through startle, tracking with eyes in the direction of the sound, and other clear changes in behavior. In order to achieve this, the infant must be comfortable, not crying, and in a state of appropriate arousal. Repeated testings are often required; the precise degree of deafness is difficult to ascertain at best, and behavioral interference may make testing invalid at worst. Early use of hearing aids is important so as to provide the infant with as close to normative experience as possible. However, the determination of which type of hearing aid to select and how loudly it should be turned up is often a matter of empiric decision.

While deaf parents automatically use their acquired skill in manual language, hearing parents' behavior in this respect depends on their advisers. Since there are two quite divergent theoretical approaches to the education of deaf children, the child psychiatrist must familiarize himself with the child's experience in this area. The oral approach is based on the conviction that if children learn sign language, they will "take the easy way out" and rely on gestural language to the detriment of acquiring skill in lip reading and sounding words. Furthermore, since verbal language is the key to competitive inclusion in the hearing world, and these educators accept the theory that verbal language is the basis of conceptual thought, permitting the child to use gestural communication will thus close his later options of functioning, limit him to deaf society, and be detrimental to his cognitive development. Parents of deaf babies are often advised to refrain even from the natural gesticulation that would ordinarily accompany their verbal interchanges.

The second theoretical approach is called *total communication* and recommends the combined use of sign language and vocalization so that language will be as rich, and will be utilized as early, as possible. Manual language, or sign, is presumed to fulfill all the criteria of language and is considered by proponents of total communication to be capable of promoting ideation and conceptualization on both concrete and abstract levels.

Whether the deaf youngster has been officially taught sign or not, he picks it up in his first contact with another child who has such competence. In an oral school, however, communicating through sign may be interdicted in the classroom and the children's unofficial use of it restricted to informal social settings. However, surveys have shown that almost all deaf adults in the United States can communicate with each other through sign. Communication through the visual route places certain restrictions on freedom of motor activity. The child's gaze must be directed toward the lips and/or hands and his attention gained through either visual or tactile means. The behavioral habits that promote communication are, in the deaf child, not indices of rigidity but rather appropriate accommodations. In addition, in the absence of sophisticated manual communication, safety rules, social strictures, and the like must often be learned through the parental demand for closer adherence to an invariant routine of carrying through actions and complying with prohibitions than would be the case for a hearing child of similar age. Children thus handled may be more insistent on following an unaltered routine and more distressed at changes of plans than would ordinarily be expected for their age. However, such behavior in a deaf child may be learned adaptation, while in a hearing youngster exposed to greater environmental flexibility, such rigidities would be more likely to reflect an intrapsychic problem.

Hearing-impaired young children employ their other senses freely, having not yet fully understood the arbitrary, selective social rules about such behavior. Thus they smell food, objects, and parts of people's bodies. They explore through touch. The presence of such behavior in sensorially intact children might imply either the failure of affective relatedness or the presence of compulsions. In deaf children, however, these are more likely to indicate an interest in exploring their world and the failure of the important people in it to have communicated social customs.

Clinical Observation. It is helpful, but not necessary, for the diagnostician to know sign. Much of the psychiatric assessment of children is nonverbal, and provided the psychiatrist speaks with clear enunciation for those youngsters who do lip-read and fully uses such nonverbal communication modalities as the glance, facial expressiveness, and gesture, he will be able to ascertain a good portion of the mental status. Affective relatedness can be determined by the child's attentiveness to the cues offered by the examiner, by his responsiveness to friendly body contact, by his facial expressiveness, and by his geatures denoting emotion and feeling. The relevance of these to the ongoing activity can be identified. As a group, deaf children are affectively well related and use every possible means of communication. The absence of such affective relatedness is not an expression of deaf mannerisms, it is pathology. One must, however, distinguish affective unrelatedness from shyness and slowness to warm up to unfamiliar surroundings and people. The affectively pathological deaf child behaves in a manner very similarly to the hearing youngster with problems in affective contact. He is oblivious to his environment except for small segments of it that relate to his preoccupations. The specific activity observed depends partially on mental ability. Such a child may sit rocking, walk about flipping an object, shriek if the ritual object is removed, and treat the examiner's hands as separate from the person. If puzzles are placed in his path, he may do them, thus showing awareness of size, shape, color, and/or content.

The level of play, motor competence, visual–motor skill, and organization of activity can be assessed if the proper materials are available. Representational toys such as furniture, trucks, and people make it possible for the deaf child to demonstrate his degree of awareness of the events in his environment through play; the level of sophistication of dramatic play can be compared with chronological age. Gross and fine motor skill and perceptual competence can be identified. In interpreting graphic productions, one should be aware that deaf children often draw human figures with a hearing aid and battery.

CASE HISTORY

Monica, age 3, presented management problems at the school for the deaf she had attended for one year. She was profoundly deaf; the diagnosis was Waardenburg syndrome, a form of hereditary deafness. There were no other defects. Pregnancy, delivery, and neonatal course were normal. Birth weight was 6 lb 6 oz. By age 4 months, deafness was suspected; by 10 months, it was confirmed audiologically. By 21 months, neurological and visual examinations were negative except for mild convergent strabismus, which subsequently disappeared spontaneously. Visual interest in the surroundings was prominent from infancy on. By age 3½, Monica's school had characterized her as "emotionally disturbed" and recommended transfer to a school for emotionally disturbed children. Complaints included repeating forbidden acts, nonparticipation in play except with a few classmates, and wandering at will when group activities were going on. She used certain skills, such a tricycle riding, only at home and refused at school.

A tall, very pretty 3½-year-old wearing a right ear-mold hearing aid, Monica's reluctance to enter the playroom was demonstrated in an orderly fashion: she walked down the hall but came back when not followed by her mother; she brought her mother's coat from the closet and put her own on. Intermittently intrigued by the equipment, she indulged in brief sequences of age-appropriate doll play and completed puzzles correctly. The diagnosis was reactive behavior disorder without disorganization.

When seen a year later, Monica, now familiar with the examiner, was affectionate, played fully and appropriately with a range of toys, and showed a long attention span and an organized approach. She followed no verbal directions and used word beginnings such as *pur* for *purple*. Meanwhile, nonparticipation at school had grown into negativism, which was also demonstrated at home and was intensified when a brother with normal hearing was born. The school was oral, but almost no verbal progress was made. Monica's temperamental qualities played an important role in her interaction problems with the teachers. A slow-to-warm-up child, her typical response to all new situations and new demands was to withdraw until she became familiar with them. In addition, she had high persistence and often preferred continuing with an ongoing occupation when changes in class activity were scheduled. Her profound deafness placed her in a group whose members, even with high motivation, failed to acquire facile oral language. The educational approach of the school was dissonant with Monica's temperamental needs. Demands were made for prompt compliance, and failure to fulfill these evoked strong disapproval. At age 7, transfer to a total communication residential school resulted in the cessation of the behavior disorder, speedy learning of sign, and progress in reading and vocal speech. A follow-up over a three-year period indicated a continuation of this positive adaptation and progress in learning.

CASE HISTORY

Nora, at age 8 years 10 months, had had fluctuating hearing because of intermittent middle-ear infections of two years' duration. With indwelling tubes for drainage, audiometric tests showed normal hearing. Loud noises made unexpectedly behind her failed to evoke a startle response. She was referred as a possible case of hysterical deafness. Pregnancy, delivery, and neonatal history were all normal, with birth weight of 8 lb 4 oz. Developmental milestones, including language, were average. Health history included many upper respiratory infections, usually complicated by middle-ear involvement. There had been a number of occasions in the period of known fluctuating hearing when alteration of hearing acuity was sudden and the child had been wrongly chastised for failing to comply with spoken requests. The parents on occasion had tried to catch her unawares with very loud noises to prove to her that she could indeed hear. In school, she did written work, recited, and maintained friendships.

Observation showed an attractive child of 8 who made use of age-appropriate materials, answered questions, and volunteered discussion. When conversing, she gazed at the examiner's mouth; when spoken to with face averted, she gave no response. However, when the examiner spoke soundlessly with proper lip movements, Nora could not follow, and the next full sentences spoken aloud by the examiner were reacted to by confusion. Her expressive language was age-appropriate and had normal inflection. The diagnosis was a reactive behavior disorder associated with chronic middle-ear infection. With the unpredictable changes in hearing ability in the past and the consequent scoldings, which she could not comprehend, the child had defensively reduced her hearing behavior to that of the safe period of total deafness. This continued even though the hearing was now normal. Since the family was moving to a warm climate, it was advised that Nora be told that this move would entirely cure her ear infection and that full hearing would return to stay. It was also recommended that no further checks on her hearing be made. The family's report several weeks after the move, and again two years later, was that Nora had immediately functioned in the new community as a hearing child and continued to do so.

Visual Defects

The classification of impaired vision is based on optimal visual correction with standard lenses for the better eye. The definition of legal blindness is "A person whose central acuity does not exceed 20/200 but is accompanied by a limitation in the field such that the widest diameter of the visual field subtends an angle no greater than 20 degrees."

Since persons with insufficient visual impairment to qualify as legally blind do in fact have difficulty in function, the National Association for Visually Handicapped (1973) classified impaired vision in functional diagnostic groupings. Blindness ranging from no light perception to central acuity up to hand movements, and with gross field loss, is considered to require the use of Braille and a dog, a cane, or other device to promote free activity. If vision permits seeing hand movements to 2/200 vision with a restricted field, the functional equivalent is defined as a marginal form of vision. Central acuity 2/200 up to 10/200 with form field exceeding 20° correlates with "travel vision" and the ability to use optical systems and TV with magnification. If vision is between 10/200 and 20/60, or there is better acuity but field is less than 20° in diameter, this is a partially seeing person who can read large print with an optical aid. Individuals within any of these classifications of visual loss are expected to benefit from reader service, talking books, tapes, and recordings.

Prevalence of Psychiatric Disorder. According to the American Foundation for the Blind (1973), there are approximately 60,000 severely visually impaired children of school or preschool age in the United States. There are no prevalence studies of behavior disorders in blind children as a total population. With the wide range in degree of visual handicap and the fact that, depending upon etiology, there may be end organ pathology only, or blindness may be associated with other defects, there is a need for prevalence data broken down by these parameters. It is assumed that there is a higher prevalence of behavior disorder among blind children than among sighted children, and autism has been specifically identified as having a higher incidence. It is not always clear, however, to what degree a differentiation has been made between the autistic-like "blindisms" such as ritualistic eyeball pressing and head weaving, which are easily abandoned in favor of human contact, and similar behaviors in autistic blind children, who prefer such self-stimulation to interaction with people. The high rates of autism in blind children with diseases such as retrolental fibroplasia and congenital rubella is likely to be the result of the accompanying brain damage—in the first case due to neonatal anoxia, and in the second due to viral infection of the central nervous system (Chess, 1971).

The presence of developmental delays in blind babies (Norris, 1956; Norris *et al.*, 1957; Adelson and Fraiberg, 1974) appears to be a crossover effect of the blindness, in which the failure of visual alerting to objects retards the motor effect of reaching or postural change for the purpose of attaining better visualization. Such delays are not necessarily an indication of retardation, and usually there is a developmental acceleration later. There is a similar temporary delay in affective development. If developmental acceleration is not evident by age 2 and motor and affective levels are still below chronological age by 5 years, intellectual retardation is to be suspected, provided that adequate stimulation has been received.

Intelligence. The distribution of intelligence has not been reported for large blind populations. The range of intellectual ability is from superior to profound retardation. If blindness is part of a syndrome in which the central nervous system is also damaged, mental retardation is likely to be among the symptoms present. In degenerative diseases such as Tay-Sachs, an autosomal recessive familial disease, the progressive blindness and mental deterioration go hand in hand. To be valid, testing of the visually handicapped should require no visual recognition and no responses to words with primarily visual association. However, tests used solely for blind children that have not been standardized on a sighted population fail to provide comparative information regarding intellectual level. Suppes (1974) summarized extensively the studies in concept formation and abstraction in blind children. To a large extent, these studies document the difficulty in making inferences as to the ability to form concepts in these subjects since the standardized tasks evaluating concept formation for normal children make extensive use of visual cues. Contrary to expectation, blind and partially seeing individuals do not have superior sound or haptic discrimination when compared with sighted subjects.

Academic Achievement. With the growing availability of Braille texts, talking books, and tapes, the educational achievement of blind children has been approaching that of sighted youngsters. Brothers (1973) studied the arithmetic computation achievement of 263 students from 42 school districts in 10 states using the Stanford achievement test. Braille students were 8% below expected achievement levels, and large-type students were 9% below. How this record compares with the largescale achievement levels of sighted youngsters across the country, however, is uncertain. Previous research had shown students in residential schools for the blind to score an average of 16–27% below norms for arithmetic achievement. Suppes (1974) reported on a 1959 study by Nolan, who found that arithmetic achievement varied to such a great degree from school to school that it reflected variables other than mental ability.

Language usage in blind children includes a high proportion of visual terms used to meet social expectations. Data on the general academic achievement of blind students are not currently available, although anecdotal reports on individual high achievers include some in postgraduate studies, including the field of medicine. There are an estimated 3,000 blind postgraduate students.

Work and Social Functioning. Blind adults work in most major job fields, although their proportion relative to the distribution of sighted adults has not been reported. The Vocational Rehabilitation Act of Congress provides federal funds to state rehabilitation programs, which include blind individuals in their training programs. The social capacities of blind children and adults vary widely and are not a direct reflection of the degree of visual handicap. With seeing-eye dogs, canes, and the training of other senses, many totally blind people travel freely alone, while others with the same degree of visual disability, or with partial sight, may be quite dependent and isolated. Training during childhood and personal temperamental qualities both contribute to this outcome.

Developmental Issues. While neonates have been shown to be capable of tracking objects briefly and young infants can show visual preference for patterns of varying complexity, the refinements of visual perception arise out of the constant interaction between environmental visual stimuli and the increase in neurological differentiation. The result is the attainment of sharper visual perception, which permits increasingly sophisticated conceptual associations in the cortical areas devoted to vision. With further maturation of the central nervous system, visual perception is integrated not only with other sensory functions but also with voluntary and reflex motor activities. In the normal infant, for example, the view of the bottle gradually leads to reaching and assuming the habitual posture for taking the bottle. Similarly the prone infant arches his back and raises his head in order to view his world; later an important impetus for sitting and pulling himself into a standing position is seeing an interesting object or hearing a noise associated with a visually important object or person. The motor development of the blind infant may be initially delayed. However, blind babies with intact or partial hearing learn to use the associations between sound and their experiences (being cuddled, fed, stroked, bathed, and played with) to alert themselves to impending positive and negative events. In an environment in which obstacles such as furniture are constantly kept in predictable places, blind youngsters can learn mobility and walk and run with spontaneity. Often the fully blind child is trained to a greater freedom of mobility than the partially blind child, who relies on his residual vision rather than having been trained to make fuller use of alternative senses.

"Blindisms," such as weaving the head from side to side and pressing the eyeballs, are more commonly indulged in when the child is unoccupied, and one may assume that they provide alternative interesting stimuli to the visually deprived youngster. Although these habits do not automatically signal behavioral pathology, they may impede the learning of more adaptive behavior and may expose the child to socially negative feedback.

The early smile of the infant is automatic. In the blind infant, the social smile and other affective behaviors whose refinements require visual feedback are delayed. When the child's maturity is such that other senses can be linked with present or impending pleasure and displeasure, and when the environment has provided rich and predictable experiential sequences, the blind child has a spurt of affective demonstrativeness. According to Norris (1956), the blind child who has no other major handicaps can be expected to be functioning up to the level of the sighted group by school age.

Clinical Observation. The diagnostician can accommodate his techniques to the limitations of the blind child with minor modifications. Communication through the verbal route is unimpaired except to the degree of limited cognition concomitant with mental deficiency or consequent to experiential deprivation. There is no special language form used by blind youngsters, and words of visual meaning are used in their colloquial sense, as "I saw my friend yesterday." The use of touch for the exploration of objects and people is purposeful and can be understood without difficulty. Facial expressions, while not showing the full range of types of grimaces or details that arise out of the imitation of visually observed facial signals, are usually clear as far as signaling mood is concerned. Affective relatedness is shown in the child's responsiveness to the examiner's auditory signals and in bodily contact, either spontaneously offered by the child or in response to the examiner's overtures. Blind children often direct their faces toward the person with whom they speak, and if there is some degree of residual vision, an affectively related visually impaired child inspects the examiner at close range and brings objects close to his eyes. However, when the blind child fails to direct his face toward the examiner during the diagnostic interview, this behavior cannot necessarily be construed as a sign of abnormal relatedness. The use of language and its content, and tonal quality also reflect affective capacities.

The affectively deviant blind child is as unrelated to people around him as the sighted youngster with affective deviance. He ignores spoken or tactile efforts or pushes off the hand that touches his head or back. His rituals differ from blindisms in that they are maintained without regard to opportunities to relate. If a ritualistic object is removed, there ensue the sounds of distress and the struggle to regain the object, but no recognition of the examiner as a person. The handling of the clinical interview depends partly on the chronological and developmental age of the child, in addition to the limitations imposed by the blindness. Discussion of play preferences is possible with children of age 2 and up if their mental age and language development are keeping pace with their chronological age. Noise-making toys, such as xylophones or rhythm band instruments, are objects of pleasure. Blind children may be interested in punching a bag once they have had an opportunity to feel it and become familiar with its action. Clearly games of skill that require visual–motor coordination, such as dart throwing, are inappropriate. Some puzzles that involve placing shapes in recessed spaces can be done by a haptic approach; these can indicate the child's competence in distinguishing size and shape and may be of interest to the child.

With the older blind child, there can be a discussion of the presence and definition of problem areas, relationships with peers and family members, fears, hopes, and plans. It is possible to inquire of the child himself how competent he feels, what his blindness prevents him from doing now or in the future, and what his attitude is about the reactions of others to him as a handicapped person. Open, unembarrassed inquiries are almost always acceptable to the child. The totality of the data thus gained indicates whether the child's interests, level of personality organization, and mode of relatedness are age-appropriate. It is possible to distinguish organized functioning from a disorganized approach to activity and disturbances of thought processes. Attention span, distractibility, motility level, and reaction to frustration can be assessed. The predominant mood and its variability and pathological behavioral qualities can be identified.

Graphic productions cannot be used to provide insight into the self-image, cognitive level, or prominent interests of blind children. However, partially sighted children are often capable and desirous of producing graphic productions, so that this instrument should not be overlooked in such cases.

CASE HISTORY

Robert, age 7, had been blind since birth because of the congenital absence of retinas. The reasons for psychiatric evaluation included a number of behavioral difficulties beyond those explicable by the blindness. From 20 months on, Robert began to react to frustration by hitting his face and biting his hands. He had worn a helmet for protection but was nevertheless constantly bruised. This behavior had gradually diminished to punching himself mildly on the forehead and chin and placing his teeth on his hand without breaking the skin. When excited, he spun about and flapped his hands at the wrists. Although the initial language development was normal, with first word at 10 months and a dozen words by 16 months, Robert then ceased to talk for a six-month period. When he began again, he would speak only to a small number of familiar people. Sleep was irregular and the total amount was only a few hours. The child would awaken during the night, and the parents heard him talking extensively to himself with clear enunciation, enumerating foods he preferred and singing nursery rhymes.

Pregnancy, delivery, and neonatal period were normal, with a birth weight of 7 lb 6 oz. At 3 weeks, the failure to focus the eyes was noted, and the absence of retinas was diagnosed soon after. The family received guidance on handling a blind child and followed the advice well. Motor milestones were delayed, with sitting at 10 months and walking by 20 months. By 2 years, coordination was good; he moved about the house without fear (furniture was always left in fixed places), and he would go downstairs by himself during wakeful periods at night and play contentedly with toys. Always a cuddly baby, Robert continued to be affectionate with his parents and sibs.

When observed diagnostically, Robert still had marks from self-hitting, consisting of thickened areas on the forehead and chin and the backs of his hands. When spoken to by the examiner, he made immediate movement to hit his face or bite his hands, which was then voluntarily aborted or minimized. Although the child replied occasionally, his tone was too low for the examiner to make out the words. He did not play with the available toys despite parental urging, except for rolling a toy car back and forth. He demonstrated affectionate contact with his parents by leaning or lap sitting and gradually responded to the examiner's physical overtures, eventually sitting comfortably on her lap. There was an occasional teasing smile in place of compliance when he was asked a question or was asked to do a task. The diagnosis was behavior disorder due to brain damage in a blind child. Because of the self-mutilation, the possibility of Leach-Nyhan's disease or some other variant of purine metabolism failure was explored, but this was ruled out.

Combined Hearing and Visual Defects

The definition of the deaf–blind child is highly subjective. Essentially a deaf–blind child is a deaf youngster whose visual defect makes it difficult for those trained to educate deaf children to use their techniques successfully, or a blind child whose deafness interferes significantly in successful integration into a facility for blind children. Children with this double handicap present very special problems of development, adaptation, and education. The largest single group of such youngsters are those whose handicaps are due to congenital rubella. When this relatively sudden influx of children came under the special education responsibility, some schools for the single defect enlarged the scope of their knowledge and accepted children with the second handicap. Many could not do so, and a National Center for Deaf–Blind Youths and Adults was established by the Department of Health, Education, and Welfare after the 1964 epidemic of rubella. It is administered by the Industrial Home for the Blind. The core of their program is parent guidance through home visits and demonstrations of techniques to establish optimum adaptation and independence. The total numbers of deaf–blind children, the prevalence of psychiatric casualty, and educational expectancies are all uncertain. Many of these children are retarded.

MOTOR HANDICAPS

The most common motor handicap in children is spasticity, with spastic diplegia or quadriplegia but usually with greater involvement of the lower extremities than of the arms (cerebral palsy). Other defects that may be encountered are muscular dystrophy, phocomelia, hypotonicity of musculature, athetosis, and surgical or accidental limb amputation. Poliomyelitis, which in the past was one of the more frequent causes of motor handicap, is now of low incidence in childhood. Each of these disabilities presents separate problems of daily management, with varying stresses and differing possibilities of successful inclusion in the mainstream of childhood experiences. The severity of the particular disorder is of great import, and in some diseases, such as muscular dystrophy, the downhill course from normalcy to death is a dominant factor. In some situations, motor pathology is a relatively unimportant aspect of a total picture, as in Down's syndrome. Some motor handicaps confer muscular weakness, which requires a different kind of accommodation than do either spasticity, with its predictable direction of distortion of an intended motion, or athetosis, with its much less predictable interference. Still another important feature for the diagnostician to bear in mind is whether and in what manner speech is affected. The "hot potato" speech of muscular atonicity creates different problems for the child in making himself understood than exist for those youngsters whose verbal productions are distorted in an athetoid manner. In each of the above types of disabilities, an important feature is the vulnerability of the child to being teased and scapegoated because of the character and prominence of distorted motility. One must remember that the term *spas* is used by children for teasing without awareness of its precise meaning.

Cerebral Palsy. Little's classical article in *The Lancet* in 1858 described 47 children with persistent spastic rigidity of one or more limbs, all of whom had had some abnormal circumstance during parturition. The term *cerebral palsy* has become a substitute for *Little's disease,* but with a much broadened definition. Cerebral palsy is nonprogressive brain damage manifested by a disorder in movement, posture, and/or coordination. Clinical manifestations, in order of frequency of occurrence, are spasticity, athetosis, rigidity, ataxia, tremor, hypotonia, and mixed forms. The brain damage may occur prenatally, during the natal period, or postnatally. The term *cerebral palsy* is generally employed up to age 21, after which the practice is to designate the specific clinical state, such as spastic diplegia. A case is considered mild if the patient needs no treatment, can function in all areas without assistance, and needs no speech therapy. In moderate cases, with some assistance, such as braces or a wheelchair, there can be independence in self-care and competence in all areas of daily living. Speech therapy is generally needed. In severe cerebral palsy, the patient is completely dependent despite the use of appropriate prostheses and aids, and there is severe involvement of speech and language.

Muscular Dystrophy. There are four separate types of sex-linked muscular dystrophy, of which the Duchenne type is most malignant and most common. These occur only in male children, and the mothers are the carriers of the gene. There are other non-sex-linked genetic types of muscular dystrophy, some being recessive. Muscular dystrophy can also occur without family history, although this is rare. The onset of the Duchenne type is in late infancy or in the preschool period. There is a progressive weakness of the muscles but not visible wasting; in fact, the appearance may be of greater bulk, so that the term *pseudohypertrophic muscular dystrophy* is sometimes employed. Death usually occurs during adolescence.

Poliomyelitis. Now an infrequent occurrence because of the effective vaccine, poliomyelitis had in the past occurred both endemically and in periodic epidemics. The lesion is in the spinal cord, in the lower motor neuron, causing weakness or total paralysis, with wasting in the particular muscle group. The paresis may affect lower or upper extremities. Bulbar paralysis can interfere with breathing, causing death or severe and prolonged dependence on an artificial breathing support (iron lung). There is no brain damage.

Phocomelia. Malformations of the long bones of the fetus have occurred sporadically for unknown reasons. The teratogenic effect of Thalidomide, a sedative available outside the United States in the 1960s and used by many pregnant women, became apparent when there was an epidemic of phocomelia in babies born in a number of countries. Some American mothers also used this drug when traveling abroad. Typically there is a shortening or absence of the long bones of the arms and/or the legs, with hands or feet attached to the stumps or to the shoulders or hips. Syndactyly and anomalous development of the facial bones may also occur. The severity of the lesions may range from syndactyly alone to severe involvement of all the vulnerable bones.

Prevalence of Psychiatric Disorder. A review of chronic disabilities reported in the United Kingdom as a whole in 1946, the Isle of Wight in 1970, and Rochester, New York, in 1970 reported the proportion of disabilities that were motor in nature to be 58%, 78%, and 67%, respectively (Pless and Roghmann, 1971). The United Kingdom study found 23% of the children with motor handicaps to have two or more behavior symptoms, as compared with 31% of those with sensory and 22% of those with cosmetic defects. In the Rochester survey, 26% of the youngsters with motor handicaps had three or more behavioral symptoms.

In cerebral palsy, prevalence data regarding psychiatric disturbance is difficult to specify. Associated defects complicate the task of knowing whether any behavior disorder, if present, is due to the motor disability. Robinson (1973) found that cases of spastic tetraplegia and of dystonic choreoathetoid tetraplegia show a much higher frequency of associated deficits than do cases of spastic hemiplegia, spastic diplegia, and atonic cerebral palsy. As Freemen (1970) pointed out, "since cerebral palsy is a heterogeneous group of disorders whose physical parameters are not yet fully agreed upon and in which associated handicaps are common, the lack of data with respect to emotional problems should not be surprising. There are no studies using sophisticated methodology, and the reports which are available seldom agree." In the adolescent age group, children with the various types of cerebral palsy must make a new type of adaptation. In the effort to make the handicap less visible, they may now refuse to wear obvious prostheses such as leg braces. They may feel, and in fact be, more excluded by their peers. Depression and suicide may be a hazard in this age period. However, no epidemiologic study has been undertaken to verify this widely held clinical impression. Qualitatively there is no specific type of psychiatric pathology associated with cerebral palsy (Freeman, 1970).

No extensive survey of psychopathology has been done in the muscular dystrophies. Coping mechanisms must deal with the awareness of the fatal outcome, frequently made quite real by the knowledge of uncles, cousins, and/or brothers who have died of this illness. Denial and hostility are often present in these youngsters. Female sibs are vulnerable to concerns about their own intactness in view of the knowledge that they can be carriers who pass the disease to their sons. This determination can now be made by chromosomal studies.

The reports on phocomelic children deal with their early childhood and it is too soon to know what their adaptations will be at later ages. The foci of the studies have largely been on development and intelligence.

Intelligence. Many of the muscular handicaps are associated with a higher rate of mental retardation than would occur by chance. Precise figures are not available. While children with cerebral palsy have mental retardation in greater proportions than the general population, every intellectual range is represented in such youngsters, including the extremely superior. In 25–50% of the cases of muscular dystrophy, there is an associated mental retardation. If mental retardation occurs in one case, it will be associated with the muscular dystrophy occurring in all members of this family.

In phocomelia, there is great difficulty in assessing intelligence. The diverse forms of malformation create varied degrees and kinds of mechanical difficulties. Gouin Décarie (1969) reported on the difficulties of ascertaining developmental and intellectual status in young Thalidomide children. Using a combination of evaluative procedures, she concluded that there is a typical profile in which language is the most retarded despite adequate hearing, and scores on the eye–hand scale are highest. One-half of her sample of 33 Canadian children followed longitudinally were intellectually within normal limits, a few were superior, and one-third were retarded. McFie and Robertson (1973) assessed 56 Thalidomide children between the ages of 7 and 10 years, of whom 4 were retarded.

Academic Achievement. Because of the great variability in motor handicaps, no overall statement can be made regarding academic achievement. Where the motor deficit is uncomplicated, learning is in general a reflection of individual intellectual ability and opportunities to attend school, providing the nature and severity of the motor limitation and the degree of prosthetic assistance permit the use of learning tools. When muscular weakness, spasticity, and/or athetoid movements prevent written or verbal communication, only the most motivated students persevere. Some individuals with very severe motor handicaps have achieved high academic status.

Work and Social Functioning. The enormous diversity in handicaps and differences in degrees to which associated handicaps are present make it impossible to attain overall knowledge about vocational success and social characteristics. Educational achievement, intellectual status, and the nonprogressive nature of the lesion all contribute to the degree to which training has been useful. Special talents and temperamental attributes can be determinative. Most reports have been anecdotal; these tend to deal with positive outcomes.

Developmental Issues. Unless they are given clear, practical guidance, the parents of children who cannot respond motorically in the expected fashion should not be expected to work out alternative modes of interacting on their own. Mothers who are devastated emotionally by the tragedy of a handicapped child may reduce their interaction to what is necessary for basic nurturing. It has been particularly noted in the limbless children that the infants were left alone for long periods of time and failed to obtain exposure to receptive language. Thus we have the crossover effect of a deficit in an unaffected area created because of difficulties in interaction caused by the affected area. The precise problems differ in each type of motor disease, and the alternative strategies developed for providing stimulation in both intact and defective systems must, of necessity, be individualized. A model of ingenuity is provided in the Gouin Décarie discussions of methods that would permit the Thalidomide babies to move upward in developmental abilities. Without such planned intervention, such youngsters cannot explore their world in the manner of Piaget's sensorimotor concept.

Clinical Observation. The clinical evaluation of motorically handicapped children requires less modifications than that of sensorially defective youngsters. Details of medical and developmental history are of specific relevance in the final overall situation. In clinical examination, the limitation of activity differs with the type of disability. At times, the psychiatrist may be in the position of being the first person to suspect a neuromuscular disease in a case referred as a behavior problem. Some children who have been referred with complaints of excessive dependency, fears of peers, or clowning and tantrum reaction to frustration have in fact had genuine helplessness due to unrecognized early muscular dystrophy or very minor athetosis. In addition, there may be overt defensive behaviors in response to the inability to compete with peers on various types of tasks requiring motor competence. Thus the psychiatrist should be alert not merely to psychological problems associated with the already-identified muscular disorder but also to the undiagnosed neuromuscular disease.

CASE HISTORY

Karl, age 11, had been showing evidences of depression. He said that he should never have been born and that no one liked him. At school, he put forth minimum effort but was nevertheless up to grade in most subjects. He had been born with spina bifida and meningocoele after a normal pregnancy and delivery. Surgery was performed in the neonatal period. Sequelae were saddle anaesthesia, lack of voluntary release of sphincters of bladder and anus, and waddling gait with feet everted and body rotating from side to side with each step. Speech had been early and perceptual abilities superior, and the child had attended the same normal school as his older sibs. While Karl was not teased or scapegoated, he was rarely included in spontaneous after-school social activities. His bowel function was maintained with enemas every other day. His bladder was emptied several times daily by manual pressure on the abdominal wall. The mother performed both tasks. She emptied his bladder just prior to his leaving for school, came to school at noon to perform this routine in the nurse's office, and emptied it again at home immediately after school. There had been no occasion of involuntary evacuation of either feces or urine in school, and the other students were unaware of the reason for the mother's daily appearance. Medical care required many doctor's visits: orthopedic evaluation to determine the advisability of prostheses and/or muscle surgery, and periodic urinary tract checkups for infection or kidney pathology due to reflux pressure. Karl refused to be taught to do his own abdominal pressure.

The history indicated an exquisite sensitivity on Karl's part to ordinary children's mutual teasing, with inappropriate hostile responses; other children then excluded him from the usual play of mutual fun insults. While he was of superior intelligence, his dependent behavior and failure to do his share made him less than desirable on schoolwork committees.

Karl was an appealing child physically, looking two years younger than his stated age. His gait was obviously ungainly, with the entire body swinging at each step to force the everted foot forward. His arm coordination was good, and his language was clear, relevant, and superior. He spoke openly and vehemently of his loneliness and his resentment of other children. The idea of assuming responsibility at any time for his bladder function frightened him. He was ready to concede that there might be something he did that "turned off" other children and hence he would wish to change this. The impression was of a reactive depression.

Treatment was direct psychotherapy in which, through combined play and discussion, there was an amelioration of the helpless attitude, achievement of greater self-esteem with increased academic output, the beginning of an ability to join in class verbal banter, and some inclusion in such after-school activities as bowling. This child is at risk for significant depression in adolescence.

Parent–Child Interaction

The birth of a baby with a visible handicap is a tragedy in several senses. If a genetic fault is implicated, the assignment of guilt, whether self-assigned or given by the other parent, creates marked marital stress at a time when the infant's needs are for cooperative parental mobilization. Often such an event brings to the surface latent maternal feelings of inadequacy. Indeed an insecure mother may be virtually immobilized. Often the presence and nature of the defect is slow to declare itself, and it may be several months or more before blindness, deafness, or certain motor handicaps are identified. Still a further waiting period may occur before pediatricians refer patients and their parents to resources that can provide specific guidance in defining the child's capacities, supplying techniques for compensating for disabilities, preventing unnecessary developmental delays, and creating opportunities for the child to develop independent functioning and smooth following of routines.

In general, parents underestimate their handicapped children's abilities and make too few demands upon them. Deaf babies' abilities to communicate through visual means, blind children's capacities to develop motor competences and affective relatedness, and motorically handicapped youngsters' abilities to interact verbally and to the motor extent possible are usually insufficiently exploited unless there is competent advice and guidance. In fact, it may often be necessary to handle the child in a manner that would be inappropriate for a child with full capacities. Schlesinger and Meadow (1972) noted that behaviors of deaf nursery children's mothers differed from those of hearing children's mothers in a number of ways. They appeared inflexible, controlling, didactic, intrusive, and disapproving; gave more constant supervision to protect; and had a narrower range of disciplinary techniques. The authors pointed out that in accordance with their study protocol, these were all hearing mothers who did not know sign, and they demonstrated feelings of frustration regarding communication with their children. However, the children themselves did not show evidence of feeling under stress at the maternal handling.

Programs to assist parents of blind babies focus on providing opportunities for safe exploration and stimulation as the initial phase of a continued emphasis on learning techniques of free motoric mobility, competence in daily routines, and development of skills. Since neither the haptic nor the auditory competence of blind children is superior to that of sighted children, these substitute modes of orientation and exploration must be taught to both parents and children. In her studies of 293 blind babies, Norris (1956) stated, "the blindness in and of itself is *not* the determining factor in the child's development. Rather, failure on the part of the adults to know what to expect of a blind child or how to encourage his optimal development creates the problems."

Motorically disabled children are realistically dependent on parents, but frequently, unless counseled, parents may foster a greater dependency than is in fact required.

In all handicapped children, there is a risk that, because of guilt, insufficient knowledge, and feelings of inadequacy, parents will give minimal nurturing and/or make insufficiently stringent demands. Behavior disorder can thus be added to the handicap itself, further compounding the stressful nature of the parent–child interaction. Thus all the measures noted above constitute primary prevention as far as behavior disorder is concerned. Where there is brain damage, behavioral symptoms directly reflecting the central nervous system malfunction may also be present, adding to the problems of parenting a handicapped child.

The psychiatric responsibility is to provide parental guidance so that shock, grief, and helplessness may be replaced by a positive program of management. If reactive behavioral symptoms are prevented, eliminated, or brought to the irreducible minimum, the potential for positive parent–child interaction over the long run can be addressed. In general, the most constructive posture is to assume that parents will be willing and skillful colleagues, if given the opportunity. Clarity on the nature of the defect and its possible outcomes, as far as is known, and on suggested management measures and the reasons behind the program, and assurances that the parental efforts may result in positive change will all go far to achieve the goal of providing an optimal atmosphere for the child patient.

20

Gifted Children

Attention to gifted children was first stimulated among educators around the turn of the century, when it became clear that the average school curriculum did not meet the special needs of children with superior intelligence. The widespread use of the IQ test as an objective measure made it possible to identify children with high scores and to devise various academic experiments to maximize these children's high learning ability. Furthermore, the large-scale, longitudinal studies of Terman and co-workers (1955) and Hollingworth (1942) provided a much-needed insight into the academic and personality development of these children.

In the Stanford study of gifted children, Terman included all schoolchildren who achieved scores of 140 and above on the Stanford–Binet test of intelligence and who resided in all the large and some of the small urban areas of California during 1921–1922. Hollingworth (1926) noted that this definition of giftedness was a matter of arbitrary decision. The top 1 or 2% of the juvenile population on any IQ test could be considered gifted. However, she was careful to point out that while these children could be considered potential geniuses, they might not fulfill the promise of their early years as they grew up. Terman's follow-up studies of the original group amply justified this cautious approach. The definitions of the two studies, based on general scores on IQ testss, do not identify children with special abilities such as music and painting.

On the whole, gifted children are distinguished by their broad attention span, speed of response, retentive memory, high ability in abstract thinking and generalization, and large vocabulary. While most studies have found these children to come from families with above-average intelligence, the role of environmental factors in facilitating the growth of intelligence among these children has not been fully explored. Much of generalization regarding children with superior intelligence comes from the studies of Terman and Hollingworth. They found these children to have shown accelerated early development. On the average, their health was slightly better than that of their peer group, and in follow-up studies into adulthood, their mortality rate was lower than that of the general population. Educationally they were above their age group, and the results of various achievement tests showed them to be even more advanced than their performance on school tests indicated. They had a large number of hobbies and interests and showed better emotional and social adjustments than children of their own age. Terman's follow-up studies (Terman *et al.*, 1955) show that as adults the group as a whole was more successful academically, had higher occupational status, and was socially better adjusted than the general population (Torrance, 1964; Getzels, 1962).

Special Problems

The superior intelligence of these children does not make them immune to the harmful influences of such factors as parental rejection or overprotection and environmental neglect and understimulation. In fact, they may become precociously aware of the complexities of human interactions that are beyond their coping abilities and are therefore sources of undue anxiety. Aside from the vicissitudes of interpersonal difficulties within the family, the most important area of the child's maladjustment relates to his functioning in school. Academic success or failure influences the personality makeup independently of the degree of scholastic achievement. When these children are not recognized as gifted, they find school programs boring and unstimulating. They become indifferent and idle, spend most of their time daydreaming, and, since they are able to meet school expectation with little effort, are led to believe that no further effort is necessary. Some children are quick to find fault with their teachers and to become disobedient toward all authority. They may become negativistic and disillusioned and may consider intellectual pursuit worthless. They become underachievers in school and drop out of college because they have not developed the study habits necessary for academic success. Other children use their high intelligence to receive approval from teachers and parents and find the uncertainties of peer relationships too difficult to cope with. They thus become isolated and harbor a deep sense of insecurity in their interpersonal relationships.

Some parents exploit their children's superior intelligence by forcing them to spend all their time in intellecual pursuits. These children do not have opportunities for interaction with their peers and remain emotionally backward. The discrepancy between their level of under-

standing and their emotional immaturity causes them to use their intelligence defensively and to shy away from human interaction. The
conflicts thus generated hinder full use of their intellectual abilities
and cause a sense of inadequacy and general dissatisfaction with life.

In comparing their study's 150 most successful and the 150 least
successful gifted children during their adult years, Terman and his associates found social adjustment to be the most important factor determining whether the subject had made use of his superior intelligence.
The absence of emotional conflicts, the ability to relate to people, and
a drive to achieve distinguished the socially adjusted group from their
maladjusted peers. Furthermore, though Hollingworth had surmised
that after the age of 12 the superior intelligence of these children may
make it possible for them to gain control of their own lives and become more independent, Terman's findings show that adolescence is
by no means an easy age of transition for the gifted group. In fact, it is
during adolescence that they may come to view themselves as inferior
and find their intellectual ability a handicap that sets them apart from
their peers. They then begin to lose interest in academic pursuits or
are so compulsive about succeeding that fear of failure immobilizes
them.

So far, we have considered all children of superior intelligence as
a homogeneous group. However, the children with a very high IQ
(above 180) present more problems in adjustment than the rest of the
gifted group. These children are a small minority even among the
gifted population (only 1 child in 1,000 is expected to have such a high
IQ). They become isolated very early in life. They may begin by participating in the games and play activities of their nursery school, but
they soon try to change the games into more complicated affairs that
other children do not appreciate and cannot follow. Thus they are soon
left out of children's activities, and since they do not easily find suitable companions, they are put in the position of having to achieve a
sense of adequacy and self-esteem with little group support. They may
in turn show intolerance and be domineering in their personal relationships and gravitate toward adults as their main source of support.

Another area of particular hazard for these children's development
is their precocious awareness of and preoccupation with such abstract
notions as life and death, the purpose of creation, and the nature of
the universe. While intellectually they can pose the questions, they
lack the emotional maturity to deal with their own intellectual grasp of
the subject. They may develop what Hollingworth has called a "negative suggestibility" in that they do not accept any direction and may
alienate their teachers and later on show disability in any relationship
that requires some degree of subordination. Some children use their

intelligence defensively, and their preoccupation with book learning becomes their main activity even from an early age. They thus fail to appreciate the emotional nuances of interpersonal relationships and deny their importance. Such children may be acceptable to their peers intellectually but are not accepted emotionally.

The families of these children may be overambitious and driving. They may use the child as a showpiece and overprotect him, or they may be angry and hostile toward the child and find his questions and acute understanding a nuisance. Some parents feel extremely insecure in relating to their highly intelligent child and become emotionally distant from him, thus leaving the child without the needed support of parental figures. When acceleration in school is the only available means for the education of these children, the gap between the child and his contemporaries widens, and the discrepancies between the emotional, social, and intellectual abilities of these children may cause extreme adjustment problems.

In studying the adjustment of a group of 12 children with IQs above 180, Hollingworth came to the conclusion that the socially optimum level of intelligence may be in the 125–155 range. Of the 81 subjects in the group of 1,500 gifted children who tested at an IQ of 170 or above, Terman *et al.* (1955) found a high percentage of severe adjustment problems, so that their rate of maladjustment was about twice that of the entire gifted group. He summarized his finding as follows:

> If the I.Q. is 180, the intellectual level at six is almost on a par with that of the average eleven year old, and at 10 or 11 is not far from that of the average high school graduate. Physical development, on the other hand, is not likely to be accelerated more than 10 percent, and social development probably not more than 20 or 30 percent. The inevitable result is that the child of 180 I.Q. has one of the most difficult jobs of social adjustment that any human being is ever called upon to meet.

Of course, it must be recognized that the majority of gifted and highly gifted children do manage to use their abilities in a creative manner and find various avenues for appropriate social adjustment and peer group interaction (Witty, 1951).

Although the gifted group comprises only 1 or 2% of the children's population and are underrepresented in psychiatric facilities, their special needs are of utmost concern to child psychiatrists. They may be referred for underachievement in school, isolation from their peer group, and a variety of interpersonal difficulties with their families or with others. It is particularly important to remember that the high intellectual ability and extensive vocabulary of these children, coupled with their advanced ability for introspection, may present a puzzling clinical picture and lead to overestimation of the degree of their emotional problems. They may be bored with the routines of school, find their classmates dull, and view their teachers with scorn. They may be unhappy over their inability to socialize with other children, or they may deny the necessity for any relationships. They are dissatisfied with the answers that they receive to questions regarding the moral and ethical issues that concern them. At times, they consider the games and physical activities of their peer group a waste of time, though they feel inadequate to compete in them. Intellectual stimulation provided in a more challenging school setting and suitable companions are the first necessary step in helping these children. However, they should be encouraged to relate to their peers on the nonintellectual level, such as through sports and games, and in the process to develop a sense of comradeship with those who are not their intellectual equals. Parents and teachers should be counseled to respect the child's intelligence without relinquishing their adult roles in providing emotional support and direction for him.

21

Normal and Pathological Behavior in Adolescence

Normal Development

The term *adolescence* is a biosocial designation that describes the developmental period during the second decade of life. It begins with the biological changes of puberty and ends when the social status of adulthood is attained.

Biological growth and pubertal changes are for the most part genetically determined and regulated, although such environmental factors as climate and nutrition play a part in the timing of pubescence and the eventual physical status of the individual. The time of onset of pubescence varies according to the criteria that are used. When menarche in girls and seminal ejaculation in boys are used as indications of sexual maturity, most studies reveal that boys achieve this stage, on the average, a year or two after girls. The average age of the first menstruation is between 12.5 and 13.5 years for girls in the temperate zones. However, the age range for the first occurrence of menarche in a group of normal girls is between 11 and 15, with 3% falling above or below these limits. The same variability of age of onset is found among boys for various indices of the biological changes of pubescence.

Some authors have used the time of maximum increment in height as the criterion for the onset of puberty. This period appears about two years earlier in girls than in boys. Longitudinal studies have placed the mean age of maximum growth for girls around 12.6 and for boys around 14.6. A comparison between the age of maximum increment in height and other indications of pubescence shows that sexual maturity occurs earlier in those children who undergo earlier changes in their skeletal growth, and conversely, later sexual maturity

375

is associated with a late appearance and a slower pace of growth spurt in height. In most cases, the rapid increase in height is about a year after the first seminal emission in boys and a year before the first occurrence of menarche in girls. Most authors believe that skeletal age, as determined by X ray, is the most satisfactory index of biological growth. The skeletal age is the percentage of the total ossified area of the wrist in comparison to the mean values for various age groups.

Although there is a sequential order in which changes in one biological aspect precede manifestations of growth in other areas, they are not necessarily completed with the same regularity. Therefore physical growth during adolescence is asynchronous and disharmonious. The wide age range for the beginning and completion of pubescence and the individual pattern of physical growth result in significant differences in the stage of physical maturity that any adolescent has attained at any given point in time. Physical growth during adolescence occurs in an accelerated fashion and is more dramatic than the gradual and steady growth of childhood. Furthermore, in contrast to the growth spurt of early infancy, physical growth during adolescence has social and psychological significance that transcends the mere fact of change in body proportion and appearance. For those adolescents whose physical growth is unusually retarded or precocious, concerns and anxieties or a sense of being estranged from peers may be a source of psychological stress.

The biological changes of pubescence are interrelated and interdependent; even though the mechanism by which any one aspect of growth is influenced by other physiological processes is not clear, their correlation is well established.

Hormonal Changes. The physiological stimulus that causes the increased activity or activation of the gonadotropic and corticotropic secretion of the anterior pituitary gland is as yet unknown. However, it is subsequent to this activation or increased activity that the primary and secondary sex characteristic appear, mature ova and spermatozoa are produced, body size and body proportion are changed, and the physiological functions of the cardiovascular and respiratory systems approach their adult state.

In prepubescent children, the adrenal cortex is responsible for the production of a small quantity of estrogen and androgen hormones in both males and females. The amount of androgen is more than estrogen in both sexes, although the ratio of androgen to estrogen is slightly higher in boys than in girls. With the initiation of puberty, the ratio of androgen to estrogen increases further in males and decreases in females, although the absolute amount of both hormones in the bloodstream rises as compared to the level in prepubescence. Fur-

thermore, stimulated by the gonadotropic secretion of the anterior pituitary, the gonads produce estrogen in females and androgen in
males, resulting in the differential pattern of sex hormones in boys
and girls. When the levels of estrogen and androgen reach a critical
state, primary and secondary sex characteristics begin to appear (Fleming, 1963).

Primary and Secondary Sex Characteristics. Primary sex characteristics include the growth and function of the genitalia and the reproductive organs. In males, the testes increase in size and volume, the
penis grows in length and circumference, and the prostate, seminal
vesicles, and epididymis undergo appropriate changes. Finally, the
evidence of the capacity to reproduce appears in the form of seminal
emission containing fully differentiated, motile spermatozoa. In girls,
the ovaries and the uterus are gradually enlarged, and ovulation and
menstruation become possible. It must be noted that the regular
rhythm of the menstrual period may not be achieved until late adolescence, and ovulation may not accompany every menstruation. In boys,
seminal emissions of the earlier years may contain predominantly immature spermatozoa, so that full sexual maturity in both sexes may be
achieved only gradually.

Secondary sex characteristics are matters of immense social and
psychological significance because they are readily observable and determine the differential responses to the sexual identity of boys and
girls. Changes in the breasts begin before menarche in girls. First, the
areola is elevated (bud stage); then, with the enlargement of the ad-
joining area by a preponderance of fatty tissue, the breasts are developed. In some adolescent boys at the beginning of puberty, the
breasts become slightly enlarged; however, this enlargement, which is
caused by the higher estrogen production by the adrenal cortex, does
not continue. The mammary glands remain underdeveloped in normal
males.

Pubic hair in girls appears shortly after the initial enlargment of
the breasts; by the time of first menstruation, the entire pubic area is
covered with pigmented, kinky hair. In boys, the appearance of the
first pubic hair predates the visible enlargement of the testes. Later on,
thicker and pigmented hair extends from the pubic area in an upward
direction. Axillary hair in both sexes appears following the growth of
pubic hair. In boys, thick, pigmented hair eventually covers the
thighs, legs, arms, forearms, and chest. In girls, pigmented body hair
is scantier than in boys. However, exceptions can be found among
both sexes.

The growth of facial hair in boys is of particular social importance.
Before puberty, there is no difference between boys and girls with

regard to facial hair. With pubescence, hair first appears in boys in the form of juvenile mustache, and gradually on the cheeks, the area below the lower lip, the chin, and the sides of the face are covered. By late adolescence, the submandibular region of the neck grows hair, signifying the growth of the beard and the attainment of sexual maturity.

The vocal chords increase in size and the larynx develops in internal dimension during adolescence. In girls, these changes are more gradual and less marked; therefore the changes in voice are not as conspicuous as in boys. The deepening of the voice and the lowering of pitch begin in early adolescence, but the characteristic tone of the adult does not appear before 16–17 years of age.

Male and female body types are differentiated with changes in skeletal development. In girls, the hips become wider; in boys, the shoulders are broadened. Body fat in girls is deposited in the buttocks, thighs, and arms, while in boys excess fat is usually located in the anterior wall of the abdomen. However, these differentiations in body type are not always present, and there are numerous variations in the extent to which any man or woman has the body-type characteristics of the opposite sex.

Sweat and sebaceous glands also increase their activity during pubescence. The sebaceous glands, particularly the ones on the forehead, on the sides of the nose, and on the chin produce larger quantities of their oily secretion. Poor discharge causes the accumulation of the secretion in the glands (blackheads), and these in turn are easily infected and produce the condition called *acne*. For most adolescents, both boys and girls, acne is an irritating and embarrassing affliction that may influence social and heterosexual adjustment. The increased activity of sweat glands in the axillary and genital regions may be accompanied by the characteristic odor of perspiration after puberty.

Skeletal growth during puberty is due to the increased activity of the growth hormone from the anterior pituitary gland. The relationship between gonadal hormones and skeletal growth is ascertained by the observation that in cases of precocious puberty due to tumor of the adrenal cortex, the individual does not attain the final normal adult status and that, conversely, when puberty is unduly delayed, a tall, eunuchoid stature results. The ultimate height attained in both men and women depends on genetic variations and nutritional factors. Children who are taller during prepubescence will eventually be taller adults. However, as mentioned earlier, the growth in height and weight is a steady process until sometime during adolescence, when a rapid increase in both takes place over a period of 6–12 months. From then on, the increment in yearly growth begins to diminish until the epiphysial cartilage of the long bones is ossified and no further increase in height is possible. The increase in the length of the long bones and the width of the shoulders and pelvic girdles is accompanied by growth in the mass of muscles and an increase in physical strength. This strength has significant social implication for adolescents and is in turn influenced by cultural traditions. In boys, the rapid increase in strength is followed by more opportunities for physical exercise in the form of athletics or occupational activities. Therefore structural changes are reinforced by functional use; in girls, on the other hand, the potential muscular strength is usually not used and tapers off quickly.

Other changes in skeletal growth are due to differential rates of growth in various parts of the body, so that the more rapid growth of the trunk changes the ratio of trunk to legs, and an increase in the size of the nose and forehead changes the facial features.

Growth in the size of the internal organs and changes in their functioning keep pace with the requirement of the enlarged body. Systolic and diastolic blood pressure rise during adolescence, with a concomitant drop in pulse rate. The respiratory capacity of the lungs is increased, although the respiratory volume per square meter per minute declines. Higher activity and enlargement of the thyroid gland cause an increase in total heat production by the body; however, because of better temperature control, the basal metabolism does not rise and, in fact, declines. Thymus and lymphoid tissues diminish in size during adolescence. Differences between male and female appear in various biological functions during pubescence and continue into adulthood. For example, the basal metabolism remains higher in men; the pulse rate is somewhat higher in women. The increment in both systolic and diastolic pressure goes in the opposite direction of the pulse rate.

The biological changes of adolescence appear over a period of seven to nine years. No one manifestation can be taken as signifying the attainment of complete physical maturity or procreative power, although they are all parts of a developmental pattern. Observations and longitudinal studies have shown that while physical maturity will eventually be achieved by the end of the second decade of life, the process of growth during adolescence is unharmonious and each individual grows according to his own unique pattern (Ausubel, 1957).

Social and Cultural Expectations. Societies and cultures differ in their expectations of and attitudes toward their younger generations. In technologically simple cultures with a high degree of social cohesion, the adolescent has easy access to adult society. His vocational choice depends to a considerable extent upon his physical strength, and the necessary skills are learned directly by gradual participation in the productive activities of family members. The social status of girls and boys is predetermined and emancipation from parental authority is not required. Furthermore, in such societies, adolescents do not constitute a separate group, and peer relationships are not expected to replace or supersede family ties. Sexual maturity is soon followed by marriage, and long periods of abstinence are not required. The value systems and religions are held as group traditions, and no individual is expected to find justification for ancestral beliefs. In most such cultures, child-rearing practices and conditionings are continuous, in that children are given an increasing amount of responsibility and the behavior that is deemed acceptable or desirable for adults is permitted during childhood (Benedict, 1949).

In more complex societies, adolescence is a protracted period because the task of acculturation and specialization requires long years of schooling. During this period, the adolescent is expected to learn and explore the scientific and moral basis of his culture and to prepare for eventual entrance into adult society by choosing a vocation and acquiring the necessary skills in educational institutions. Before the eventual goal is achieved, the adolescent remains financially nonproductive and is discouraged from engaging in a marriage contract and sexual behavior that may force the young man or woman into unwanted and unregulated parenthood. The high concentration of adolescents in school settings and their common status provide the impetus for the development of group mores and standards that influence their behavior. Acceptance or rejection by the peer group and the degree that this group's values parallel or diverge from parental value systems are potential sources of strain in intrafamilial relationships. However, group values are, for the most part, a reflection of the social and cultural tradition, and the process of socialization and acculturation of the young continues even though the central authority shifts from adults to age mates (Caplan and Lebovici, 1969).

Within the context of the complex industrialized societies, the course of adolescent development is viewed as a gradual progression toward the establishment and exercise of volitional, financial, and emotional independence from the family and adaptation and adjustment to social expectations. Changes in the parent–child relationship are initiated by the gradually rising expectations of the parents that the adolescent will take more responsibility in managing his own affairs. Reasoned arguments replace the earlier reliance on authority; rewards and punishments are explained on the basis of the seriousness of the infractions of the rules or the exceptional quality of the achievements. Differences in opinions and questions regarding parental beliefs and attitudes are tolerated and discussed. Adolescents, in turn, become more sensitive to their own wishes and more assertive with regard to their own preferences. Their cognitive development makes it possible for them to entertain various points of view and become aware of contradictions and inconsistencies in the value system of their culture or their particular group. Because they are most familiar with the value system held by their own families, their debates and arguments are first and foremost directed toward parental beliefs. The opinions or deeds of peers, other parents, teachers, and others are presented as examples to be followed and values to be espoused. Extreme positions are advocated and alien ideologies sponsored even though the eventual outcome may be sharing of parental values (Offer, 1969; Offer and Offer, 1971).

Vocational interests and planning for a future occupation become more crystalized during adolescence. The development of a self-critical ability allows the adolescent to make a more realistic assessment of his own potentiality and limitations and to become aware of the range and scope of the opportunities available. Income, prestige, and a host of other environmental factors are viewed as relevant parameters in the choice of a future career. Once the options are narrowed down, the adolescent sets out to acquire the necessary qualifications for his future occupation. He begins to shape and construct attitudes and standards compatible with his choice, and his activities—academic or otherwise—are directly or indirectly related to this goal. The emerging sense of social identity in the adolescent is partially anchored to the productive role that he hopes to undertake in society.

Peer relationships acquire particular importance during adolescence as every adolescent begins to realize that he must seek emotional support and intellectual understanding from his contemporaries, whose lives will run parallel to his own. The fear of rejection and striving for acceptance by peers are strong motivational forces underlying the conformity of adolescents to peer group standards, such as manner of speech, style of clothes, or fascination with some ideologies. Heterosexual interest is in part initiated by the biological changes of puberty; however, sexual role acceptance is fostered by sociocultural expectations transmitted by family and peers. Adolescents are perceived as members of a male or female group and are expected to engage in culturally appropriate feminine or masculine behavior. Even though they may not be sexually active, they are encouraged to participate in such socially approved heterosexual behavior as dating. The acceptance of sexual role and mastery over the nuances of heterosexual relationships are important steps toward the establishment of an individual identity for adolescents (Chess *et al.*, 1976).

The multitudes of developmental tasks facing adolescents and the varieties of demands placed upon them make this developmental period a potentially stressful one. Asynchronous physical development, biological changes within the body, shifting relationships with family and peers, and concerns over future roles are all possible sources of anxiety, disappointment, and even depression. However, the majority of adolescents are capable of coping with the conflicts and stresses of their particular status without experiencing more than mild to moderate degrees of anxiety and depression. This conclusion, which stands in contradiction to the statements of earlier authors in the field, is substantiated by longitudinal studies of nonpsychiatric populations of adolescents (Masterson, 1968). Data from the long-term follow-up of Offer and Offer (1971) have revealed that the psychiatrically normal group of freshmen high school students who were first evaluated in 1962 and have long since entered adulthood achieved emotional independence from their family "without total devaluation of parents" and established a sense of identity and developed vocational goals with little experience of confusion and disorientation. Some personality characteristics and styles of interaction remained relatively unchanged, while other coping mechanisms appeared in response to the challenges of new situations.

The adolescent's sense of insecurity, his fear of social slighting, and his great distress in response to the fluctuations of attention he receives within his own group are consequences of what Lewin (1939) called the marginal status of adolescents in society and are therefore transitory in nature. They may color the kind of psychiatric symptomatology that is exhibited during adolescence, but adolescence *per se* cannot be considered an etiological factor in various psychiatric problems.

Psychiatric Problems

A sizable minority of children come to psychiatrists' attention during their pubescence for problems ranging from neurotic, maladaptive behaviors to overt psychosis. A problematic adolescence may be presented as an exaggeration and intensification of the common concerns of adolescents or as a clearly deviant and pathological behavior. For example, the struggle for volitional independence may, under certain circumstances, lead to a total estrangement of the child from his family and an identification with people from a group or subculture that is despised and disapproved by the parents. Such identification may be the motivating element behind some adolescents' running away from home, their truancy from school, their lack of academic interest, and their involvement in delinquent activities. This state of affairs, although disturbing to the parents and detrimental to the adolescent, is not qualitatively different from the more common conflicts between generations, although the intensity and extent of the conflict is symptomatic of long years of a distorted parent–child relationship. Depending on the nature of their deficiencies and the unavailability of socially acceptable alternatives, they may no longer be capable of finding a compromise solution and, as a result, experience crippling anxiety, depression, or an extreme degree of anger and dissatisfaction. Their subsequent activities may be motivated by the phobic avoidance of tension-producing situations, such as school, or their need for discharging their hostility through antisocial behavior. They may try to change their moods by abusing drugs or alcohol or may seek a temporary state of heightened vitality by engaging in dangerous adventures (Thomas and Chess, 1976).

Because society considers adolescence the end of irresponsibility and indulgence, it expects the adolescent to take charge of his own destiny, to compensate for his own deficiencies, and to judge the appropriateness of his own behavior in accordance with cultural norms. When children have failed to master the developmental tasks of earlier years, they lack the necessary cognitive and psychological equipment to achieve this higher degree of social effectiveness and competence. Their sense of defeat at the threshold of adulthood frightens them about the future, and their bitter memories of past failures kill any desire for a sense of continuity with their past. They are thus deprived of the necessary elements for the establishment of an independent identity. They are outraged, anxious, and depressed. This sense of confusion and lack of clarity within them is reflected in unstable relationships with their contemporaries, ambivalent interactions with their families, and thoughtless experimentations with sexuality. The adolescent's "turmoil" is experienced not only by the individual himself, but also by all who come into contact with him. He is unpredictable, moody, unable to accept the standards of the group that he has chosen to join, and unwilling to take responsibility for his own actions. He may be brought to the psychiatrist's attention because he has made suicidal attempts or has shown such violent rage that he is feared as a possible danger to others. His suicidal communication may turn out to be a genuine desire to die or a manipulative maneuver to control his parents or friends. He may excuse his aggressive behavior as a justifiable response to environmental provocation, or he may be puzzled by its intensity. The overall impression given by such an adolescent is that of an individual who feels incapable of coping with his own desires and anxieties and fulfilling the expectations of his environment.

To the extent that such a clinical picture is the end product of the smaller failings of childhood years, the designations of *adjustment reaction of adolescence* or *adolescent turmoil* are misleading. However, such terminology is indicative of the belief of some clinicians that a good percentage of these adolescents will manage to overcome their difficulties and develop adaptive behavioral patterns in later years. This point is of particular importance in relation to the psychiatric evaluation and treatment of adolescents. When deviant behaviors are considered phase-specific and dismissed as something that the adolescent will outgrow without any outside help, the patient is deprived of treatment that may be vitally necessary for him. On the other hand, when the behavioral manifestations are viewed with great alarm and undue pessimism, the patient is either under- or overtreated. The possibilities and potentials for change and continuity inherent in adolescence require therapeutic approaches that aim at revitalization and redirection of basic strengths of the patient and minimization of the effects of his deficiencies.

Some psychological reactions in adolescents may be directly traced to the incongruity and disharmony of their physical development. Early-maturing girls and late-maturing boys may find their social relationships hampered or distorted by their physical status. Boys who mature later are not able to compete with their peers in sports and are usually ignored by girls who are interested in heterosexual relationships. Early-maturing girls, on the other hand, are neglected by their same-sex friends and are perceived as heterosexual partners by older boys earlier than their emotional development would allow for such commitments. These adolescents experience feelings of loneliness and depression and become oversensitive in regard to their position among their peers. Assurance, understanding, and support from adults, be they teachers, parents, or psychiatrists, are necessary to alleviate the present distress and promote understanding, acceptance, and appreciation of individual differences in the rate and timetable of physical maturity.

Distorted parent–child relationships, in the form of rejection, neglect, over- and underdomination, and long-standing parental disharmony, may all show their cumulative effects during adolescence. These children have failed to develop a sense of self-esteem and are insecure. Their past achievements have fallen short of arousing parental interest, or their failures have been treated as parental betrayal.

They have come to fear failure so intensely that they do not dare undertake any new tasks, or they have never learned to draw self-satisfaction from the learning process. They are unable to regulate their own lives since they have never been allowed strict limits from the environment. They are in conflict with their peers because they cannot cooperate or compete without guilt and resentment. They are inept in heterosexual relationships or engage in various sexual activities without a concomitant tenderness toward their partners. Their academic performance deteriorates because they are expected to work more diligently and with a lesser degree of parental involvement or because in rejecting their parental values they have also rejected school as oppressive and irrelevant. Chronic guilt, anxiety, anger, and depression engendered by conflictual relationships with parents are at the root of neurotic and aggressive–hostile (delinquent) behavior of adolescents. The clinical picture in these disorders is not as fixed and crystallized as the same conditions in adulthood. However, psychiatric intervention is necessary not only to relieve the immediate distress but to prevent the unwanted consequences of maladjustment during the crucial formative years of adolescence (Weiner and Del Gaudio, 1976).

Psychotic Disorders. The introduction of the term *démence précoce* by Morel in 1856 focused psychiatric attention on the long-observed fact that the first manifestations of the illness that later came to be known as the group of schizophrenias may be seen during adolescence. In the present state of ignorance regarding the etiology of schizophrenia, it is not possible to state whether the hormonal and other biological changes of pubescence play a causative role or even act as a triggering mechanism for the initial expression of a schizophrenic disorder. The clinical picture of schizophrenia during adolescence may appear as an acute process and may run a course marked by remission and exacerbations, or it may be present with insidious onset and slow progression. Sometimes acute exacerbation suddenly changes the course of a slowly progressing illness and leaves the patient with incapacitating defects.

The clusters of symptoms most frequently noted are withdrawal, decrease in energy, unstable mood, and obsessive preoccupations. Other symptoms include aggressive and impulsive behavior, depersonalization, hallucinations, and thinking disorder. The most important characteristic of adolescent schizophrenia is that the symptoms may be episodic, transitory, and fragmented, except for a withdrawal and a decrease in energy, which may dominate the life of the adolescent. Withdrawal may be first manifested as a reluctance to attend school and refusal to associate with friends that are rationalized as a lack of a common interest or embarrassment over the inability to go to school. Decrease in energy is sometimes justified by adolescents as their unwillingness to conform with the demands of society or their boredom with schoolwork. Schizophrenic preoccupation with abstract and at times obscure ideas must be differentiated from the normal adolescent's propensity for thinking about such philosophical concepts as life, death, and man's place in the universe. In normal adolescents, such a preoccupation does not interfere with the individual's ability to carry on his daily life, while the morbid obsessions of the schizophrenic patient replace other forms of intellectual activity.

Longitudinal studies of the course of schizophrenic illness have not as yet provided any explanation for its variable course in different individuals. It still remains perplexingly true that of two individuals with the same diagnosis, one may continue to function in a relatively intact, though marginal, manner, while the other may deteriorate rapidly and become demented.

Manic–Depressive Psychosis. Reported cases of manic–depressive psychosis during adolescence are very few as compared to schizophrenia. The clinical picture of manic psychosis may resemble that of schizophrenia or acute toxic psychosis, and only follow-up studies will differentiate and clarify the diagnosis. Diagnostic difficulties in adolescence are reported for both inpatient and outpatient populations, and mixed symptomatology is noted in all categories of psychiatric illnesses. Hudgens (1974) studied a group of 110 adolescent psychiatric inpatients and compared them with the same number of adolescents in medical–surgical wards. Of the 110 psychiatric patients, 29 were called "undiagnosed, unclassified." This designation was given to cases who had a variety of psychiatric symptoms but no cluster of symptoms so dominant that the illness could be classified as a probable case of a defined syndrome. Another group still undiagnosed was classified as resembling major psychiatric illnesses. In this study, 14 out of 110 psychiatric inpatients and 13 out of the 110 control group were described as "undiagnosed, most like depression." Of the 110 psychiatric patients, 13 were diagnosed as "bipolar manic–depressive," while "unipolar depression" was found in 14 psychiatric subjects and 8 controls. Comparison of the two groups of "undiagnosed, most like depression" and "unipolar depression" revealed a preponderance of vegetative symptoms, death wishes, and hopelessness in the depressed patients, while the "depressionlike" syndrome was accompanied by more irritability and crying spells. The depressed group reported a longer history of psychiatric problems and dysphoric mood during the premorbid stage.

Suicidal behavior and suicidal communication did not differentiate the two groups. In fact, suicidal behavior appeared in all categories of psychiatric disorders, diagnosed or undiagnosed. More than half (67%) of the patients in the psychiatric group had exhibited some form of suicidal behavior. Among the control group, only those with psychiatric illness had made any suicide attempts or threats. The diagnosis of psychiatric illness in nonpsychiatric controls was based on symptoms other than suicidal behavior.

Masterson (1964) studied a group of 110 adolescents who were attending a psychiatric outpatient clinic and a matched control group from a school population. The patients and the controls were, on the average, 16 years old at the beginning of the study and were periodically evaluated until 21 years of age. Of the 72 patients who were given psychiatric diagnoses at the end of the five-year follow-up, 43 were diagnosed as having personality disorder, 18 as having schizophrenia, and 11 as having character neurosis. The author reported that some diagnostic difficulties were resolved only with the passage of time, when the clinical picture of mixed symptomatology "gradually tended to differentiate more clearly into the usual diagnostic categories."

Diagnostic ambiguity and uncertainty are present in regard to all behavior problems of adolescents. Thus drug abuse, excessive alcohol intake, unusual sexual activities, or violent temper outbursts may be presented as part of a clinical picture that on follow-up may be diagnosed as psychosis, personality disorder, or neurotic behavior. Serious consideration and attention must be paid to all behavior problems of the second decade of life, and psychiatric treatment and supervision must be instituted with the view of limiting the functional impairment at the time of initial consultation and as the process unfolds.

IV
METHODS OF PSYCHIATRIC INTERVENTION

22

Treatment

All psychological treatments are based on a number of implicit or explict philosophical and social assumptions regarding the nature and process of human existence. The foremost among these is that the basic human condition is that of a solitary, self-contained unit, enmeshed and interacting within a social network, and that feeling ill at ease in, dissatisfied with, and incapable of harmonious functioning within such a framework is the cause or the inevitable outcome of psychiatric problems. Although some degree of subjective and intrapsychic distress is compatible with effective social functioning and, conversely, social situations with limited conflicts may not cause intrapsychic distress, the interpenetrating nature of the various facets of human existence is such that regardless of the original source, conflicts and distress lead to social maladjustment and individual suffering. While changes in the values and demands of the social network are desirable and occur continuously, in the final analysis it is the individual's perception, his mode of communication, and his style of interaction that are more susceptible to modification at a rate that could make a significant difference within his lifetime.

Psychotherapy, whether in group or dyadic and regardless of the theoretical background of the therapist, is based on the belief that man's perception, his emotional state, and his thinking are modifiable within the context of interpersonal relationships. Within such a context, the therapist provides a nonthreatening and accepting atmosphere where the patient can have the courage to reveal his thoughts and express his emotions. For some patients, this opportunity is a liberating experience, whether or not the therapist chooses to emphasize the patient's statements and reflect his feelings, as is done in nondirective, supportive psychotherapy. Other patients are in need of a cohesive pattern for their varied experiences. The therapist's questions help these patients articulate their tentative hypotheses, contradictory feelings, and sensibilities in and out of the treatment situation. The emerging patterns are then examined, possible motivating factors are discussed, and a unifying framework is presented. Psychoanalysis is the prototype of this kind of treatment. Another group of patients are locked in a rigid, maladaptive chain of action and reaction with their environment. They need help to break their chains and to learn to communicate in a more productive and less alienating manner with others. The therapist tries to heighten their awareness of the impact of their behavior and uses the therapeutic situation as a laboratory for teaching them new techniques. Behavior therapists find this method of great value with some patients.

Delineation of problems, examination of maladaptive patterns, confrontation, clarification, interpretation, and finally, presentation of alternative strategies of interaction are components of all psycho-therapeutic relationships. The degree of emphasis on each element differs in various methods. Psychotherapy can be conceptualized as a corrective interpersonal experience by which a more accurate way of evaluating self and others is learned and unambiguous communication promoted, although the why of behavior may or may not be clarified. It is the reintegration of the individual within the community of his fellows and the acceptance of this community by the individual that is the common purpose of all psychological healing methods, be it the absolution of the sinner, the appeasement of the tribal spirits, or the work of psychotherapists. The frequency of sessions, duration of treatment, and techniques of intervention are strategies by which the goal is achieved.

As far as the aim of psychotherapy is concerned, the treatment of children is not different from the treatment of adults. Of course, children may not be convinced that they need help. They may consider their visits to the psychiatrist punishment for their nonconforming behavior, or they may insist that they are blamed for their justifiable responses to environmental provocations. Therefore they need to be motivated at the onset of their treatment, while in adult psychotherapy resistance to change appears after treatment is under way. Young children do not have the capacity for introspection that develops with age. They do not differentiate between their feelings and their actions and cannot offer tentative formulations of their problems. It is the responsibility of the psychiatrist to discover their maladaptive behavior by observing them in action and to infer their anxieties from their expressed wishes. Children do not store bits of psychological insights and information in their memory for future reference; thus confrontation and clarification can be useful to them only when they are simple and situationally relevant. Whether the psychotherapy is of the expressive or suppressive type, the therapeutic relationship with a child is expected to aim for age-appropriate correction in reality testing, self-awareness, interpersonal skills, and sensitivity to the environmental consequences of one's actions. The child who has suppressed his emotional reaction to a trauma needs an opportunity to unburden himself, while an impulsive child must be helped by clear messages of disapproval. Children who have been censured and rejected must be encouraged and accepted generously, while children whose upbringing has led to an uncompromising, selfish orientation toward others are in need of specific guidelines as to the kind of response that they can expect from their environment and the ultimate loneliness that such a posture will impose upon them.

Due to the limitation of verbal communication and cognitive sophistication in children, techniques that are less dependent on verbalization and closer to naturalistic observation are used in diagnostic and therapeutic work with children. Play, drama, and the graphic arts are the techniques best suited for this purpose.

Play

The interest of psychologists in children and their play activities dates back to the latter part of the 19th century. The early studies were mainly concerned with the observation, categorization, and classification of play activities and their forms and structures. When psychoanalytic treatment, with its emphasis on the childhood origin of adult neurosis, was logically extended to the treatment of children, analysts soon realized that the most fundamental tool of psychoanalysis—namely, free association—could not be used with children. Children are either incapable of or unwilling to associate freely, and their anxieties, feelings, and thoughts cannot be uncovered by the analyst's attentive ears. Melanie Klein (1932) was the first analyst who argued that because children's play activities are free from the demands and censorship of reality, they can be considered equivalent to adult free association and can be used for the purpose of psychoanalytic treatment. This view soon gained popularity among students of child psychology, partly because the psychoanalysts were in the unique position of having a ready-made system of symbolism and meaning, developed on the basis of adult memories of childhood, to superimpose on children's play. Even though much of psychoanalytic theory has been questioned, modified, or discarded, the historical background of the use of play has continued to exert a powerful influence upon the interpretation of play activities of children, and alternative systems of interpretation have not been fully developed. In play therapy, even when the psychoanalytic symbolism of every act is disregarded, the idea persists that, like adult thinking, playing is the child's way of problem solving.

Piaget (1962) divides play activities into three categories: sensorimotor games, symbolic games, and games with rules. Sensorimotor games involve the child's body. They are exercises of motor functions that search for and maintain various sensations. During the preverbal stage, almost all play activities are of this kind. As the child grows older, his sensorimotor games become more complex, but their basic structure and aim remain the same. For example, a child who has just begun to run enjoys being chased and runs even when she is told not to do so, while a 6-year-old child competes in a running race with a classmate. A 2-year-old child enjoys playing with sand and water; a few years later, he may engage in creating a design with finger painting.

The second category of games is symbolic games. Children between 4 and 8 years of age are particularly interested in these make-believe games, during which objects represent other objects: a stick becomes first a horse, then a sword, then a hunting rifle. A piece of paper is an airplane. Puppets are the feared teacher and the innocent student. Toy soldiers die and are resurrected to take revenge. Reality is distorted, then corrected, and the consequences of each alternative are played out. The new baby of the family is eaten by dogs, burned in the oven, and then taken for a walk by his loving brother. Wishes are fulfilled, only to be discarded. Deficiencies are compensated for and the gains are neglected. Symbolic games are the most revealing games of children in that they represent the child's concerns and anxieties, his wishes and longings, and his attempts to gain mastery over the perplexing world of interpersonal relationships, with its ambiguous characters and puzzling logic.

While some children may choose to play out a version of their actual experience on a small scale, the majority of children's games are the child's concrete understanding of the highly abstract messages that abound around him. A 6-year-old boy who had heard his teacher telling his mother that he had made progress while he was drawing a picture, called his drawing a "progress." A 5-year-old girl who heard her father referring to a business loss by saying "I got burned" had the father doll going to the office and being set on fire by his boss, though he returned home all cured. Children whose games are full of violence and aggressive interactions may indeed be very well socialized or even timid and fearful. Conversely, children who have their dolls in jail and tortured by enemies may be those who are most aggressive. Erikson (1963) contends that children's play may be disrupted by internal anxiety created by a traumatic experience and that when the child is able to complete the game, the resolution of the conflict has been achieved.

Creative and imaginative games are more cognitively controlled and imitative and therefore are not as revealing as symbolic games. Even when symbols are used, they are usually collective symbols and cultural stereotypes, such as superheroes.

The third category of games is games with rules, such as chess, checkers, and the like. These are social games that provide children with well-defined forms of social interaction. From these games, something can be learned about the child's style of playing, whether he cheats to win, is devastated by a loss, or arranges to lose consistently. During a play session, a child may engage in one or more varieties of games. He may be comfortable only with stylized social games; he may engage in sensorimotor games, such as throwing darts, punching the punching bag, threading beads, or water play; or he may choose to discuss important subjects while busy with some toys. The child's play may remain unchanged for what seems to be an interminable time to an adult. It may be obsessive repetition of one form of activity or a ritualistic ordering of toys without any obvious purpose. Each situation presents a unique problem in diagnosis and must be understood by collecting all information about the child, not only from his play, but also from his general behavior, his views about coming to the sessions, and his activities and experiences outside of the treatment situation.

Play Material. Even in the world of make-believe, the physical properties of play materials exert an influence over what the child can do with them. While chairs can be used as cars, trains, or airplanes, the toy car is rarely used as a birthday cake. Toy guns do not lend themselves to representing friendly dogs. Clay materials provide an opportunity for three-dimensional representation, while with paper and pencil no more than two dimensions can be represented. Baby dolls are easier to spank and feed with a bottle, whereas toy soldiers may facilitate stories about defense and aggression. Some children are intrigued with the squiggle game; others like to outdo the therapist in the mutual storytelling technique. Some children prefer to reveal their thoughts in the use of costumes and in role playing. As a general principle in working with children, any game and any harmless material that could make a child comfortable and provide him with the security to reveal himself are acceptable.

Some children are too inhibited to engage in play; others come from backgrounds that have not provided them with the skills necessary for the imaginative use of toys; and still others find any office, even a playroom, too confining or threatening. Child therapists may go to playgrounds, play basketball, or just walk on the street with their patients in order to establish a relationship with them. Competency in child psychiatry is highly related to flexibility and the use of every technique to meet the child on the level that he has managed to reach.

Types of Psychotherapy

Psychoanalysis

There are disagreements among child analysts as to the degree of similarity between the psychoanalytic treatment of children and adults. Melanie Klein (1932) contended that the play activities of children can be used as free association similar to that of adults and that transference neurosis can be worked through in the same fashion. Anna Freud (1964) questioned the strength of transference neurosis in childhood since the original parents are still very much in the picture and in constant interaction with the child. Furthermore she emphasized that instead of free verbalization, the not-so-free action and play has to be accepted in children.

Child analysis can be conceptualized as occurring in two stages. The first stage is the preparatory phase, during which the analyst tries to establish a relationship with the child by providing him with a supportive, need-gratifying, steady figure. This may take anywhere between six months and a year. During the second phase, cognitive elements play an important part in the child's comprehension of the analyst's comments, interpretations, and clarification, and the analysis is carried out in much the same way as adult analysis. Symbolism in play and dreams is interpreted, and the unconscious elements are made conscious. The goal of psychoanalysis in children is to work through the Oedipal complex and to resolve the genital conflict. The process of child analysis usually takes between four and five years, with four to five weekly sessions. The most likely candidates are children with circumscribed neuroses based on internalized conflicts for whom one can safely count on continuous support from a normal environment.

Psychoanalytic psychotherapy is a more modest and limited version of psychoanalysis. The patient is seen two to three times a week for two to three years. The goal is to alleviate neurotic symptoms and reduce anxiety. Although the dynamically relevant materials are interpreted according to psychoanalytic theory, there is no systematic uncovering of the unconscious material. Children with mild phobic symptoms, mild depression, and mild conduct disorder are candidates for psychoanalytic psychotherapy, since psychoanalysts believe that disturbances of more intensity should be treated with intense classical analysis. As can be noted, the theoretical orientation and frequency and duration of treatment sets child analysis apart from nonanalytic treatment, although the techniques used, the manner by which the child is motivated, and even the periodic meetings and exchange of information with parents are similar in all therapeutic endeavors with children.

Nondirective Play Therapy

Nondirective play therapy is an extension of the Rogerian school of psychotherapy with adults. The atmosphere is that of total permissiveness; only actions that may be injurious to the child or the therapist are not allowed. The therapist is a nonparticipant observer, encouraging the child to use whatever material is available according to his own wishes and for as long as he desires. The therapist listens to the child's verbalization, with particular attention paid to the feeling tone, and conveys his understanding to the child without any attempt to interpret the message. He is neither critical nor approving. The reflection of the feeling is the only task that the therapist undertakes. Decisions are left to the child, including the decision to terminate treatment. The basic assumption of the nondirective school is that the drive for self-realization motivates all behavior in children as well as in adults and that every individual, given the opportunity to think or play through his own emotions and conflicts, will manage to arrive at a constructive solution. Complete freedom in the therapeutic sessions gives the child an opportunity to experience the feelings, wishes, fears, and perceptions that emanate from his own life experiences and enables him to gain a sense of confidence in himself and to master his own conflicts.

Nondirective therapists report that while at the beginning of treatment a child's emotions are negative, diffuse, and undifferentiated, with the passage of time anger becomes more focused and related to specific individuals and experiences. The intensity of negative feelings slowly diminishes, some ambivalence appears, and the child gradually becomes more capable of experiencing positive feelings. This state, when the child can experience both positive and negative feelings under appropriate circumstances and with well-modulated intensity, is the desirable outcome of the treatment. Nondirective play therapy is deceptively simple in that the child sets the pace and the therapist need only reflect the child's feelings. However, the sensitivity and disciplined responsiveness required from the therapist differentiate the positive outcome achieved by skilled therapists from the failures of inexperienced enthusiasts (Moustakas, 1973).

Behavior Therapy

Behavior therapy is the name given to methods of treatment that are based on the concepts of learning theory. Although the language of the behavior theorist is new, the concepts are not. Learning and teaching have taken place for centuries as the result of interaction between men and their inanimate and human environment. Experiments with laboratory animals have helped to uncover and articulate the laws governing limited aspects of the learning process. Learning by imitation, modeling, and identification is not easily observable, yet these kinds of learning comprise a large part of learning by socialization. Behavior psychologists have attempted to generalize the simple, fundamental laws of learning by trial and error to account for the complexity of human psychology. They have met with limited success and much opposition.

Objections to behaviorist theory and its application come from two divergent groups. On one side is the school of psychology that contends that the laws of learning applicable to the controlled situations of laboratory animals are too simplistic to have much value with regard to human interactions. On the other side are those who fear that techniques based on behavior theory may become so successful in manipulating human behavior that a small elite of manipulators could control the majority of the people. In actual practice, the application of behavior modification techniques, even within the controlled environment of the special units of various institutions, has not produced generalized and permanent changes in the behavior of all subjects. While such failures may not negate the soundness of the theoretical basis of behavior theory, they reveal that total programming of the human environment is not an easy task. Even if one accepts the unfounded assumption that the preexisting psychological state and experiential background of the individual are irrelevant to his present interactional strategy, the inflexible response patterns fostered by behavior modification techniques may not be adaptive in a different environmental context.

A realistic appraisal of behavior therapy shows that successful application of its methods can replace a series of circumscribed, rigid, and maladaptive response patterns with more adaptive ones without any guarantee that a new set of stimuli may not elicit another kind of maladaptive behavior. Behaviorists have not been more successful than nonbehaviorists in explaining the etiology of behavior disturbances; however, they have brought new insights into the study of psychopathology by delineating the environmental factors that help maintain behavioral patterns. Their insights in the functional relationship between organismic actions and environmental responses has added a much needed dimension to the individual-centered tradition of psychology and psychiatry.

Behavior therapists have used Pavlovian conditioning along with the instrumental or operant conditioning of Skinner in efforts to remove symptoms and to change unwanted behavior. They have defined behavior as whatever an organism does, be it action, verbalization, or the expression of feelings. The behavior of an organism operates on and influences the environment, leading to changes that, in turn, affect and modify the subsequent behavior of the individual. The environmental factors in this process of interaction are called *stimuli*, while the organismic actions and reactions are referred to as *responses* or *response patterns*. A change in interaction can be brought about by changing the response or the stimulus. Responses that are positively reinforced or rewarded tend to occur more frequently than those that are ignored or discounted by the environment. In fact, nonreinforcement of a response leads to its eventual extinction. When a response is severely punished, it is suppressed but not extinguished and may be repeated in another context. Another way of extinguishing or suppressing a response is by stimulating a diametrically opposite response in the individual, such as simultaneous presentation of an anxiety-provoking and an equally strong relaxing stimulus (Marks, 1976; Wherry and Wollersheim, 1967).

The principles and methods of behavior therapy have become incorporated into the child-rearing practices of parents, the management strategies of child care workers and teachers, and the discussions of parental counselors. Ignoring the temper tantrum of the toddler, withholding attention from a disruptive pupil when he is out of his seat, and lavishing praise for the futile attempts at group participation of a withdrawn child are all examples of behavior modification techniques.

While other schools of psychotherapy have concentrated on changing the individual's perceptions, feelings, and thoughts, behavior therapists have emphasized the impact of the activity on the environment and the reactions perceived by the individual from his surroundings. In devising a therapeutic plan, behavior therapists try to define the undesirable behavior operationally and observe and analyze its frequency of appearance, the circumstances that seem to induce the particular behavior, the goal that is achieved by it, and the factors responsible for its termination. If sets of environmental reactions are identified as reinforcers of the behavior, the treatment consists of withholding the reinforcers while helping the patient develop more acceptable ways of receiving environmental feedbacks, such as care, sympathy, and attention. When, on the other hand, there is a lack of proper response, the plan for treatment consists of identifying the reinforcing factors for the subject and rewarding responses that may approximate the desirable behavior until the pattern is learned and the behavior is well established.

The timing and frequency of the positive reinforcers, or rewards, that follow a desirable act are important components of any treatment schedule. It has been shown that successful modification in behavior can be best achieved by a discontinuous reward schedule and periodic maintenance reinforcement. Positive reinforcers may be such things as candies, toys, tokens to buy desirable objects, trips, praise, adult attention, and physical contact. The negative reinforcers that precede the desirable response and their termination are what motivate the emission of a specific behavior. For example, a child is not allowed to play or watch television until he has finished his homework. Punishment is an aversive reaction that follows an undesirable behavior. A child is expelled from school following assaultive behavior, or a child loses his weekly allowance because he has broken his sibling's toy. However, under laboratory conditions punishment does not extinguish the response and only temporarily suppresses it. For this reason, and because of the potential for misuse, punishment is used only in limited situations in behavior therapy. Punishments range in severity from loss of privileges, "time-out," or short periods of exclusion from social interaction, to the application of electric shock for cases of intense self-destructive activities. Various forms of behavior therapy have been used in the treatment of behavior disorders of children, and reports of improvement abound in the literature. In the following discussion, some examples of the application of behavior therapy techniques are reviewed.

Desensitization. This technique, developed by Wolpe (1958), is used in cases of specific phobias, such as fear of animals, closed spaces, and high places. Some clinicians have used this method in treating children with school phobia. Children who develop anxiety symptoms when it is time to go to school are at first encouraged to accompany the therapist or the parents to the school building without entering the school. Once the sight of the school no longer causes anxiety, the child is taken inside the building for a few minutes. Still later, he is required to remain for longer periods within the school and, while his mother waits for him, is encouraged to spend a few minutes in his classroom. This time in the classroom is slowly increased until the child can tolerate a whole day in class without undue anxiety. The final step is to have the child attend school without his mother, though he may be allowed to make one phone call to her at lunch break. Some therapists use relaxation training concomitantly with this desensitization schedule. Others may use tranquilizers as an adjunct in the treatment.

When the child is afraid of an animal, talking about the animal, drawing pictures of it, looking at its picture, playing with a toy animal, and imagining himself at various distances from the animal can slowly desensitize the child to the point at which he can face the animal without fear. Necessary time should be allowed for each stage so that lack of anxiety and total relaxation may be ensured at each level before the next step is taken. Some behavior therapists have used reciprocal inhibition technique by introducing the anxiety-provoking stimulus along with pleasurable activities, such as showing the picture of the feared animal while the child is relaxing in his mother's arms. Others have used the modeling technique of Bandura (1967) by including fearful children in groups of children who are not afraid of a particular situation in order to facilitate the learning of a different set of responses instead of the customary avoidance behavior. When lack of skills and unfamiliarity account for the child's fear, teaching the necessary skills and playacting in a supportive surrounding help the child overcome his fears (Rachman and Costello, 1961).

Conditioning and Operant Conditioning. In the treatment of enuresis, an aversive reinforcer in the form of a bed-buzzer apparatus has been found useful. A loud noise is produced by the apparatus when the child begins to micturate, interrupting sleep. Reported cure rates have ranged from 30 to 90%, although some children revert to enuresis after they have become dry with this schedule. The timing of the aversive reinforcer and its frequency and periodic application are the subjects of continuous research.

Temper tantrums, fainting spells in adolescents, and food refusal in children may all be treated by withholding the intense attention that these behaviors customarily receive from the environment. In anorexia nervosa, care and sympathy are given only when the patient eats, and the patient is informed that he can gain privileges such as visitors, television, and reading materials only when he gains weight. In elective mutism, the child is informed that unless he has uttered a particular word he cannot leave the school at the end of the day. His efforts to communicate by gestures are ignored, while he is praised whenever he verbalizes his wishes.

The parents of encopretic children are advised to begin a behavior modification schedule in which, at first, the only requirement of the child is to change his soiled garment and clean himself. His compliance is verbally praised and his failures are ignored until the procedure has become routinized. The next step is to demand that the child limit his soiling to the bathroom. This will indirectly focus the child's attention on his bodily cues for elimination. Once he has successfully managed this stage, he is rewarded for refraining from soiling his clothes. For some children, encopresis has become an unfailing method of attracting parental attention. The impersonal manner of behavior therapy deprives the child of such environmental reinforcement, while assuring the parents that something is being done to remove the symptoms. In all these situations, it is of the utmost importance to identify the conditions that have led to the choice of the particular behavior and to remove the cause in conjunction with the symptom (Ullmann and Kasner, 1965).

The principles of learning theory have been used in classrooms to control the disruptive activities of hyperactive children by withholding attention when the child tries to attract attention and by praising and attending to the child when he is quiet, by giving tokens, points, or gold stars for good behavior and imposing a fine when the child misbehaves. Token programs have been used with delinquent children as a reward for appropriate behavior and control of impulsive activities and as a motivating agent for school attendance (Schaefer and Martin, 1969).

With Psychotic Children. Behavior therapy with psychotic children is aimed at eliminating repetitive, self-stimulating rituals that interfere with social interaction and at fostering cooperative, socialized behavior. Children are rewarded for their slightest move toward people, and their self-stimulating behavior is repeatedly interrupted by whatever activities the particular child finds pleasurable. By the use of the technique of successful approximation, socialized behavior is slowly shaped and attachment to adults is reinforced. Language training is of particular importance in providing these children with communicative skills. They are rewarded for the emission of spontaneous sounds and are prompted to combine different sounds, to repeat a word, to learn the names of various objects, to pay attention to verbal directions, and finally, to express their needs by verbal communication.

The self-destructive activities of some children are life-threatening, and their suppression by punishment may be the only choice available to therapists. Restraining the child, engaging his attention away from the mutilating behavior, and finally applying electric shock are methods used to eliminate such behavior. The results of intense treatment programs for psychotic children so far have not been highly

encouraging. Even when a high level of motivation is created by isolating the child and arranging for his daily intake of food and drink to
be given in small amounts following the emission of specific behavior,
it has been found that the response capability of some of these children is quite limited (Churchill, 1969). But it has also been noted that
children who are involved in these programs develop attachments to
adults, and as long as they experience some success in their attempts
in learning, they are more attentive to their environment and less
likely to engage in their rituals. On the other hand, when the level of
task complexity is raised and failures are more frequent, the children
withdraw and their bizarre behavior reappears.

With Mentally Retarded Children. Learning principles are used in
teaching retarded children skills such as self-care, skilled motor activities, and verbal communication. Reinforcers in the form of candies,
toys, physical contact, and displays of affection are paired with verbal
praise to encourage the child in each small step toward the complete
mastery over the required task. Tasks are graded by degree of difficulty and are analyzed as to the components that have to be learned.
Each child is started at his level of competency. The components of the
task are introduced according to the logical manner in which they
combine to produce the final result. Care is taken to make learning as
easy as possible and to provide for steady progress. Once a skill is
acquired, the child is encouraged to practice it as often as possible,
and parents and caretakers are dissuaded from doing for the child
what he can do for himself, even if his accomplishment falls short of
adults' expectation. The more necessary skills are taught first, and
various elements of learned patterns are combined to form a new skill.
For example, it is more necessary for the child to learn to put on and
take off his shirt than to tie his shoelaces, and when he has learned to
put on his shirt, he can easily apply the same skills to putting on his
jacket or raincoat.

In behavior therapy with children, regardless of the nature of the
reinforcer used, it is important to aim at bringing the child's behavior
under the control of verbal cues, since negative or positive verbal
statements are the most frequently used reinforcers in human interaction, and children need to modify their behaviors on the basis of such
social feedbacks. Of course, nonpsychotic children also learn to detect
approval and disapproval from the tone of voice or the facial expressions of others and modify their behavior accordingly. Although behavior therapists are concerned only with what the individual does, it
is quite apparent that changes in behavior influence the child's relationship with his environment, the kind of experiences that become

possible for him, and consequently his feelings about himself. In this sense, the ultimate result of successful treatment with behavior therapy is not different from that of other forms of psychiatric intervention. Furthermore, at least as far as treatment of behavior problems in children is concerned, changing the environment of the child through parental guidance and/or appropriate school placement is necessary if the new patterns of behavior are to be maintained.

Eclectic Psychotherapy

All psychotherapeutic interventions with children require flexibility of approach based on the accurate diagnosis of the child's deficiencies and assets, his most central problem, and the identification of those deviations that are most amenable to intervention. A permissive, nonthreatening atmosphere is the first requirement of any therapeutic situation; the therapist may choose to combine the principles of various schools to help the child achieve an understanding of his behavior and to educate the child in decoding the messages that he receives from his environment. Imparting new knowledge, explaining, clarifying, and reality testing are all an important part of treatment and provide a sense of relief for the patient in the same way as do abreaction and the expression of anxieties and concerns. A corrective emotional experience, which includes approval and disapproval, encourages identification with the therapist, and helpful suggestions and persuasion make it possible for the child to experiment with new modes of interaction. The therapist's responses in a treatment situation ought to be dictated by what is helpful to a particular child at the specific point in his development rather than by tenets of a theoretical school of psychology or psychotherapy. A pragmatic orientation requires continuous vigilance and reassessment of the child's needs and the stage of development that he has reached. Some behavioral deviations that may be particularly disturbing to the parents are remarkably short-lived, and their disappearance cannot be credited to therapeutic intervention. On the other hand, the modification of some behavioral styles that have far-reaching, negative consequences for the child should be the goal of psychotherapy even though the parents seem to be unaware of their content and implications (Carek, 1972; Anthony, 1964).

Effectiveness and Duration of Psychotherapy

The length of time for which any therapeutic intervention must continue should ideally be dependent upon the disappearance of all symptoms or the achievement of the goal envisioned for treatment. Although there is very little disagreement about the presence or absence of well-defined symptoms, the issue of the therapeutic goal is not as easy to define or measure. Analysts who define their objective for the child as "having reached and worked through his Oedipal conflicts" give a time span of four to five years of visits five times a week to achieve this purpose. The nondirective school is dependent upon the child's interest for continuation of treatment and reports good results within a few months of therapy. Winnicot (1971) believes that when the child's environment is free of gross abnormality, the question the therapist should ask should be "How little need I do to make a bridge between conscious and unconscious as soon as possible?" Winnicott went on to describe his intervention during two or three therapeutic interviews with a 12-year-old child who engaged in stealing.

Research studies with dropouts from clinics indicate that some parents found the diagnostic interviews to have had such a salutary effect that they did not feel the need for returning to the clinic. Others withdrew after a few sessions of treatment and were satisfied with the result. Some clinicians have specifically limited their intervention to brief periods (8–12 sessions) and have reported good results with this method (Rosenthal and Levine, 1971). Meanwhile, follow-up studies have failed to show any difference in outcome between children receiving short- or long-term treatment. Taken together, these reports seem to indicate that when the child's problem is of recent origin and appears in the background of a previously healthy adjustment within a supportive environment, brief intervention with the child and minor modification of the family attitudes are all that is needed to reestablish the child's previous adjustment. Such a plan is most effective when all the involved members, the child, the therapist, and the child's caretakers are motivated to work toward the earliest possible termination date. When the child's problems are of such crippling magnitude that no significant change can be expected within 10–12 sessions, it is still necessary to reevaluate the results and the objectives of the treatment every few months and to terminate treatment when it is clear that further improvements are of such a nebulous character that they do not justify the investment of the therapist's time and the expense incurred by the family.

Some children may need periodic evaluations. Others may feel that the availability of the therapist is an essential part of their security. For these children, it is usually enough to assure them that they can return for one or a few sessions whenever they feel the need. The same kind of reassurance is helpful for parents who express their anxieties over the possible return of the symptoms and are in need of periodic consultation and validation of their child-rearing practices and decisions. The effectiveness of various psychotherapeutic interventions has been the subject of a few follow-up studies (Levitt, 1971; Shephered *et al.*, 1971). In these and similar studies, dropouts from psychiatric clinics or children with behavior problems who had not been referred for psychiatric evaluation were compared with those who had received psychiatric care. The results have so far failed to show any significant difference between the two groups in follow-up. However, research on the effectiveness of psychotherapy is fraught with methodological problems. Even when the two groups of children are controlled for a variety of socioeconomic variables, the question of the intensity of the problem behavior and the implications of any item of behavior deviation have not been settled. Furthermore, neither the kind of treatment nor the type of therapeutic results can be evaluated by the results of questionnaires listing the presence or absence of particular symptoms.

It is a well-known fact that some behavior symptoms abate with age and that some psychiatric syndromes show a remitting course over time. However, it is difficult to measure the amount of subjective distress and adverse environmental reaction that is generated by any particular behavior, and even though given time a disorder may subside, one cannot cite such statistics as justification for lack of intervention or the ineffectiveness of treatment. If a well-planned and appropriate treatment strategy, designed and executed by a skillful therapist, can be shown to shorten the duration or decrease the intensity of the behavior problem of the child and the concomitant stress in the family, no other proof of its effectiveness is needed. On the other hand, unsubstantiated claims of beneficial results for vaguely defined problems brought about by unspecific methods over unspecified time cannot be accepted as psychotherapeutic intervention and compared for effectiveness with no treatment at all. Psychotherapeutic interaction is a learning experience aimed at the removal of symptoms. Whether or not the goal has been achieved is easily verifiable, but the more subtle effects of the interaction are not quantifiable. This factor accounts for criticism leveled at researchers by clinicians. More recently, it has been noted that future investigation in this area should be directed at devising a research strategy with the more circumscribed goal of finding out what kind of treatment, by what kind of therapist, for what period of time, and with what kind of patient would be most effective. Such a strategy would require definable goals; planned treatment; an awareness of the therapist's personality, style, and skill; and, most importantly, homogeneous groups of patients with similar problems. Before such answers can be found, the results of psychiatric treatment remain dependent on the clinical impressions of therapists and the vague reports of improvement or lack of it by patients and their families, without objective verification (Frank, 1968).

Group Therapy

Psychodrama, the earliest form of group therapy with children, was initiated by Moreno first in Vienna (1911) and later on in the United States (1927). Since then, various kinds of group therapy for different ages and diagnostic categories in and out of institutions have been devised. The results are not easy to assess, although the reports from the practitioners of group therapy tend to support their contention that for some children group experience, with or without individual psychotherapy, can be of therapeutic value. Group therapy for preadolescents is usually focused on nonverbal activities, while older children and adolescents can participate in more verbal interchange. Although some clinicians specifically exclude children with certain problems—such as disruptiveness and aggressive behavior—from the group, others have found that in smaller groups of four to six children, the therapist or group leader can manage to provide a helpful atmosphere for all and at the same time protect the nonaggressive children from the aggressive ones (Abramovitz, 1976).

The primary advantage of group experience is to give the child an opportunity for socialization with group members and to facilitate self-awareness and sensitivity to others. Interpretations in the form of clarification of communication and identification of the environmental feedback, whenever possible, add valuable dimensions to the process of group participation. When children do not show severe behavior deviation, group modeling is of particular advantage to children who are mildly phobic and tend to withdraw from active competition and group participation. In adolescents, particularly juvenile delinquents, group therapy has shown good results since the peer orientation of adolescents makes the responses of group members an effective vehicle for changes in behavior and perception, and the presence of the therapist hampers the dominance of one person over others (Ginott, 1961). The results of sporadic attempts at treating young psychotic children in groups are open to question, although Speers and Lansing (1965) considered group therapy a helpful method of treatment for these children.

Family Therapy

All forms of therapeutic intervention in child psychiatry involve some degree of change in the psychological equilibrium and transactional patterns of the family. Even in those instances in which chemotherapy is the main form of treatment, the expectations of family members and their perception and accommodation to the child's emerging pattern of behavior are important factors in the success or failure of the therapeutic endeavor. Unless one espouses the extreme view that all behavioral problems of children are created or maintained by, or are symptomatic of, parental discords, there is little justification for the inclusion of all family members in the treatment of a youngster. However, parental involvement is a necessary part of psychiatric work with children.

Sometimes one or both parents may be helped to become the primary modifier of the child's behavior. On other occasions, counseling, clarification, and guidance can maximize their parenting functions. The numerous half-hearted attempts of parents in maintaining discipline and the subsequent conflictual relationships either between the two parents or between the child and both his father and his mother may be at the root of a child's disobedience. Rigid adherence to the abstract principles of a professional authority on child rearing may lead to behaviors that are clearly maladaptive. In all these situations, discussion with parents may be the only necessary step in ameliorating the distress that is experienced by all members of the family, including the patient, or may be an adjunct to individual psychotherapy for the child.

Parental psychopathology, although it may be a contributing factor to the child's problem, is not always the causative agent, nor can it be assumed that when such parents are referred for treatment for their own emotional disorders, the child will no longer require individual psychiatric work. Furthermore, even when one or both parents are in treatment, it must be remembered that in psychotherapy with adults, the therapist's knowledge about the children in the family is based on reports by the parents alone, and therefore even if suggestions and clarification are offered, they may not be appropriate or useful for a particular child. It is thus necessary for the child psychiatrist to meet with such parents periodically and to provide concrete guidance and information about the needs of the child and the best way that they can be met and handled.

Children with various disabilities and defects are at a higher risk for the development of maladaptive behavior. Parental couseling may be the most effective preventive measure available to these patients and their families. When the child psychiatrist is a member of a treatment team caring for children with a physical illness or disability, the staff of the hospital or school as well as the parents are in need of support and guidance regarding the child's behavioral peculiarities and emotional needs. Consultation and discussions with the child's caretakers are an important part of the psychiatric care provided for the patient, and the skill with which psychiatric knowledge is imparted to the caretakers is a decisive factor in the outcome of the child psychiatrist's work with the patient. It must be emphasized that for parents or other caretakers, diagnostic labels or psychodynamic formulations are of little practical value in dealing with the child and may, in fact, be quite confusing. Rather, it is the implication and meaning of the child's behavior and suggestions for effective management and a corrective plan of action that are helpful and appreciated.

Family therapy as a distinct treatment modality evolved during the 1950s from the original experimentations of child psychiatrists who began to note the significance of observing the child in interactions within his customary human milieu. The evaluation of the family was soon followed by a desire to treat deviant families, and further theoretical justification for family therapy was provided by the system theory, which maintains that any change in one part will influence the other components of the presumed system. The patterns of interactions and transactions within the family were thus conceptualized as comprising a system. Efforts at change and correction were directed at the family with the hope that the accrued benefits would result in the extinction of the maladaptive behavior patterns and the development of appropriate modes of interaction in all family members.

Some family therapists further postulated that even though individual members, particularly children, may be presented as the patient, it is always, or nearly always, the family that is in trouble and that the patient is only the designated symptom of the disordered family. Akerman (1963) defined the aim of family therapy as helping the family to achieve a clear definition of the "real content" of their conflict and as counteracting the displacement of the conflict onto the victimized member. Family therapy sessions usually include all members of the household. In theory, all members are expected to participate in discussions and express opinions and feelings, while the therapist clarifies the intent of the messages and offers interpretations as to the meanings of the interactions. At times, the therapist tries to encourage the children to freely indicate their opposition to parental opinion; however, taking sides with the children evokes resentment on the part of the parents, who consider their authority undermined. On the other hand, sometimes children feel even more victimized when their misdeeds are publicized. The parents may be reluctant to discuss sensitive, personal issues in the presence of a child, while these may be precisely the subjects that underlie a significant portion of their conflicts.

Insights gained during a successful therapeutic session may be so distressing to the parents that they engage in excessive acknowledgment of guilt or apportionment of blame or other indications of their psychological stress. Exposure of the children to such emotional outpouring is at best unnecessary and at worst harmful. While it is undoubtedly true that some children are scapegoated and victimized by their parents or other family members, in practice children's behavioral problems are not always solved by changes of parental attitudes or other transactions within the family. Even though the diagnostic interview of the family may provide important insight into the nature of ambiguous communications, "double-bind" messages, and parental prejudices or, conversely, may shed light on the nature of the child's provocative and irritating behavior, such evaluations are best used for further delineation of the basic problems confronting the child and his parents. Knowledge thus gained can be used in devising a treatment strategy for the child and as a point of discussion and guidance for the parents (Haley, 1970).

Family therapy for the purpose of helping the troubled child must be limited to those circumstances in which the child has achieved a degree of cognitive sophistication and a tolerance for frustration sufficient for participation on equal terms with the parents in the process of self-examination and self-expression. Furthermore, the problem behavior must be shown to be caused by a breakdown of communication among the family members and its generalization to other areas of the child's life referrable to the child–parent interaction. Akerman (1963) summarized the indication for family therapy as "those psychiatric disorders in which intra-psychic conflict is not a major problem, or where the disturbance is not of long standing." Very young children are unable to maintain an attentive posture for the lengthy sessions of family therapy, and even when they do so, they cannot be expected to understand the nuances of the abstract language of adults, with its emphasis on feelings and ideas. Some family therapists provide toys and games as an acknowledgment of the child's limited attention span and his special needs for expression through play (Zilbach *et al.*, 1972). However, reports of such treatment processes fail to specify the particular advantage that children received from attending such sessions and only emphasize the better understanding of the family dynamics that was gained by the therapist and presumably imparted to the parents.

Home visits for the firsthand observation and evaluation of families with multiple social and psychiatric problems have been advocated to broaden the understanding and outlook of psychiatrists whose professional training had been heavily weighted toward the study of intrapsychic and interpersonal phenomena. Community psychiatry, with its public health orientation, has given impetus to experimentation in family therapy and on-the-spot intervention at the time of family crisis, usually at the home of the patient. Such psychological first aid or attempts at reaching out to a population that is reluctant or unable to seek help from conventional institutions are important steps in psychiatrists' efforts to fulfill their obligations to care for all those who are in need. However, regardless of the location and mechanics of service giving, the evaluation and diagnostic workup, as well as the individualized treatment plan for each child, must remain the cornerstone of the child psychiatric endeavor (Speck, 1964; Freeman, 1967).

Compensatory Education

A sizable majority of children with behavior disorders present deficits of varying degrees in academic performance, which may be one of the etiological factors or the result of their maladaptive behavior. Because of the central role of education and educational institutions in the process of socialization and personality growth of children, failure in school is associated with maladjustment and distress in all areas of a child's functioning. A complete psychiatric evaluation of a child must include an assessment of his educational status, and the treatment plan for the disturbed child must provide specific recommendations for remedial efforts toward optimal learning. Underachievement in school may be due to motivational factors, oppositional attitudes toward parents and teachers, interference with learning based on a high level of anxiety or other negative mood states, interrupted schooling, chronic truancy, or organismic factors such as attentional deficits, perceptual problems, and language or other cognitive disabilities.

Psychotherapeutic work with the parents and the child may be needed to prepare the child for engaging in the learning process. However, such preparation must be concurrent with an appropriate teaching strategy to help the child acquire the necessary learning set and academic skills for handling scholastic tasks. Teaching strategies for compensatory education with children are based on a few general principles that provide the individualized framework within which each child has to be taught.

Underachievers have had a long history and repeated experience of failure. They are self-protective and fearful of any new commitment to learning. Teaching them requires sensitivity to their pessimism, strong faith in their ability to learn, and continuous support and reward for their modest achievement without reinforcing their low level of expectation from themselves. A positive personal relationship between these children and their teacher is even more important than the interpersonal relations between teachers and normally functioning pupils. Such affectional bonds make the teacher's commands and suggestions more effective and criticism less alienating. The span of attention of the child, rather than the requirement of any institution, must dictate the instructional program, although the ultimate goal is for the child to attend to any academic task for as long as is expected from his normal peers. Children who become perseverative should not be left to engage in nonproductive activities, while for those who are excessively distractible, the amount of external stimuli must be carefully controlled.

When one or more sensory modalities are impaired, instruction must at first be carried out through the nonimpaired sensory channels. In children with impaired vision, oral teaching should be emphasized, while with children who have disorders of auditory functions, visual presentation of material is necessary. Combining several modalities, such as tactile, kinesthetic, and audiovisual, is called for when the child's problem lies in his difficulties with intersensory integration and deficits of auditory and/or visual perception. Specific exercises should be designed to facilitate concept formation, language function, perceptual differentiation and discrimination, motor coordination, and spatial orientation (Gallagher, 1962).

Finally, the child should be taught methods by which he can use environmental cues for independent self-evaluation and constructive self-correction.

For some children, remedial education may be all that is needed to alleviate the anxiety, depression, and anger that underlie much of their deviant behavior. In other children, the feeling of mastery and self-esteem gained through school achievement provide the strength and motivation necessary for psychotherapeutic commitment by the child and complement the efforts of the therapist concerned with the child's emotional growth and the resolution of his conflicts.

INSTITUTIONALIZATION

The psychiatric institutionalization of children may be a carefully planned intervention or a response to an emergency; it may be for a short period of up to three months or for a long period of two to three years. Differences in the organization and philosophy of various centers are usually dictated by geographical location, source of financial support, and other factors extraneous to the needs of the patient population. However, these differences are reflected in the type of children that a particular center will serve. Centers with an on-campus school facility are more likely to accept children with severe behavior disorders, while centers that are dependent on the community school deal with children with milder disturbances.

The staff of most centers come from such varied educational backgrounds as psychology, child psychiatry, social work, education, child care, nursing, and activity therapy. The inpatient units of the hospital usually function along a medical model and are headed by a psychiatrist. In other institutions, the child psychiatrist functions primarily as a consultant and a supervisor of the overall treatment plan, with other professionals as the primary therapists. Diagnostic evaluation is the joint effort of a team that includes a pediatrician, a neurologist, a psychiatrist, a psychologist, a social worker, and an educational diagnostician. In some centers, children are assigned to counselors, social workers, or psychiatrists for individual psychotherapy. Other centers consider the experiences within the milieu sufficient for therapeutic purposes.

Although there are some subtle theoretical differences between various centers, all institutions are devised to provide for the social, educational, and interpersonal needs of children. The goal of providing corrective emotional experience, even in hospital units, is to a large degree achieved by the child's daily interactions with his caretakers rather than during individual psychotherapy sessions. The therapeutic interaction is a continuous process created and maintained by all staff members who come into contact with the patient. The quality of psychiatric care in any institution is directly related to the sensitivity, intelligence, and professional skills of the staff and the degree to which the treatment philosophy can be translated into actual practice. While the ratio of professional staff to patients is likely to be higher in the more therapeutically effective centers, the quantity cannot compensate for the quality of treatment rendered.

Because there is, as yet, no yardstick by which the quality of treatment can be measured, it is not possible to assess the effectiveness of institutionalization in the treatment of psychiatric problems of children. The reports of successful outcome of treatment from some institutions have not been duplicated by others, in part because the criteria for admission to most institutions are set by each admission committee in generalized terms that allow the center to accept or reject particular referrals. Discharge from the institution is also based on numerous factors independent of the child's psychological state. Children with interested parents may be prematurely withdrawn from an institution, while children from fostering agencies, who comprise more than half of the institutionalized population, are more likely to remain months after the treatment centers deem their stay unnecessary.

The decision to institutionalize the child must be based on an evaluation of the child's needs at the time of referral as well as on those factors that may influence his future life following the stay in an institution. For some children, separation from the family may seriously jeopardize their chances for reintegration within it, and the disadvantages of a long career in a succession of institutions and/or foster homes have to be weighed against other alternatives.

Emergency Hospitalization. Emergency hospitalization for children and adolescents is usually brought about by self-destructive or assaultive and aggressive behavior and acute psychotic episodes. In a majority of cases, the disturbed behavior is of long duration and the crisis is a reflection of the sudden alteration of the family's support for the child or pressure from the community. The chronic disruptive behavior of a child becomes intolerable when he assaults the teacher and is expelled from school; his repeated fire-setting is taken lightly until a big fire has caused substantial damage; his poor judgment is ignored until he is caught walking on the railroad track. Although all suicidal and destructive acts of children and adolescents require immediate psychiatric attention, emergency hospitalization should be recommended only when there is substantial danger and failure to hospitalize the child would endanger the physical and psychological health of the child or his family.

Emergency psychiatric hospitalization is a potentially traumatic experience for the young patient and his family. It generates guilt and anxiety in parents and feelings of abandonment and victimization in children. Young children are frightened by their belief that they are being punished for their past misdeeds, and adolescents fear the implication of hospitalization in terms of their sanity. The state of family crisis preceding the emergency hospitalization, and the anxiety and helplessness following the patient's admission, diminishes the family's effectiveness in reassuring the patient and places a heavy emotional burden on the hospital staff.

The child's immediate reaction may be that of panic or frustration and rage; some children are unable to sleep, and other lose their appetite or refuse food in the hope of forcing their parents to have them released or the doctor to discharge them. They may be negativistic and hostile to other patients and staff, may try to run away, or may cry and act helpless. They may exaggerate the real or fancied hardships of the hospital life, complain to their parents of mistreatment by the hospital staff, or tell stories about the forbidden activities of other children. Some children try to induce guilt in their parents by accusing them of rejection and lack of care; others perceive their parents' ambivalence and insecurity and try to make them unhappy by comparing them unfavorably with the hospital staff. A minority of children react to hospitalization with relief, only to become depressed after a few days.

During the first few days of hospitalization, the child's mood and his behavior are influenced by the experience of separation from the family and the unfamiliarity of the new situation and therefore cannot be considered typical of his pattern of response under ordinary circumstances. Although such behavior can give valuable information regarding the child's repertoire of coping behavior and his ability to master his anxiety and relate to a new environment, the more in-depth assessment must await the emergence of the child's customary pattern when he has made a reasonable adjustment to the hospital setting.

The parents need to be reassured repeatedly that their decision to hospitalize the child has been in his best interest, and they must be helped to mobilize their psychological resources to plan for the child's future. Contacts between the child and the parents, at first in the hospital and later on at home, will convey to the child and his parents the message that they are expected to remain involved with each other and that their affectional bond is not disrupted. This is particularly important for families who tend to reorganize and reinstitute their emotional balance once the child–patient has been excluded, and the child's reentry is experienced as another major trauma.

Both family and child should be given enough advance warning as the time for discharge approaches. Concrete plans for follow-up based on the diagnostic workup and the response to treatment should be recommended in order to prepare the way for needed continuity in psychiatric care and to channel parental anxiety into constructive use. For some children, the idea of discharge reactivates some of their original apprehension, and for a few days, they exhibit symptoms of excessive anxiety, such as irritability, temper outbursts, and sleep difficulties. These symptoms are usually transient and no change in plan is warranted. Regardless of the original reason for hospitalization, any child who has been exposed to the experience is entitled to a complete physical, psychiatric, and educational evaluation before discharge. This requires that the child remains for three to six weeks in the hospital in order to be observed in a variety of situations and roles and to give the psychiatrist a reasonable opportunity to make realistic recommendations for the child's future. The parents and the patient should be informed at the time of admission of the minimum time required for an evaluation in order to prevent premature withdrawal of the child and to provide the child with a time limit to counteract the sense of aimless confinement (Gair and Solomon, 1962; Atkins and Rose, 1962).

Planned Institutionalization. Planned institutionalization may be for diagnostic and/or treatment purposes and may last between a few weeks and a few years. Although the diagnostic evaluation cannot be strictly separated from the treatment of the behavior problem, there are occasions on which the observation of the child away from his parents is necessary in order to separate out the environmental contributions to the causation and maintenance of a particular behavioral deviation. Inpatient evaluation of the child is indicated when reports from community, school, and home do not seem to describe the same child, and the psychiatrist's limited contact does not allow for a formulation of a diagnosis that could account for the contradictory information, or when problem behavior remains unchanged or worsens despite all therapeutic efforts. Not only does inpatient observation provide a more accurate clinical picture, but the child's response to treatment can also be assessed, and in the case of chemotherapy, the kind and dosage of medication can be regulated.

Institutionalization for treatment purposes becomes necessary when the severity of the disturbance requires intensive corrective experiences or when the behavior problem is maintained or aggravated by pathological interactional patterns within the family. Anorexia nervosa and severe school phobia belong in the latter category. The case of a severely disturbed child may tax the family's emotional resources to such a degree that other children of the family are emotionally neglected; or a family that has managed to care for the disturbed child may no longer be able to do so because of another member's medical or psychiatric disability. Severely retarded and psychotic children may have to be institutionalized because their management requires professional care around the clock or because their abnormal behavior and poor judgment endanger the lives of themselves or others.

A sizable number of children in residential treatment centers come from foster homes and institutions for dependent children. Even a mildly disturbed or behaviorally deviant child may not be tolerated for long in a nonspecialized foster home. These children usually are placed in a succession of foster homes, and more often than not, their behavior deteriorates as the result of multiple placements. Therefore, unless foster parents can be motivated and supported to continue to care for a disturbed child or unless an appropriate foster home is found to accept the child with the knowledge of his behavior problems, these children are placed in residential treatment centers before further attempts at boarding with foster families are made.

Children's attitudes toward the staff and their behavior within the therapeutic settings change several times during their stay. At the beginning, the patient may be cooperative and abide by the rules with no difficulty, but before very long most children go through a period of rejecting the institution. They become hostile to the staff, try to run away, withdraw from interaction with peers and caretakers, and are depressed. As the child becomes more dependent upon the institution, he is more discriminating in his relationship with the staff, becomes fond of some persons, and may dislike others. When the discharge date is set, he once again begins to withdraw and prepare emotionally for the separation.

Peer interaction is at times colored by the child's relationship with adults. Children may become jealous of another child whom they perceive as receiving special treatment. Strong sibling rivalries may be fostered by the staff's reactions and the amount of their personal attention to some children (Montalvo and Pavlin, 1966). Because in most institutions children are grouped according to a reasonable age range and are housed at times in cottages or small units, the opportunity for peer interaction is more or less limited to the members of the group, and though this arrangement has the advantage of providing a more intimate atmosphere, it is also conducive to stronger positive or negative emotional reactions among the children in each group. When individual psychotherapy is a regular part of the residential treatment program, not only the child's past conflicts but his current interpersonal relationships are discussed, with the goal of fostering better adjustment to the present circumstances and making the child more sensitive to the nuances of his relationships with others (Sonis, 1967).

Disturbed adolescents are in need of a high degree of flexibility and understanding from the staff. They can be extremely provocative, sexually or otherwise, and are more prone than younger children to active and open defiance of authority. Their physical strength, coupled with poor impulse control, can make their outbursts frightening to peers, caretakers, and themselves. Their desire to impress their peers may at times lead them to engage in hazardous behavior, and in their search for an environmental response, they may imitate the self-destructive behavior of another member. In therapeutic centers for adolescents, the program must include vocational guidance and training besides the regular school curriculum, and adolescents must be encouraged and allowed to participate in various aspects of planning and executing the daily activities of the center.

Drug Therapy

The clinical application of psychoactive drugs in the treatment of behavior disorders in children began over 40 years ago. Since then, researchers with more sophisticated methodology have been engaged in a continuous assessment of the effects of pharmacological agents on the behavioral problems of children. However, psychopharmacology in child psychiatry has remained more limited than in adult psychiatry. Drug research with children is more difficult than with adults for a variety of legal, ethical, and psychiatric reasons. The physiological and behavioral consequences of the drugs in normal subjects cannot be evaluated because experimentation with normal children is ethically abhorrent and parental consent for such purposes is of questionable legal value. The diagnostic categories of childhood psychiatric disorders are even less defined than in adult psychiatry. In very young children, because of their limited repertoire of responses, distinctions between such psychiatric entities as adjustment reactions and neurosis, or organic brain syndrome and developmental deviations, are not easy to make. Developmental disorders may present as a generalized inability in interpersonal relationships, or, conversely, emotional problems arising from interpersonal difficulties may adversely affect the acquisition of age-appropriate skills.

Furthermore, drug treatment, like all other forms of treatment in children, is carried out in the context of family relationships and attitudes. The acceptance by and the expectations of significant members of the family of the prescribed drug exert a powerful influence over the perceived or reported outcome of the treatment. Even when drugs are used in an inpatient setting, it is not always possible to relate the improvement or deterioration of the child's behavior to the pharmacological agent that he is receiving. Maturational factors and environmental changes cannot be controlled, and their influences on the child's behavior are not separable from the effects of medication. Many of the reports regarding the effects of various drugs in the treatment of children's behavior disorders are contradictory or inconclusive because the subjects are heterogeneous, the number of children is too small, and the criteria for improvement are not well defined. A child reported as improved by the parents may be considered the same or worse by teachers. Or the conflictual relationship with the parents continues while school performance is improving. Or the earlier reports of improvement are replaced by complaints, even though the medication has not changed (Fisher, 1959).

The biological individuality of each child, as well as the unknown maturational and experiential variables, makes the comparison between two groups, or even two children, a difficult task. In some studies, children with seizure disorders, mental retardation, or structural damage of the central nervous system are excluded, while it is precisely in these children that environmental manipulation and/or psychotherapy often fails to produce a substantial change in disturbed behavior. In psychosis of early childhood, the effectiveness of biochemical agents has so far been limited to reduction in anxiety and hyperactivity and improved sleep rather than changes in psychotic symptomatology. On the other hand, tranquilizers, antidepressants, and stimulants have all resulted in some improvement in children with anxiety, depressed mood, or hyperactivity. From the published reports of some studies, it is impossible to know whether or not a drug that proved effective over the short period of experimentation continued its beneficial influence in controlling the particular symptoms over a long period. Nor can it be ascertained if the reduction or removal of a symptom was maintained once treatment was discontinued.

The preceding remarks are not intended as a negation of the value of psychopharmacological agents as useful adjuncts in psychiatric treatment of the behavior disorders of children. Rather, it is our contention that the awareness of these issues is a prerequisite for the judicious selection and prescription of drugs.

Principles of Psychopharmacotherapy in Children. Whenever the use of a drug is contemplated in child psychiatry, the parents' opinions and attitudes should be sought, their questions answered, and their full cooperation enlisted. If disagreement between the parents and ambivalence regarding the use of medication are not resolved beforehand, these factors may mitigate the effectiveness of any therapeutic agent. Some parents accept medication with reluctance, do not follow directions, and find every excuse to discontinue the regimen. Others come to expect drugs to be a panacea, are disappointed and disillusioned with the results, and demand a change in medication when the child is not cured of a problem that they find particularly distressing. Although children themselves accept drugs as an inevitable outcome of going to a doctor, they are quick to sense their parents' disappointment in the drug or their disapproval of it and thus become unwilling to take the medication, giving their parents an excuse to justify their own noncompliance.

Parents should be informed about the reasons for drug therapy, the particular target symptom that is likely to be reduced or removed by the medication, the most common side effects of the drug, and the measures to be instituted if unwanted side effects develop. The time necessary for evaluating the effectiveness of the medication and some indication as to the length of time that a child may need to remain on a maintenance dose must be given to the parents. Older children should be informed about the reasons for drug therapy in concrete and practical terms, preferably with their own complaints used as a basis to explain the decision. However, both the parents and the child must know that the medication is not a substitute for their own efforts in trying to solve the problems but rather may make it easier for them to do so.

Drugs should be selected on the basis of their effectiveness for specific target symptoms. No drug in child psychiatry has proven to be beneficial for all children with certain disorders. Medications that have been available for longer periods of time and whose relative safety has been established are preferable to newer products because it is only with the passage of time that the long-term consequences of chemical agents come to light. The beginning dose should be between one-third and one-fourth of the total contemplated dose, and the necessary increment should be added every two to three days until the maximum effects are achieved. Unless the severity of the side effects requires a change of medication, a therapeutic trial of three to four weeks is necessary before it can be considered ineffectual. The timing of administration needs careful regulation; for example, drugs with sedative effects can be initially given at bedtime for a few days to minimize sleepiness during the day, while stimulants that may interfere with sleep are given in the morning. The observations and comments of parents, teachers, and the patient regarding the effects of the medication should be actively and regularly solicited. Life events, affective states, and physical conditions influence the child's response to psychopharmacological agents; consequently it is not unusual to see a child who is more sleepy or more hyperalert with the same dose of medication on different days. Unless the child is physically ill or the unwanted effects last more than a few days, no change in medication is necessary.

Once the effectiveness of a drug has been clearly established and the child's behavior improved, the daily dosage should be gradually decreased and the drug discontinued—if not permanently, at least so that the therapist may find out if the continuation of chemotherapy is justified. When children report that they forgot or refused to take their medication, it is important to seek their opinions regarding the drug, to clarify any misconceptions that they may have about the effects and the side effects of the medication, and finally, to reconsider the necessity for the continuation of chemotherapy. It is not uncommon to discover that children who have forgotten to take their medication are no longer in need of it.

The psychoactive drugs used in child psychiatry can be divided into four categories: stimulants, major tranquilizers, antidepressants, and minor tranquilizers.

Stimulants

In 1937 Bradley published the result of his investigation of the responses of a group of children with chronic behavior disorders who received Benzedrine (amphetamine sulfate) in a residential treatment center. According to this report, about 50% of the 30 children in this sample showed marked improvement in their schoolwork, gained an increased sense of well-being, and became more interested in their environment. Furthermore, some children who had been hyperactive became subdued. Bradley was impressed with the observation that a drug that is a stimulant and an energizer had a calming effect on these children, and he considered this a "paradoxical" effect. Following Bradley, clinicians in other centers began experimenting with Benzedrine and Dexedrine (dextroamphetamine sulfate) in children with a variety of behavioral disorders, with varying results.

In 1957 Laufer and his co-workers introduced the term *hyperkinetic impulse disorder* to describe a constellation of symptoms that includes hyperactivity, impulsivity, short attention span, and distractibility. Because some of these children had histories of pre- and perinatal problems that could conceivably have resulted in brain damage, and because some children with known histories of structural damage to the central nervous system showed a similar constellation of symptoms, the term *minimal brain damage* or *dysfunction* gained currency. Researchers began to use dextroamphetamine in the treatment of children designated as hyperkinetics or those with minimal brain dysfunction. The results of these investigations have provided sufficient evidence to conclude that stimulants are effective drugs in the treatment of some, but by no means all, children with "minimal brain dysfunction" and with or without hyperactivity. The most impressive change in behavior following the administration of these drugs is in the areas of attention and responsiveness to environment. Parents and teachers report an increase in the child's ability and willingness to engage in the goal-directed activities demanded by the school and overall improvement in their attitude toward their peers, teachers, and other authority figures.

The reported improvement in school performance is most likely due to a more focused attention and other motivational factors, though Conners (1971) found improvement of perceptual–motor functioning in one subgroup of hyperkinetic children who had shown poor eye–

motor coordination. In another subgroup with good spatial orientation and poor perceptual integration, only the performance on the Bender–Gestalt test improved following administration of the stimulants. Fish (1971) has pointed out that the response to the stimulants is not limited to children with minimal brain dysfunction and that, in fact, these drugs can have beneficial effects in some children with mild neurotic disorders. The search for amphetamine responders has focused on such characteristics as the presence or absence of nonfocal neurological signs and EEG abnormalities. The results so far have been nonconclusive.

Pharmacology. Amphetamine is a sympathomimetic phenylethylamine that was first synthesized as a substitute for ephedrine. There is some evidence that amphetamine causes the release of norepinephrine in the brain and influences the metabolism of serotonin. The site of action is believed to be in the reticular activating system, which plays an important role in regulating the state of consciousness and is possibly involved in maintaining the drive state. The behavioral consequences of amphetamine ingestion in children may or may not be due to the action of the drug on the reticular activating system; however, our limited knowledge regarding the neurophysiology and neuropsychology of the psychoactive drugs does not allow for the formulation of any alternative hypothesis.

After 30 years of experimentation with amphetamine, it is now believed that the action of the drug in reducing hyperactivity is not a "paradoxical" effect; rather, when the child's attention span is increased, the reduction in aimless motor activities follows. Furthermore, it is still unclear whether the beneficial effects of central nervous system stimulants on attention are limited to children with minimal brain dysfunction or whether normal children can also show such increment (Eisenberg, 1972; Grinspoon and Singer, 1973).

Dosage. The effective dose of dextroamphetamine (Dexedrine) and methylphenidate (Ritalin) has to be regulated on an individual basis. The use of amphetamine in children under 3 years of age and of methylphenidate in those under 6 years of age should be avoided because side effects are more likely to appear and anorexia may interfere with the normal intake of foods. In older children, the recommended strategy is to begin with 5 mg of dextroamphetamine or 10 mg of methylphenidate once a day before breakfast and to increase the dosage by the same amount every two to three days. The maximum dosage of amphetamine is between 30 and 40 mg/day and of methylphenidate between 60 and 80 mg daily. The total daily intake may be divided into two or three doses, and the timing should be selected with the goal of maximizing the beneficial effects and minimizing the untoward reactions, so that in children whose sleep is disturbed by the medication, the final dose of the day should be given before 4 P.M., and those who lose their appetite should take the drugs after rather than before meals. The choice of methylphenidate or dextroamphetamine is dependent upon the clinician's preference and the child's responsiveness. Some children may respond to one drug and not the other.

Side Effects. The most frequently encountered side effects are anorexia, mild gastrointestinal disturbances, and insomnia. In most cases, these disturbances disappear within a few days with no intervention. When anorexia persists and results in weight loss, the dosage must be reduced. Some recent reports have indicated that the long-term use of stimulants may have an inhibiting effect on growth; it is therefore advisable to discontinue the medication during school holidays and summer vacation. In some children, the therapeutic dose of stimulants may lead to the deterioration and disorganization of behavior; others become agitated and irritable. The withdrawal of the drug results in remission of these symptoms. In psychotic children, stimulants have been ineffective and it is best to avoid their use. So far, there is no indication that the use of stimulants during childhood increases the risk of later drug abuse. Accidental or intentional overdose in children may have very serious results. Treatment includes acidification of the urine and the use of chlorpromazine or other neuroleptic drugs to prevent hypertension. Acute toxic psychosis due to amphetamine is manifested by confusion, panic, restlessness, delirium, and peripheral symptoms of sympathomimetic activities.

The duration of drug treatment depends upon the individual child's responsiveness. In some children, treatment may have to be continued for a few years. Others do not need the drug for more than a few months. Discontinuation of the drug during summer months provides a good opportunity to assess the necessity for further treatment when the child returns to school.

Major Tranquilizers

The first neuroleptic agent, phenothiazine, was introduced to psychiatry in 1952. Since then, the number of psychotropic agents has multiplied, and the search for more potent, safer, and more specific drugs continues. New compounds are first used in adults so that their safety and effectiveness may be assessed before their application for children can be recommended. Some drugs that have met the safety requirements of the regulatory agencies for use in adults and adolescents are still in the experimental stage for children, and special permission is needed from the regulatory agency before they can be pre-scribed for children.

Among the neuroleptic drugs, phenothiazine derivatives are the most widely used in child psychiatry. The site of action of these drugs is subcortical, in the mesodiencephalic area of the central nervous system, including the reticular formation, where the monoamine neuro-transmitters are concentrated. Phenothiazines exercise an inhibiting effect on these neurotransmitters. The sedative and antianxiety effects of these drugs, with little or no interference with state of conscious-ness, are due to their subcortical sites of action. The antipsychotic ef-fect of neuroleptics in psychosis of early childhood is not as remark-able as in older children and adolescents. In most investigations, phenothiazines have been used to counteract specific target symp-toms, such as hyperactivity, aggressiveness, and anxiety. The results have shown the effectiveness of the drugs in these situations (Camp-bell, 1973).

Of the phenothiazine group, chlorpromazine (Thorazine) is the agent with the longest record of therapeutic trial, and the immediate as well as the long-term side effects are well known. Very young chil-dren respond with excessive sleepiness to the drug, while school-age children have a higher tolerance than would be expected on the basis of the milligram per kilogram dose in adults. Trifluoperazine (Stela-zine) is about 18 times more potent than chlorpromazine and has a less sedating effect. It is particularly useful in younger children who become sleepy and unresponsive to their environment on therapeutic doses of chlorpromazine. Thioridazine (Mellaril) is similar in its effec-tiveness and potency to chlorpromazine, while perphenazine (Trila-fon) must be used in much smaller dosages. Haloperiodol (Haldol), one of the newer neuroleptics, is not as yet released for children under 12 years of age, though the drug has been found useful in psychosis of adolescents and adults.

There is no consistent evidence to support the superiority of one drug over another. The use of psychotropic drugs in children is essen-tially dependent upon clinical judgment and the degree of familiarity of the clinician with the particular drug. Because the reactions of chil-dren to any medication are more varied than those of adults, the type of drug and its dosage must be individualized and carefully titrated. Some children do not respond to one drug but are responsive to a chemically related agent. Others show the desired response on a very low dosage of one medication, and increasing the dose may in fact cause a deterioration in their behavior.

In prescribing major tranquilizers for children, the target symp-toms must be clearly delineated and the particular drug dosage slowly increased until the desired effects are achieved. This usually takes between three and four weeks, and during this time, a change to another drug is unwarranted unless the side effects make the continuation of the drug hazardous. As a rule, more disorganized children are in need of more potent drugs. However, the presence of some residual symptoms does not justify an increase of medication beyond the safe limit. Furthermore, it must be remembered that drugs cannot replace other forms of management in child psychiatry. Children still need appropriate class placement, remedial education, and the resolution of conflictual relationships with parents and other family members. Drug therapy in child psychiatry is seldom the only necessary treatment modality, and the more disturbed and disorganized the child's behavior, the less can one depend on medication alone to remedy the situation.

The safe dosage of various medications may depend on the individual child and his idiosyncratic reaction. Most reports in the literature have indicated that chlorpromazine can be safely administered up to 400 mg daily to an average child of school age (range between 50 and 400 mg). Mellaril may be effective in a much lower dosage, though daily doses of up to 300 mg have been used with no untoward reaction. Stelazine is the most potent drug of the tranquilizers used in children. The dosage must be carefully regulated. More than 20 mg/day is not considered necessary or safe. The total daily dose of neuroleptics may be given at one time or divided into three to four doses. In practice, it seems more beneficial to give the larger portion of the drug at bedtime and smaller doses in the morning and at noontime. This regimen causes the least amount of sleepiness but allows for the curtailment of hyperactivity and aggressive outbursts during the day, when the child is in interaction with his environment.

Side Effects. The most common side effect of tranquilizers is sleepiness, which usually disappears in a few days with no intervention. Extrapyramidal symptoms are relatively rare in children and can be effectively treated with diphenhydramine (Benadryl). Orally administered doses of 25 mg Benadryl one to three times a day for two to three days are all that is needed. Anti-Parkinson drugs are not recommended and may cause agitation in children. Hematological side effects are very rare, though when children are on a maintenance dose, a periodic complete blood count is advisable. Endocrine disorders in adolescent girls in the form of amenorrhea, lactation, and false positive pregnancy tests have been reported. Withdrawal of the drug leads to the disappearance of these symptoms. Photosensitivity has been reported and parents must be cautioned against allowing excessive exposure to sunlight, particularly in the summer months. Weight increase has been noted in children and adolescents on long-term treatment with Mellaril and Thorazine. In several cases of long-term treatment with tranquilizers, corneal and lens stippling have been seen in children without any detrimental effect on vision. The drugs must be discontinued when such side effects are encountered.

Tardive dyskinesia—the rhythmical and myoclonic-like movement of the distal portion of the upper extremities, with protrusion of the tongue, chewing movement of the chin, and contraction of the upper lip—have recently come to light following the rapid or sudden discontinuation of tranquilizers in children. The symptoms usually disappear in between 3 and 12 months without any treatment. From the limited reports in the literature, tardive dyskinesia does not seem to be as refractory in children as it is in adults (McAndrew *et al.*, 1972).

Antidepressants. These groups include tricyclic (amitryptiline and imipramine) and the monoamine oxidase inhibitors (phenelzine and isocarboxidase). Of these drugs, only imipramine (Tofranil) is approved by the U.S. regulatory agency for treatment of enuresis in children. The recommended dosage is 1–2 mg/kg/day (between 50 and 75 mg/day for children between 6 and 8 years of age, given in one single dose).

Researchers in the United States and Europe have used antidepressants in the treatment of a variety of clinical conditions, such as school phobia, hyperactivity, and depressed mood. The results of these studies have provided some evidence of the effectiveness of these drugs, although there is no uniformity of opinion as to their specific actions (Frommer, 1968). The dosages used in these studies have ranged from 5 to 14 mg/kg/day (Elavil or Tofranil). Side effects have included convulsion, cardiovascular problems such as tachycardia, hypotension, and abnormalities on EKG such as bundle branch block. Overdoses of these drugs have resulted in cardiac arrhythmia and cardiac arrest.

Minor Tranquilizers. This group are used for their mild sedative and antianxiety effects. Diphenhydramine (Benadryl) is particularly helpful in the treatment of sleep problems and irritability in preschoolers. The drug has a wide safety range and up to 300–400 mg/day can be given in divided doses. Chlordiazepoxide (Librium) and diazepam (Valium) are of value in the anxiety reactions and hypochondriacal preoccupations of school-age children. Some children may complain of sleepiness on the therapeutic dose of these medications. Others may show excitation. The usual dose for children between 6 and 12 is between 10 and 50 mg of Librium and 10 and 30 mg of Valium.

Anticonvulsive medications and barbiturates have not been useful in the treatment of children with behavior problems, and barbiturates have on occasion resulted in agitation and disorganization of behavior (Fish, 1966).

23

Prognosis and Prevention

Prognosis

Historically, psychiatric theoreticians conceived of failure to develop a moral conscience and higher intellectual abilities as a partial explanation for mental deficiency and psychopathy. However, the notion that the psychiatric disorders of adulthood are a continuation of the behavioral deviations of childhood or that they are etiologically related gained currency following the introduction of psychoanalysis. Retrospective studies of the life histories of adult patients and follow-up investigations of children with behavior disorders have so far failed to substantiate the assumption of the continuity of behavior in spite of the logical appearance of the hypotheses. Furthermore, although it has been established that children with identified behavioral disorders have a three to four times higher risk of becoming psychiatric patients as adults than the general population, no differential pathognomic patterns have been found to signify the nature of the future psychiatric illness (Mellsop, 1972). For example, in some studies timidity, shyness, and social isolation are found as precursors of adult schizophrenia, while in others aggressive and antisocial patterns of behavior have been noted in the childhoods of patients later diagnosed as schizophrenics (Rutter, 1972). Some behavioral symptoms associated with anxiety—such as nail biting, thumb sucking, and tics—are not more prevalent in the background history of adult neurotics. Nor do phobias and anxiety attacks of childhood necessarily lead to neuroses in adult life. Diagnostic and prognostic uncertainty continues into adolescence, so that ambiguous terms such as *adolescent turmoil* have been used to describe the clinical picture of psychiatric problems with varied course and outcome in this population (Pichel, 1974). The affective disorders, which comprise a significant portion of the psychiatric illnesses of adults, have not been identified in childhood, which has led some researchers to postulate a phenomenologically different picture of behavioral deviation in early life as the precursor of affective illnesses. On the other hand, the future of children with the hyperkinetic syndrome, a frequently diagnosed entity during childhood, remains uncharted.

Uncertainty regarding the natural course of the behavioral deviations of children and adolescents makes prognostication an extremely difficult task in child psychiatry. Follow-up studies of children with various psychiatric disorders have failed to identify variables of predictive value, and this failure, in turn, has made it impossible to assess the effectiveness of any therapeutic endeavors. In psychosis of early childhood, high scores on IQ tests have been shown to be associated with better prognosis; however, in some children the scores begin a downward trend during adolescence, and these patients' adaptations deteriorate; therefore IQ score and related functions such as academic achievement can be considered of prognostic importance only when no deterioration has taken place. One-half of the children with antisocial and aggressive behavior are expected to become well-functioning adults, but present studies have not identified the factors that are responsible for or associated with this favorable outcome (Robins, 1966).

Attempts at the construction of measures to predict future maladaptive behaviors have been disappointing in that they have not significantly improved on the clinicans' educated guesses or the teachers' evaluations and predictions. In a prospective study, Roff (1972) found that the majority of children with good peer relationships were free from antisocial behavior at the time of the follow-up, while children with poor social relationships were engaged in a variety of delinquent activities. However, in children of the lowest socioeconomic class, which is overrepresented among the delinquent population, the quality of peer relationships did not differentiate between the delinquent and nondelinquent groups. The investigations of treatment in child psychiatry clinics have repeatedly revealed that children with neurotic problems are more likely to receive individual psychotherapy than children with mental retardation, organic brain syndromes, and severe conduct disorders. Concomitantly follow-up studies have shown that children with neurotic disorders and adjustment reactions have a good prognosis for later adaptation and adjustment. Two alternative conclusions with vastly different implications can be drawn from these observations. Either neurotic disorders and adjustment reactions are self-limiting, or, conversely, psychotherapeutic efforts are effective methods of treatment and should be extended to children with more severe behavioral deviations. In the present state of psychiatric knowledge, neither one of these two hypotheses can be discounted.

Retrospective studies have attempted to define correlational tendencies between the diagnostic categories of adult psychiatric disorders and such familial factors as the presence or absence of similar or dissimilar psychiatric illnesses in biological relatives, and, environmental occurrences, such as separation from the parents, broken homes, and educational attainments. The statistical correlations have so far failed to provide a reliable measure of predictability in regard to the psychiatric outcome; however, they have generated some hypotheses as to a variety of at-risk factors that need to be tested through longitudinal studies of children deemed vulnerable. Descriptions of patterns of child-rearing practices, which are theoretically an important variable in shaping the personality and styles of adaptive and maladaptive behavior, have proved to be too vague and overgeneralized to be of any predictive value with respect to the development of psychiatric problems. However, there are some clinical indications that tolerant families who are not overwhelmed by the child's deviancy may contribute to a better prognosis (Rutter, 1972).

Prevention

The design and application of preventive measures are dependent upon the knowledge regarding the etiology and the natural course of an illness and the availability of effective therapeutic methods and intervention strategies. However, some preventive work is undertaken solely on the basis of clinical impressions and statistical correlations without any firm proof of cause-and-effect links among various factors.

In public health work, preventive activities are divided into the primary, secondary, and tertiary categories. Primary prevention involves the application of those measures that are expected to stop an undesirable process from developing in an individual or a group of individuals. In child psychiatry, so far such activities have been directed at trying to lower the rate of mental retardation in the child population (Stein and Susser, 1971).

Artificial limitations on reproduction and the termination of pregnancies have become two major preventive tools. Genetic counseling requires diagnostic studies of the affected individual; a review of the medical records of the biological relatives suspected of having a similar disorder; chromosomal analysis of the parents, siblings, and the patient; and the statistics of the occurrence of the specific anomaly in the general population (Crandall, 1977). For example, it is known that 1% of patients with Down's syndrome have an affected sib; however, this rate is operative when both parents have normal karyotype and the child's chromosomal pattern shows a trisomy 21. On the other hand, if the mother has a D/G translocation, the risk for the recurrence of Down's syndrome among children is one in three, or 33%. The termination of the pregnancy is usually recommended in the presence of prenatal complications, such as infection or irradiation, proven to have a high probability of affecting the fetus, or when anomalies are discovered following diagnostic amniocentesis. In this procedure, 10–20 cc of amniotic fluid are withdrawn from the expectant mother between the 12th and 16th weeks of pregnancy. After the separation of fetal cells from the fluid, the cells are cultured and suspected anomalies are searched for. So far, more than 55 different genetic defects have been identified, and although not all lead to mental retardation, a significant portion of them have been implicated. Therapeutic abortion in these cases relieves the family of a future burden and lowers the rate of mental retardation or degenerative diseases in the child population.

Prenatal care—with early diagnosis and prompt treatment of maternal malnutrition, infection, toxemia of pregnancy, immunologic reactions, and metabolic disorders—is expected to decrease the number of reproductive casualties and consequent intellectual and behavioral deficiencies. However, the causes of premature birth are still unknown, and no direct benefit has come from proper prenatal care in lowering the rate of prematurity. Parental education and consultation regarding child-rearing practices have not been researched enough to rank as a primary preventive measure, although the issue remains a theoretical possibility.

Secondary prevention includes the early identification and remediation of problem areas. On a biological level, the diagnosis of such disorders as Rh incompatibility, phenylketonuria, and thyroid deficiencies shortly after birth, and appropriate treatment such as exchange transfusion, restricted diet, and addition of thyroid extract will prevent or at least minimize the risk of kernicterus and mental retardation. In the psychological areas, measures such as preschool enrichment programs and perceptual training have been designed to counteract the effects of experiential deprivation and/or developmental lags (Blank, 1970). The results of such programs have been disappointing, at least insofar as the favorable outcome has been defined as an increase in test-measured intelligence or higher reading proficiency. Follow-up studies have not substantiated the earlier claims to beneficial effects of many of these early interventions (Belmont and Birch,

1974). Psychotherapeutic efforts at the time of crisis and in the treatment of early behavior disorders in the acute stage have been shown to be of value, although their long-term effectiveness has not been established.

Rehabilitative endeavors, or tertiary prevention, are undertaken to maximize the child's potentials for normative experiences, to increase the acquisition of necessary educational and social skills, and to neutralize the pathogenic potentials of disabilities and defects. Because secondary and tertiary preventive efforts are directed toward the individual patient, their effectiveness cannot be measured solely by statistical proofs and experimental programs. Clinical impressions and subjective reports of improvement by families, patients, and teachers are valid parameters, even when changes cannot be verified by objective scales.

Some authors have conceptualized the subject of prevention as activities that promote mental health rather than those that are expected to influence the rate of mental disorders (Berlin, 1975). The implications of such a conceptualization are not substantially different from prevention, although the standards of effectiveness are less clear and more theoretical. According to these authors, obviating organic problems, enriching the social and psychological milieu, and correcting a depriving or traumatizing situation are the basic tasks of child psychiatry. Even though various modifying contingencies may influence the eventual outcome, such a lack of certitude is not an excuse for nonintervention.

24

Patterns of Delivery of Services

There are a number of organizational patterns through which psychiatric services can be provided for children. These fall into the general categories of clinics and other outpatient services, inpatient units, liaison functioning within pediatric care facilities, liaison with child rehabilitation units, units within community health centers, and liaison with schools.

Within each of these formal structures, there has been great diversity in the precise manner in which psychiatric care is given. Some services providing diagnostic workups may not offer treatment and refer the children elsewhere for the carrying out of their recommendations. Others provide only psychotherapy. For the most part, however, clinics attempt to carry a child patient from diagnostic evaluation through whatever management and/or treatment is deemed necessary. A group of services have been organized by special interests to meet needs considered inadequately fulfilled, such as those of children with mental retardation or infantile autism. The theoretical orientation of the psychiatric facility may be a factor limiting patient care. Some facilities provide long-term analytically oriented psychotherapy, while others focus on behavior modification. The element of timing is another differentiation. The psychiatric facility may be organized in such a manner as to provide crisis intervention or some other speedy response. On the other hand, it is not unusual to find a clinic so organized that its formal intake and extensive routine evaluation procedures result in a long waiting list; waits as long as two years from the time of initial application to the first visit have been reported (Bazelon, 1974).

Clinics and Outpatient Facilities. The terms usually employed for children's ambulatory psychiatric care facilities are *mental hygiene* or *child guidance clinics.* These may be free-standing or may be one of a medical center's many outpatient clinics. Since child psychiatry is a subspecialty, not all medical centers with adult psychiatric outpatient services have provisions for children. Many child guidance clinics were originally organized by local communities or private agencies. In the current period, the trend has been for such free-standing child guidance centers to arrange for an affiliation with a hospital or a medical center in order to obtain accreditation. While it is customary for the psychiatrist in charge of the clinic to be certified in child psychiatry by the American Board of Psychiatry and Neurology in Child Psychiatry or to be board-eligible, it is not required that all of the psychiatrists working with the child or the family have formal training in this discipline. Often it may be the psychologist or the social worker who carries out the treatment under psychiatric supervision. In a medical center with an accredited training program in child and adolescent psychiatry, residents and fellows in training are responsible for carrying out diagnosis and treatment under the supervision of trained child psychiatrists. In sum, whether the clinic is hospital-based or run by an independent voluntary agency, the manner in which a clinic is conducted depends upon its theoretical orientation, purpose, and manner of organization.

Inpatient Services. Inpatient units for children and adolescents are scarce relative to their need. Many psychiatric hospitals do not have children's divisions, and many training programs for child and adolescent psychiatrists have no residential accommodations for these age groups. Adolescents are often sent to adult inpatient units. There are some residential hospitals and schools exclusively for children and adolescents with psychiatric disorders. These either are under psychiatric auspices or maintain regular psychiatric consultants on the staff. Depending upon the degree of psychopathology of the youngsters it serves, an inpatient facility or residence may have its own school or send its children to a neighboring educational program.

Children's and adolescents' residential units require a higher ratio of caretakers per child than do inpatient facilities for adults and are consequently more costly. Children and adolescents need more medical attention than most adults, and they also require a higher degree of individual attention. Since a unified approach by the whole staff is essential for successful milieu therapy, an important feature of the inpatient care of psychiatrically ill children or adolescents is planned and frequent consultation among those who come into daily contact with the patients at various levels of interaction. The provision of recreational opportunities for child and adolescent patients is also a fundamental aspect of their care.

Pediatric Liaison. Centralized facilities for the physical health care of children are not in general use, nor are they available in all geographic areas. However, those that are in use can provide the largest samples of children to be found anywhere except in the schools. Hence they are a logical locus for case finding and the effective delivery of psychiatric services. The personnel in baby health stations and pediatric clinics and pediatricians in private practice have the opportunity to monitor babies' developmental sequences and to note deviancies in behavior in terms of either the attainment of normative milestones or the qualitative aspects of functioning. The pediatric facility can thus be the first psychiatric screen. Traditionally, once the personnel of a pediatric facility are convinced that a behavioral deviance requires full psychiatric evaluation, a formal referral is made to a psychiatric unit or a private practitioner.

In a liaison service, psychiatric consultation is provided at the pediatric facility itself. This may range from seminar-type discussions given to the staff, on-site consultations to parents and children at regularly designated times, or a full psychiatric–pediatric liaison service working within a pediatric in- and outpatient hospital unit. The functions of such units may range widely. One pattern provides on-site case finding and preliminary assessment, with selective referral to the child psychiatry department for further diagnostic study and appropriate intervention when deemed necessary. Other units carry the full responsibility, including orienting pediatric personnel, case identification, evaluation, and management. In concert with ongoing pediatric care, the psychiatric treatment is given through a combination of environmental manipulation, parental guidance, special services such as tutoring or recreation, and, if necessary, individual or group psychotherapy.

While the medical model is common to both pediatric and psychiatric personnel, it is nevertheless necessary for child psychiatric personnel to modify their traditional referral mechanism in order to function within the context of the pediatric service. The success of the liaison unit depends in great measure upon this accommodation. The pediatrician, the nurse, and other associates are pursuing the child's physical care. To an increasing extent, they include psychological well-being in their care, but this attitude is far from universal. More often, there is the orientation that once they have identified the possibility of behavior deviance, the rest of the task of diagnosis and intervention belongs to the psychiatric unit. This attitude is justified in the same way as a referral of a visual or orthopedic problem to a specialty clinic. However, when the pediatrician remains the primary physician and maintains the basic continuity of the child's total health care, he should be kept abreast of the psychiatric findings and recommendations by the liaison unit. The fact that the pediatric patient has an ongoing relationship with his primary physician adds to the probability that he will continuously receive the needed psychiatric services. The positive attitude that parents have toward the pediatric facility is transferred to the psychiatric unit, which is correctly perceived as one of the pediatric specialties. Missed appointments can be rescheduled, and a shaky rapport can be repaired by meeting the patient and parents at the next pediatric visit. A further benefit of the psychiatric liaison with a pediatric service is that it becomes possible to follow children over time and obtain longitudinal pictures of their functioning, thus permitting assessments of the impact of psychiatric intervention (Chess and Lyman, 1969).

Another extremely important element in the delivery of psychiatric service at the pediatric locus is that psychosomatic problems may be identified early and chronicity prevented. There is a steady stream of problems in which psychological stress is presented as somatic complaints in the absence of organic pathology. The identification of such a possibility is usually made by the pediatrician, who notes the frequency of complaints in the absence of identifiable organic disease. Psychiatric treatment may then begin without delay. In some cases, organic etiology is finally found, and it is necessary to determine whether psychological stress caused the organic pathology or the symptoms are solely the reflection of an underlying disease. The more frequent psychosomatic issues are those in which stress is created by a disease that involves chronic pain, episodic frightening symptomatology, painful and disruptive treatment, and/or disabilities that prevent the pediatric patient from participating in normal experiences. In each of these instances, parental handling of the ill child may be a crucial factor in the degree to which the noxious psychological consequences of physical illness can be prevented or minimized. A joint effort by the pediatrician and the psychiatrist may be achieved in individual situations in the ordinary pattern of psychiatric care, but such an effort can become routine only in a pediatric–psychiatric liaison model of service delivery.

Rehabilitation Liaison. The principles and ongoing function of the rehabilitation liaison organization are similar to those of a liaison with a pediatric unit, as discussed above. The psychiatrist's manner of relating to the patients and the staff should fit into the organization and style of the rehabilitation center. It is also essential that the psychiatric staff be familiar with the course and consequences of the diseases and disabilities themselves and that they become knowledgeable regarding the direct and indirect behavioral concomitants of the particular physical and social stresses involved.

Community Health Centers. There has been a succession of concepts regarding mental health networks: community mental health centers, health maintenance organizations, and university-affiliated services. Discouragement with established patterns of service delivery that fail to meet the needs of children has led to the formulation of "innovative" patterns. To some extent, these patterns are based on the belief that any new and different method will, like a new detergent, be better than the old. However, the packaging of such services has not proved to transcend their actual day-to-day functioning (Hetznecker and Forman, 1971; Panzetta, 1971; Rafferty, 1975). Some mental health centers have become active, useful, and important psychiatric facilities, accepted by their communities and well utilized. Others have spent much of their personnel's time in diffusely focused meetings with community representatives, draining time and effort from the actual giving of service.

The basic idea behind the community-based mental health facility is to establish a network of services that provides comprehensive care for a geographically specific catchment area. Provisions for caring for children as well as adults are included in the guidelines, and it is also specifically mandated in the United States by federal provisions for community mental health care centers that the psychiatric needs of mentally retarded children be met. Because of the arbitrary nature of the geographic boundaries mandated for some catchment areas, there is often overlapping with, or fragmentation of, previously established networks of service given by either community agencies or hospitals. Furthermore, the number of trained child psychiatrists is insufficient for a countrywide network of comprehensive community health centers. The mandating of the programs also failed to take into account the differing needs of urban centers and rural areas. While an initial group of such centers were built and staffed in various parts of the country, the full program has not been implemented, especially for children. As a result, the community mental health center has not become a major provider of children's services in the United States.

Paraprofessionals. Among the proposed methods of extending mental health care to larger numbers of children, the use of paraprofessionals has been presented as an innovative approach. In such programs, individuals selected for their personal capacities rather than for their formal academic credentials are trained to recognize behavioral deviances and are given varying degrees of responsibility for participating in the diagnostic process. In some settings, paraprofessionals are assigned aspects of direct therapeutic intervention, such as play therapy and discussions with patients and parents.

This is a controversial area. On the one hand, since paraprofessionals have been used almost exclusively for patients at the lower socioeconomic levels and since the virtues of such programs include the fact that they cost less in staff salaries, the suspicion has been voiced that they exemplify giving poor service to poor people. The proponents, on the other hand, point to the alleged inability of middle-class professionals to communicate successfully with members of the lower socioeconomic groups. In addition, because of the budgetary savings, it is argued that services can be extended to a large patient group at equal cost. As with other innovative programs, the initial application showed greater potential than the later, more widespread functioning of the program. It is still necessary to determine to what degree, and with what training, specific aspects of diagnosis and therapeutic response can be enhanced by employing paraprofessionals in child psychiatry.

Liaison with Schools and Child Care Centers. While the school is organized primarily for the acquisition of academic skills, the child's emotional and social development are decisively affected by the events of the school day. The school is the place where children learn to relate to authorities other than their parents and to cope with successive learning and task performance demands. The school also provides an opportunity for even the most home-bound children to develop relationships with peers. The degree of success or failure in each of those areas determines, in large measure, a child's estimate of his own capabilities and his feelings about himself. Those children who have developed maladaptive patterns at home may, in school, develop alternative cooperative ways of relating to authority figures and friends, or they may continue the unsocialized, aggressive, or overcompliant attitudes that characterize their behavior at home.

Since the tasks of the early grades are the acquisition of the basic skills of reading, writing, and computation, upon which the rest of the curriculum is based, learning disabilities, while basically a responsibility of educators, have such a far-reaching impact on emotional status that they are a legitimate area of psychiatric concern. The child who cannot learn to read at the expected age will develop other symptoms that can transform an initial learning problem into a psychiatric disorder, which may sometimes reach major proportions. Defensive attitudes of denial or avoidance and distracting maneuvers such as clowning and aggression may in fact so overshadow the original problem as to appear to be themselves causative. A fallacious assumption that the reading failure is derivative sometimes results in a decision to send the child for psychotherapy rather than the remedial teaching he needs. In some children who have both learning and behavior problems, the primary problem may be emotional and the learning difficulty a secondary consequence. Thus, the diagnosis of psychiatric status and its relationship to the learning failure are essential elements in planning an appropriate program of both educational and psychological intervention. It is pertinent not only to determine which problem came first but also to institute a total program involving simultaneous or sequential interventions, depending upon the actual deficiencies in achievement and motivation.

The diversity of developmental rates among young children is particularly pertinent to the psychiatric dialogue with educators. Instruction is usually geared to the mean capacity of a class but may, in certain circumstances, be aimed at the highest achievers. Those whose abilities, such as perceptual discrimination, attention span, or fine motor control, are immature may be perceived by the teacher, their classmates, and themselves as failures, when in fact they are "late bloomers." For such children, there are the twin dangers of a self-view as "stupid" and a permanent reduction of education expectation on the part of the teachers. These derogatory self-judgments and lowered expectations are then reflected in a decreased capacity and skill in the children, leading to a self-fulfilling prophecy despite their high potential.

Since there is universal education by law, finding cases of children with psychiatric disorders is possible in the school setting. The practicality of such an endeavor, however, depends on two factors: (1) the availability of psychiatric personnel, either in the schools or in backup facilities, to complete the evaluation and implement the needed intervention within a brief time span; and (2) the degree to which the mental health worker is viewed by the parents as a concerned and helpful individual, as opposed to one merely interested in labeling children as abnormal for the purpose of excluding them from the usual educational track (Bower, 1969).

Psychiatric projects in the schools have usually been selective in their efforts—serving one or a number of schools rather than the whole system, focusing on a specific segment of the educational hierarchy, or a combination of these two strategies. Thus some programs choose to work through seminars attended by guidance counselors, with the idea that in this way the psychiatric effort will have the greatest impact by eventually filtering down to the classroom teachers. Another pattern has been for a professional member of the backup psychiatric facility—a psychiatrist, a psychologist, or a social worker—to be in the designated school on scheduled days, when parents, children, and teachers can be seen for the identification of problems, diagnostic evaluation, interpretation, consultation, and individual and/or group meetings with children and parents. The option to refer a child to the psychiatric facility is usually included in such a program at any point in this diagnostic–therapeutic chain.

The key to the success or failure of such programs is the ability of psychiatric workers to accommodate to the structure and the needs of the educational institution. To begin with, it must be recognized that the school personnel have different concepts and criteria than mental health professionals for designating behavioral pathology and emergencies. Furthermore, the traditional referral model must be abandoned. In the traditional model, the school refers individual children who present behavior difficulties in the classroom to clinics for diagnosis and treatment. Although many children demonstrating behavior disorders in school are referred for psychiatric evaluation, a large portion of those who are told to go to psychiatric clinics do not keep the appointments. From the point of referral on, the school regards the mental health of the child as being the clinic's responsibility. Communication takes place primarily through written reports, following a bureaucratic model that is fragmented, slow, and inefficient. The school sends a request for evaluation along with information as to academic status and a translation of the teacher's complaints into psychopathological terms, such as "anxious" or "aggressive." Often, unfortunately, these reports fail to give the clinic a real picture of the child's life during the school day. The clinic then evaluates the child in its own setting. While the basic psychiatric diagnosis may be accurately defined, the differences in the demands and the general atmosphere of the two settings make it unlikely that the psychiatrist will observe those behaviors that were the school's reason for referral.

The report of the clinic to the school is often couched in psychiatric jargon, and it is extremely difficult for the teacher to understand its implications for the educational setting. In addition, the same term may have a different meaning for clinic and school when applied to a specific child. For example, the clinic's recommendation for "individualized attention" may mean an approach to the child that takes into account his special problems and vulnerabilities. The school, however, may have referred this child to begin with because he was demanding excessive "individualized attention" from the teacher.

It is this "Alice through the looking glass" aspect of traditional school–clinic interaction that a liaison program in the school needs to change. An "emergency" in a classroom means that the child's behavior is either disruptive to teaching or harmful to other children, while to the clinic it may refer only to suicidal danger or serious aggression.

The severe problem in the classroom is the disruptive child, while to the clinic it is the youngster with thought disorder. The mental health worker in the school can observe the child in the classroom and show the teacher and the guidance counselor how to make and record behavioral observations that are meaningful to the diagnostician and how to state the referral questions pointedly. Similarly, with an ongoing relationship at the site of the school, it becomes more possible to translate the clinical findings into terms relevant to the instructional approach and classroom management.

The principles discussed above relating to psychiatric efforts in the schools and in health care settings are equally relevant to recreational and day care centers. Each of these has its own purposes, yet each has concerns about and difficulties with children demonstrating deviant behaviors. Day care centers for working mothers may, in fact, be the place where the children spend a majority of their waking hours on workdays. Hence the issues of appropriate developmental expectations, affectionate interrelationships, and continuity of caretaking personnel may be fundamental to the young child's healthy psychological development. Recreational centers often provide role models for children that diversify and enlarge their experiences. Where parental models are constructive, the diversification merely enhances the child's exposure. If the child–parent interaction is a noxious one, recreation leaders can have a corrective influence, showing alternative modes of interrelating and gratifying experiences of cooperative versus antagonistic functioning.

It is for such reasons that it may be desirable for psychiatry programs to provide on-site service to child care and recreational centers. Such consultation may range from an orientation of staff regarding child development in general, to a discussion of individual children, to the diagnostic evaluations and treatment of individual youngsters who are identified by the center or by the mental health workers as showing deviant behavior. The general principle holds here as in other settings: the psychiatric mode of procedure, language of discussion, and attention to presenting problems must be in the context of the purposes and needs of the program to which it is providing service (Allinsmith and Goethols, 1962; La Vietes and Chess, 1969; Lawrence, 1971; Forman and Hetznecker, 1972).

25

Children and the Law

In most societies, including the United States, there are no, or very few, laws governing the rights of children. Historically children have been viewed as the property or extensions of their parents. Those born to privileged situations inherited their parental status and fortune, while the children of serfs and slaves belonged to their masters. The subject of most existing children's laws was the age at which contractual relationships were valid or a child could manage his own property. In feudal societies, when minor children inherited property, the state found it necessary to appoint a "guardian" for the child in order to assure the collection of taxes in the social interest and to assume responsibility for the care of the child. The doctrine of *parens patria*, thus came to define the state as the guardian of all those who cannot protect themselves and has been the legal guideline most frequently used in relation to children.

The awareness that children are the human resources of the future and the belief that fulfillment of their developmental needs is in the best interest of society have provided the state with the legal power to require compulsory education and universal vaccinations and to intervene on the child's behalf when the parents are neglectful, abusive, or otherwise unfit. More recently in the United States, various litigations have resulted in the direct or indirect assertion of the applicability of some constitutional rights to children. Thus the provision of "equal protection under the law" has been the basis of judicial orders to boards of education to provide handicapped children with appropriate education equal to that of the nonhandicapped in duration and quality. The constitutional right to "protection from harm," which is based on the Eighth Amendment prohibition against cruel and unusual punishment, has been invoked by the court to mandate individual plans for the education and treatment of mentally retarded institutionalized children.

In the *Kent* and *Gault* decisions, the Supreme Court of the United States extended the right of due process to all children who appear before the juvenile court. In these proceedings, children are now guaranteed the right to receive a specific notice of the charges against them, to be represented by counsel, to confront their accusers, and to avoid self-incrimination. The right to privacy and the prohibition against cruel and unusual punishment are the bases of litigation that has sought to curtail parental rights to volunteer their children for nontherapeutic medical experimentations and sterilization in the cases of mentally retarded individuals. In cases of child custody, the principle of the "child's best interest," enacted into a law in some states, requires the court to pay specific attention to the child's needs rather than to the competing claims of the parents.

The role of the mental health professional in legal proceedings relating to children is that of an expert witness who is expected to assist the court by providing an assessment of the child's emotional and intellectual status and outlining his specific developmental needs. Suggestions and recommendations as to the therapeutic or preventive course of action comprise part of such assessments. The court may accept or reject the plan on substantive grounds; or it may agree with the substantive issues but be unable to implement the recommendations because of the unavailability of particular facilities.

Because a sizable number of children are involved in legal proceedings, no child psychiatrist can remain aloof from the legal establishment. As a consultant to the court, the child psychiatrist is expected to express his opinions in nontechnical terms, to be prepared to clarify his implicit assumptions, and to enumerate the observations, facts, and theoretical inferences upon which his conclusions are based. In advocating a particular intervention, he must be sensitive to issues such as parental rights and the right of the community to be protected from further harm by the child, as well as to the legal and practical limitations of the court. Statements about prognosis must be based on the collective knowledge within the field that is applicable to the specific child. Vague threats of future disasters or ambiguous promises of reformation and change do not serve the best interests of the child or the community. When psychiatric opinions are based on accurately observed behaviors and empirically substantiated interpretations, the consultant is secure in the knowledge that his conclusions represent the best-informed psychological assessment of the situation and that any decision founded upon his evaluation is likely to benefit the child. This security is of the utmost importance when the child psychiatrist appears in the unfamiliar forum of the court and is confronted with the adversary process of fact finding that is the underlying orientation of the lawyers challenging the consultant's views and recommendations.

Juvenile Delinquency

A juvenile delinquent in New York State is legally defined as a child between the ages of 7 and 16 who has committed an act that would be considered a crime if committed by an adult. Roman common law did not hold children below 7 years of age responsible for their activities. This view still prevails in that age 7 is the lower age limit for the definition of juvenile delinquency. The societal response and reaction to young offenders above the age of 7 has undergone numerous changes over the centuries. Most societies throughout history have refrained from the imposition of maximum penalties on young people on the grounds that since their insight and understanding are limited, they cannot be held fully responsible for their behavior.

In Western cultures, the 19th century brought a fundamental change in the legal philosophy: punishment was found to be ineffectual both as a deterrent and as a retribution for crime, and the concepts of crime prevention and the rehabilitation of criminals gained acceptance. Attention was thus focused on children who had exhibited disregard for authority and/or broken the law. The majority of young offenders were found to have been raised under adverse environmental conditions with little or no supervision and care from their families. Dealing with them called for a new legal principle and separate legal proceedings. The first juvenile court in the United States was established in 1899 in Chicago, and its philosophy was formulated by the Chicago Bar Association as follows: "The fundamental idea of the Juvenile Court Law is that the state must step in and exercise guardianship over a child found under such adverse social or individual conditions as to develop crime." In 1938 Congress passed the first federal law pertaining to juvenile delinquency. The purpose and aspiration of the juvenile court were restated by Justice John Warren Hill as "reclaiming for society those children who are neglected or delinquent." In order to carry out the mandate of the juvenile court law and to provide for the individual needs of children, the office of probation, state training schools, and mental health clinics were created.

Over the years, the original optimism of society regarding crime prevention has been replaced by a more somber outlook, and the legal profession has become skeptical about society's willingness to provide the necessary manpower, financial support, and facilities to deal with juvenile delinquency. Civil libertarians have questioned the appropriateness of depriving citizens of their liberty when the state training

schools do not provide the treatment and habilitative programs prom-
ised to the children who were remanded to them. Others have questioned incarcerating those children who have not committed criminal
acts, which is the case of most children labeled *PINS* (persons in need
of supervision). Citizens concerned with the safety and protection of
the community criticize the juvenile court judges for their alleged leniency in regard to youngsters who commit violent crimes. According
to their view, the gravity of the criminal offense and the juvenile's
prior history of delinquent activities are factors that must be taken
into consideration as well as the needs and interests of the offender.
These new developments may change the laws pertaining to delinquents. At the present time, the legal proceedings in juvenile court are
informal, the names of the offenders are not a matter of public record,
and the adjudication of delinquency is not equal to a finding of guilt
in criminal courts. In some states, in cases of serious crime, the juvenile can, under some legal provisions, be referred to criminal court to
stand trial.

Following the *Kent* and *Gault* decisions of the Supreme Court of
the United States, minors who are charged with delinquent behavior
are entitled to the constitutional guarantee of due process during both
the first phase of fact finding and the second stage of disposition. During the fact-finding stage, information regarding the alleged offense is
presented to the court. Law guardians, who are the legal representatives of the child, may provide additional information to the court,
advise their client of his right to withhold self-incriminating evidence,
and challenge the adequacy of the evidence of the alleged offense.
Once the finding of delinquency is made and the child is adjudicated a
delinquent, another legal conference is held to decide on a proper disposition. During this stage, the probation officer and/or the law guardian presents the court with the child's background history, social adjustment in the school and the community, and prior history of antisocial activities. A report on the child's environmental conditions and
the other social agencies involved with the child and his family is also
made. In preparation for this dispositional hearing, a psychiatric consultant may be called upon to provide the court with an opinion of the
child's psychological state, his intellectual functioning, his diagnosis,
and the needed treatment.

The psychiatric assessment may require one or a series of interviews with the child and his family or observation in an inpatient setting. Various laboratory and psychological tests may be needed in
order to exclude or verify a possible diagnosis. Although all such children have engaged in antisocial activities, their personality makeups
and motivations and the nature of their deficiencies are not the same.

In some children, delinquent behavior is the direct result of intrafamilial tension, while others have never been sufficiently socialized. In some, psychosis, mental retardation, or brain injury has limited the appreciation of reality by the youngster or his capacity for impulse control. Blind rage against significant family figures may be generalized by some youngsters to include the whole society, while others may be calculatedly trying to receive what they have been deprived of or are not entitled to. Families or gangs may encourage their members to engage in social misconduct by rewarding them for their daring and assuring them that they will be protected from the consequences. Some children commit delinquent acts only in the company of other offenders, while others may be the leaders of such groups. Violent crimes may have been committed in a state of disorganizing panic or may be the outcome of vicious premeditation.

In devising a strategy for treatment and intervention, the child psychiatrist must be sensitive to the implications of the youngster's behavior for the community. When social resources are not available and assessment of the family reveals their unwillingness or inability to provide support and supervision for the child, plans for outpatient treatment are doomed to failure. On the other hand, when there is equal likelihood for successful intervention in and out of an institution, the child is entitled to receive treatment in the least restrictive environment. Educational backwardness, physical defects, and intellectual subnormality, although they are not causes of delinquency, may play a large part in creating the feeling of incompetency and low self-esteem that may be a component of the delinquent's psychology. The alleviation and correction of modifiable deficiencies and compensation for the nontreatable ones must be an important part of any plan for intervention.

Acute psychoses are best treated within a hospital or a residential treatment center, while the socialization of nonpsychotic delinquents may be best achieved within other types of structure milieu. For some young offenders, a period of supervisory interest by the probation officer is enough to allow other measures to take effect. Others are willing to avail themselves of psychological and educational help only following a court order. Some families are awakened to the gravity of their children's behavior only when legal intervention has become necessary, and they can be counted on to cooperate fully with the spirit and the letter of the court recommendations. Other families may sabotage the chances of the youngster's rehabilitation or remain uninvolved. For these juveniles, foster home placement is the first therapeutic step if they are to remain in the community. Group therapy, behavior modification techniques, and individual psychotherapy may be carried out on an out- or inpatient basis, depending upon the child's needs and the legitimate concerns of the offender's community.

While psychiatrists may overestimate the potential for dangerous behavior in adult patients, they may be more accurate in evaluating the gravity of an adolescent's impulsiveness and the paucity of his psychological resources for coping with them. However, such assessments and opinions must be presented to the court in carefully reasoned language, and the observational and historical bases must be expressed and exposed in such a fashion that the law guardians can provide contrary evidence and the necessary rebuttal and challenges, so as to assure that the final decision by the court is in the best interest of the juvenile offender and protects the communal rights of safety and security from harm. Although it is the judicial decision that formulates the nature of the compromise between society's claims and the developmental needs and civil rights of the individual delinquent, the duty of the psychiatric consultant as an advocate of all children is to define the most desirable treatment plan, regardless of the inadequacies of society's provisions and facilities, and to recommend the most appropriate alternatives within the existing situation.

An awareness of social psychology and the reactions of victims and the victimized community is an indispensable attribute that will eventually determine the success or failure of any rehabilitative effort. Even when it is clear that a juvenile rapist is in a misguided search for love and affection or is longing for acceptance by the opposite sex, it is unrealistic to expect a sympathetic welcome or unrestrained approach from his community upon his return. When the young offender returns to an environment that is overtly hostile, active rejection is added to prior causal factors as motivational forces impelling his aggressive behavior. While families and communities no longer seek revenge by physically endangering the lives of those who have wronged them, subtle hostile reactions, such as rejection, distancing, and refusal to hire an individual or to rent an apartment to his family, await those who are considered undesirable. The youthful delinquent thus faces more alienation and hostility subsequent to the antisocial activities that brought him to juvenile court. When treatment in the community is the chosen course, insight into the community's reactions must be imparted to the delinquent child in the early stages of treatment if counteraggression by him is to be prevented.

"Person in Need of Supervision"

A "person in need of supervision" is legally defined in New York State as a boy or a girl under 16 years of age who is out of the control of the parents or other lawful authorities. The child's behavior may not be considered a criminal offense if committed by an adult but is in direct conflict with the social expectations and standards for children. Habitual truancy, if against parental wishes, would qualify the child as a person in need of supervision, while parents who actively encourage truancy or do not discourage it would be charged with neglect. Children who are in conflict with their parents, run away from home, keep late hours, engage in sexual activities, use alcohol or other intoxicants, or sniff glue and other inhalants have been variously referred to as incorrigible or unruly or in need of supervision. Parents, guardians, or social agencies may petition the juvenile court to make a finding on the basis of the child's behavior. If the child is found to have exhibited behaviors that require treatment or supervision, the court makes a disposition in view of the child's needs. The court has the discretionary power to place the child with public or private agencies, in or out of his own home; to remand him to a state training school; or to keep him under the supervision of the probation office. Because such proceedings may result in the loss of personal liberty, law guardians are appointed for children to protect their constitutional rights in every step of the process and to assure that their needs are met, with the least possible interference with their civil rights.

Psychiatric consultation is expected to assist the court in weighing the multitude of organismic and environmental factors that have contributed to the child's conflictual relationships with his own family and to his rebellious attitudes toward, or disregard of, social standards. The mere fact of habitual truancy, in and of itself, does not reveal the motivational factors involved. Children may be truant because they are unable to follow what goes on in the classroom, or they may find the pace of instruction too slow for their quick grasp of educational materials and therefore view compulsory attendance as foolish. Some anxious or depressed children have learned of the mood-changing properties of alcohol or other drugs and use them for the temporary relief of their unpleasant feelings. For some young people, running away from home is the unmistakable expression of their desire to escape abusive or neglectful parents, while others run away out of fear of anticipated consequences of some behavior disapproved by parents. A child may run away from home in search of an unknown place where he hopes to feel less restless or in order to escape from his fancied enemies and persecutors. Sexual activities may be the expression of neurotic needs or psychotic disorganization of a young individual, or they may be the means by which emotional and/or financial supports are gained. Mentally retarded youngsters may be unable to appreciate the prohibition against sexual activities when their physical maturity confronts them with the impulse for sexual discharge.

An evaluation of the child and his family should provide a clear idea of who the child is and why he has failed to adjust and of the circumstances that have brought about the expression of maladjustment at this particular juncture in the child's life. Parental divorce cannot be reversed because the child's behavioral difficulties are traced to his unhappiness over the breakdown of his family, nor can stepmothers and stepfathers be replaced because the child is actively or passively in conflict with them. However, in each situation, the child needs help, and the attitudes and activities of various adults may be amenable to some modification. For some children, treatment must be carried out in a setting away from home. Some youngsters find the court a forum for expressing their views and becoming aware of the opinions of others about them. The legal process itself may be instructive and therapeutic for all the involved parties. When a recommendation is made to place the child in a restrictive environment, the psychiatrist must be familiar with the nature and actual functioning of such facilities. A child whose running away from home is motivated by his inability to tolerate the average amount of anxiety and anger engendered by interpersonal conflicts does not stop his behavior when placed in an unfamiliar situation. A youngster who uses alcohol or other drugs to be relieved from depression or extreme anxiety may decompensate if he is placed in a strict environment among individuals who are capable of threatening his physical and emotional safety. Furthermore, some institutions, while set up to provide treatment, do not actually have the manpower and financial resources to do so, and a recommendation to place a child in need of treatment in such an institution is contrary to the ethical principles of medical practice.

Child Neglect and Child Abuse

For centuries, the only official attention paid to the plight of children who were abandoned by their parents or who lost their family through wars, natural disasters, or death came from religious organizations. During the 19th century, children came to be viewed as potentially important for the welfare of the state, and social legislation was enacted to assign to the state the responsibility for the ultimate protection of the child's welfare. Neglected children thus became the wards of the state, and the conception of neglect was broadened as new ideas regarding the needs and interests of children were incorporated into the legal definition. Today neglect of the physical care, medical necessities, educational needs, and emotional well-being of children is one of the issues in which the family court, as the representative of the state, can intervene on the child's behalf and permanently or temporarily suspend the parental rights of guardianship.

Maltreatment of children had been justified for centuries as a necessary measure to maintain discipline, expel evil spirits, or transmit educational ideas. In this country, the Society for the Prevention of Cruelty to Animals was founded long before the Society for the Prevention of Cruelty to Children, which began functioning in 1871. Through the diagnostic use of X ray, radiologists began to report in children fractured bones caused by trauma, and in 1961 the American Academy of Pediatrics, in a symposium on child abuse, alerted its members to the prevalence of the battered-child syndrome. Although the provisions of criminal law can be invoked to punish those who have harmed children, the substantiation of evidence against parents is extremely difficult. Furthermore, such provisions do little to protect the child victim or to assure his future well-being. It has therefore become necessary to provide special legislation to deal with the problem. Because child abuse is a nationwide problem found among all social classes, most states have passed laws requiring teachers, nurses social workers, and doctors to report cases of suspected child abuse. The reporters are immune from liability and are not required to provide proof of their suspicion. In some states, failure to report a suspected case of child abuse is punishable by law. The New York Family Court Act of 1973 defined an "abused child" as a child under 16 years of age whose parents or other legal guardians have inflicted physical injury or sexual abuse on him, have allowed such injuries and abuses to be inflicted upon him by others, or have directly or indirectly created a substantial risk to his physical safety. *Maltreatment* has replaced the term *neglect*, and a "maltreated child" is defined by law as a child under 18 years of age whose parents have failed to provide him with adequate food, clothing, education, shelter, or medical care, even though they are financially able or have been offered help to do so. Failure to provide supervision and guardianship, excessive corporal punishment, the habitual use of alchhol and addictive drugs that create substantial risk for the child or lower the parental capacity for care, and the abandonment of children are covered under this definition.

The report of child abuse or child neglect is given first over the phone to the special division of public child welfare services. A written report is requested when the reporter is a person who is by law required to inform the authorities of suspected child abuse. The role of the protective service division is to make a prompt investigation of the report and to assess its veracity. If it is determined that a child is probably neglected or maltreated, the investigators must decide whether the child is in such "imminent danger" as to necessitate his removal from home at that time or whether the family can be helped to care for the child according to his needs. Some parents can be persuaded to accept the offered help for themselves and their children; others surrender the child for adoption or temporarily relinquish their right to custody and allow the child to be placed. Parents are represented by counsel in neglect and abuse proceedings. Evidence pertaining to the specific allegation of abuse or neglect (such as the child's physical and emotional status), and factors that may impair the parents' capacity to function (such as alcohol and drug abuse) are presented to the court. If the parents are found guilty of the charges, the court then attempts a disposition according to the specific needs of the child and the capacity of the parents. Thus parents may be ordered to undergo treatment, the child may be temporarily placed, or parental rights may be permanently terminated.

Most neglected children come from families with multiple and complex problems. Their fathers tend to be unemployed, alcoholic, and physically or psychiatrically ill, and tend to have a history of institutionalization or imprisonment. Some have deserted their families or are irregularly in and out of the family picture. The mothers are young, inexperienced, and overwhelmed by the responsibilities of a large number of children. Some families belong to ethnic groups that are unable or unwilling to enter the majority culture and suffer from overt and covert discrimination. They may have sought companionship among other socially incompetent groups and may be involved with alcohol or drugs or suffer from various chronic illnesses. Pregnancies are unwelcome, although tolerated, and concern for children is not translated into appropriate care for them. Some mothers find it easier to care for smaller children, who do not baffle them with their behavior. Others are less troubled by older children, who can be entrusted with some responsibilities. Some mothers favor their female children, while others find taking care of their sons a better investment for their future.

A neglectful parent is usually a person whose incompetence in the parenting function is only one among many indications of inadequacy. When it is possible to treat and help such a parent, the particular child or children may be more appropriately cared for in their own home. Compensatory socializing experiences, remedial education, and medical or psychiatric treatment can be arranged to assure that the child's needs are met. On the other hand, when parental inability seems to interfere so seriously with the child's functioning that he is in danger of continuous exposure to distorted and harmful influences, the well-being of the child dictates his removal from the home. At times a recommendation for the child's removal does little more than end his residence in a highly pathological environment, since temporary shelters are not the warm, accepting, and well-ordered institutions that such children need. In addition, even the most carefully selected foster homes may prove to be unsuited for the particular child. Nevertheless, in every stage, the psychiatric consultant is expected to base his judgment and recommendation on carefully drawn conclusions from his observations of the child, his knowledge of the known facts in the field, and his familiarity with the available options in the community.

The literature regarding abusive parents is limited, to date, to those parents who have been identified as abusive by the courts, by social agencies, or by medical and psychiatric groups. Although most authors contend that child abuse cuts across educational and social class barriers, the cases discussed are usually from lower socioeconomic groups and families that use public educational and health care facilities. In this group, the abusive parent is more often the child's mother. The father is unemployed or under financial strain. The child is the product of an unwanted pregnancy and presents the family with an emotional burden. At times, the mother's tolerance of the frustrating circumstances surrounding child care chores is at a low ebb because of personal problems unrelated to the child. On other occasions, the parents' unrealistic or irrational demands regarding the child's responsiveness and behavior are the factors that precipitate the maltreatment of the child. In any event, there is little disagreement regarding the undesirability of child abuse and its detrimental effect on the child's personality development, even when the consequences for the child's survival and physical health are not disastrous.

Psychiatric consultation in cases of child abuse must be addressed to an evaluation of the child, an assessment of the child–parent relationship, and a delineation of the factors in the personalities of the parents and the child that create the conflictual relationship and lead to violent attacks by the parent on the child. If the parents can be helped to change their response pattern to the child and if his deviant behavior—if any—can be remedied, there is the possibility of saving the family as a unit. Some parents need to be relieved temporarily from the constant presence of the child before they can be helped to develop a more constructive response pattern; at other times, the child's life is in such danger that removal from home is mandatory. When children are frankly unwelcome and unwanted, no purpose is served by attempting to force them on their parents; but when parents are disturbed by their own violent reactions to their children, they can be motivated to reestablish control over their own temper. Some guilt-ridden parents, while sufficiently receptive to recommendations and guidance, are in reality unable to overcome their ambivalent attitudes toward the child or to maintain control over their hostile reactions and therefore continue to be abusive.

Battered children may be frightened, nontrusting, or provocative and cannot be expected to change their behavior as soon as they are placed in a new environment. Foster parents or other caretakers must be sensitive to the effects of the abusive background of these children and must base their responses on this insight rather than on the immediate reaction of the child.

The decision to return an abused or neglected child to the parents requires a total reevaluation of the child and his parents. When the original factors contributing to neglect and abuse are clearly delineated, a reassessment of the total picture is easier than when no attempts were made to provide a basis for future comparison. For example, if it is felt that a particular parent finds the vigorous crying of an infant especially irritating and it has become unbearable to her as a result of her own depression, one may assume that when the mother's depression has been treated and the child is capable of expressing his desires through verbalization, the child's return to the mother may be indicated. Because psychiatric consultations have far-reaching consequences for the child and the family, the logical links between psychiatric findings and recommendations must be unambiguously stated, even though many of our assumptions and predictions are based on clinical and empirical impressions.

Child Custody

In every society, there are some traditional or legal provisions for the continuous care and guardianship of children following the dissolution of families due to the divorce, death, or disappearance of the parents. In some societies, a child's blood tie to the father is of prime importance, and the father or his relative becomes the automatic guardian. In other communities, the continuity of the mother–child relationship, at least during early childhood, is considered crucial, and the mother is the preferred guardian. The sex of the child may play a role in such matters, in that some children are given to the same-sex parent. In almost all instances, the unofficial arrangement between two parents regarding custody goes unchallenged because of the notion of the rights of natural parents over their children.

The dispute over custody arises when both parents present the court with competing claims about their own suitability and the unfitness of the other party to be the guardian of the child. Acrimonious allegations and counterallegations may develop during the divorce process or at any point following the official dissolution of the marriage. While some parents may be genuinely concerned about the well-being of the child, others exploit the subject of custody and visitation rights to carry their marital conflicts into the postdivorce stage. The divided loyalty of the child may provide the necessary weapons for such struggles, since in their attempts to maintain the love and affection of each parent, children tend to be sensitive to the desires of each parent and to give the reports that they perceive to be required of them. The outcome of such a process is psychologically devastating to the child, in that his basic trust in both parents is undermined and his perception of interpersonal interactions is distorted. Alternately guilty and angry, he cannot feel close to either of the two parents and feels insecure because he has betrayed them both. His anxieties, anger, and confusion may be expressed in his relationship with the environment or in his disturbed subjective experiences. He may come to view himself as "bad" and disloyal and withdraw from the company of his friends, or he may develop an exaggerated sense of his own power and thus alienate others. Regardless of the etiology of the parents' disagreement and their possible individual psychopathology, it is obvious that such situations are detrimental to children's development.

Lawyers and judges involved in questions of custodial disputes have long been aware of the plights of children in custody cases, and the consensus of opinions in this country was formally articulated by the family law section of the American Bar Association in 1963 as the doctrine of "The best interest of the child." According to this principle, legal decisions regarding the custody and visitation rights must be based on what is beneficial to the child's development rather than on the time-honored tradition of parental privilege. One of the consequences of this new approach to awarding custody is the implicit inclusion of mental health professionals in the decision-making process. In Michigan, the first state to enact the "best interest of the child" principle into law, evaluation and consideration of 10 factors by the court is necessary as the basis of a legal decision. The 10 factors as follows:

- The nature of the interpersonal relationship and emotional ties between the child and each parent.
- The capacity and willingness of competing parents to provide the child with food, shelter, clothing, and any necessary medical care.
- The desirability of maintaining the child in a satisfactory and

stable environment and the length of time that the child has spent in such circumstances.

- The likelihood that the child's present home or the proposed custody home will function as a family unit.
- The nature of the child's adjustment in his present school and community.
- The moral fitness of each parent.
- The physical and mental health of each parent.
- The child's preference, provided that the court is satisfied that the child is capable of making a reasoned decision.
- All other factors that may be deemed relevant to the custody dispute.

Although the above list is not exhaustive, it is sufficiently broad to include most factors that can influence the child's development. The child psychiatrist's function in cases of custody is to evaluate the child's developmental level, the quality of his relationship with both his parents and his peers, his academic and social standing in his group, his reasons for any stated preference, and his perception of his surroundings. Some children may perceive the nonguardian parent as more permissive because during their short visits no altercation occurs. The preferences of others are based on neurotic reasons. For example, a highly anxious child who worries about the safety of the absent parent may feel that his anxiety will be relieved when he goes to live with her or him. Children who have school problems may come to believe that going to live with the other parent will give them a respite from scholastic demands. For other children, the idea of a change is appealing, or they believe that they can maintain the most desirable aspects of their present situation while ridding themselves of those they do not want. At times, the nonguardian parent believes that an undesirable aspect of the child's behavior is a direct consequence of his life with the other parent and is therefore accepting only the non-problem part of the child.

It is the duty of the psychiatric consultant to bring the child's problems and the need for specialized care to the attention of the court. Some competing parents coach the child to reflect their views and try to influence the psychiatric and judicial opinions in their favor. However, such parroting of parental ideas does not survive close scrutiny, and when the child is asked to expound on his rationale, it becomes clear that his statements are learned responses. Under ideal circumstances, the psychiatric consultation is requested by both parents, their lawyers, or the court, and the child psychiatrist is given the opportunity to interview both parents and the child in order to arrive at an unbiased decision. However, most custody disputes are an emotional battleground between warring parties. Each parent decides to seek advice and an opinion from a different child psychiatrist, and at times, the contradictory opinions of the experts becloud the issues. Therefore behavioral manifestations and descriptions of the child's feelings and thinking must be carefully recorded, and reports about the child's behavior must be collected from as many sources as possible before the child psychiatrist can reach a diagnostic conclusion and venture a particular recommendation. Even if various consultants draw different conclusions from their evaluation of the child, a clear presentation and a reasoned interpretation of the facts make it possible for the court to weigh the evidence and award the custody according to what it perceives as the best interest of the child.

When evaluating the parents' relationship with and perception of the child, the child psychiatrist's opinion must be limited to those views and behaviors of the parents that affect their parenting functions. Diagnostic labels are not, in and of themselves, very revealing. For example, the label of *schizophrenia* does not necessarily imply that a parent cannot care for the child unless it can be shown that this particular disability would hamper the child's adjustment and well-being. The moral fitness of the parents is a social, not a psychological judgment, and therefore only those parental behaviors with direct psychological implications for the child may be discussed by the child psychiatrist consulting with the court.

Visitation rights are customarily granted to the nonguardian parent, and only when they can be clearly shown to be harmful to the child are they restricted or eliminated. Whether the frequency and the duration of the visits are privately arranged or defined by the court, the most important factors from the child's point of view is that they are predictable and regular and that the child's time is not spent in discussions of the faults and follies of the guardian parent. Some children may decide to discontinue their visits. This decision may result in a series of accusations, counteraccusations, and retaliation by the rejected parent, such as the nonpayment of child support. When the court is convinced that the child's decision is based on his own reasoned preference, both parents are directed to respect the child's right to be left alone.

The principle of "the best interest of the child" has been directly or indirectly used to settle the competing claims of foster and adoptive parents versus biological parents. However, in these cases, the prior rights of the natural parents must also be considered, and the compromised solutions do not always work to the child's advantage.

The conflict of interests between the child and parents, guardians, and institutions standing *in loco parentis* is a subject of concern to advocates of the civil rights of children. Parents exercise guardianship over children usually up to 18 years of age and, in cases of mental incompetency, for life. They can therefore commit their children to institutions, volunteer them for research purposes, and in the case of mental retardation, petition the court for sterilization. In those cases where a judicial decision is necessary, the courts have recently maintained that when there is not convincing evidence that the interests of the child are served by a particular course of action, the parents cannot waive their children's constitutional rights. For example, parents may not give prmission for the sterilization of a child, even if mentally retarded, without provision for due process. However, since children cannot initiate legal action on their own behalf, a child cannot contest his parents' decision to institutionalize him, nor, once in the institutions, can he refuse to accept a particular form of treatment, because the institution acts in place of his parents. These considerations have led some civil libertarians to suggest a system of child advocacy in which the child advocate could intervene on behalf of children in a variety of circumstances, including any complaint regarding parental behavior, school policy or institutional practices. Such advocates would theoretically be able to initiate legal action on behalf of the child to secure his personal constitutional rights and thus define the extent to which parents can make decisions for their children. Such actions would presumably clarify the issue of whether parents can withhold their consent for a lifesaving operation when the newborn baby is mentally retarded, or whether adolescents can request contraceptives without parental consent. The logical place for such an advocate's operation would be in schools, hospitals, and other institutions that deal with children. The existence of the advocate would be made known to the children, who would be allowed to consult with him and request his services.

References and Bibliography

Chapter 1

Anthony, E. J. (Ed.) (1974). *Explorations in Child Psychiatry.* New York: Plenum Press.

Campion, E., and Tucker, G. (1975). A note on twin studies; schizophrenia and neurological impairment. *Arch. Gen. Psychiatry* 29:460–464.

De Sanctis, S. (1906). On some varieties of dementia praecox, in S. A. Szurek and I. N. Berlin (Eds.), *Clinical Studies in Childhood Psychosis.* New York: Brunner/Mazel, 1973.

Eysenck, H. J. (1952). The effects of psychotherapy: An evaluation. *J. Consult. Psychol.* 16:319–323.

Group for the Advancement of Psychiatry (1957). *Clinical Psychiatry: Problems of Treatment, Research and Prevention.* New York: Science House.

Healy, W., and Bronner, A. F. (1948). The child guidance clinic: Birth and growth of an idea, in L. G. Lowrey (Ed.), *Orthopsychiatry 1923–1948: Retrospect and Prospect.* New York: American Orthopsychiatric Association, pp. 14–49.

Kanner, L. (1949). *A Miniature Textbook of Feeblemindedness.* New York: Child Care Monographs, No. 1.

Kanner, L. (1957). *Child Psychiatry.* Springfield, Ill.: Charles C Thomas.

Langmeier, J., and Matejcek, Z. (1975). *Psychological Deprivation in Childhood.* New York: Halstead Press.

Maudsley, H. (1867). *The Physiology and Pathology of the Mind.* London: Macmillan.

Rie, H. E. (1971). Historical perspective of concepts of child psychopathology, in H. E. Rie (Ed.), *Perspectives in Child Psychopathology.* New York: Aldine-Atherton.

Sechzer, J. A., Faro, M. D., and Windle, W. F. (1973). Studies of monkeys asphyxiated at birth: Implications for minimal cerebral dysfunction. *Semin. Psychiatry* 5:19–34.

Wade, H. (1976). IQ and heredity: Suspicion of fraud beclouds classic experiment. *Science* 194:916–919.

Wolff, P. H. (1970). "Critical periods" in human cognitive development. *Hospital Practice*, November.

Chapter 2

Arasteh, J. D. (1968). Creativity and related processes in the young child: A review of literature. *J. Gen. Psychol.* 112:77–108.

Bank, S., and Kahn, M. (1976). Sisterhood–brotherhood is powerful: Sibling sub-systems and family therapy, in S. Chess and A. Thomas (Eds.), *Annual Progress in Child Psychiatry and Child Development*. New York: Brunner/Mazel.

Bell, R. Q. (1968). A reinterpretation of the direction of effects in studies of socialization. *Psychol. Rev.* 75:81–95.

Berlyne, D. (1960). *Conflict, Arousal and Curiosity*. New York: McGraw-Hill.

Birns, B., Blank M., Bridger, W. H., and Escalona, S. K. (1965). Behavioral inhibition in neonates produced by auditory stimuli. *Child Dev.* 36:639–645.

Bowlby, J. (1969). *Attachment and Loss*, vol. 1. New York: Basic Books.

Brazelton, T., Koslowski, B., and Main, M. (1974). The origins of reciprocity: The early mother–infant interaction, in M. Lewis and L. A. Rosenblum (Eds.), *The Effect of the Infant on Its Caregiver*. New York: Wiley.

Brown, R., and Bellugi, U. (1964). Three processes in the child's acquisition of syntax. *Harv. Educ. Rev.* 34:133–151.

Bruner, J. (1973). Organization of early skilled action. *Child Dev.* 44:1–11.

Bruner, J., Oliver, R., and Greenfield, M. (1966). *Studies in Cognitive Growth*. New York: Wiley.

Cairns, G. F., and Butterfield, E. C. (1975). Assessing infants' auditory functioning, in B. F. Friedlander, *et al.* (Eds.), *Exceptional Infant: Assessment and Intervention*, vol. 3. New York: Brunner/Mazel.

Chomsky, N. (1957). *Syntactic Structure*. The Hague: Mouton.

Clements, S. (1966). *Minimal Brain Dysfunction in Children*. National Institute of Neurological Diseases and Blindness, Monograph No. 3. Washington: U.S. Department of Health, Education and Welfare.

Deutsch, M. (1965). The role of social class in language development and cognition. *Am. J. Orthopsychiatry* 35:78–88.

Emde, R., and Harmon, R. (1972). Endogenous and exogenous smiling systems in early infancy. *J. Am. Acad. Child Psychiatry*, 11:11–200.

Fantz, R., and Fagan, J. (1975). Visual attention to size and number of pattern details by term and preterm infants during the first six months. *Child Dev.* 46:3–18.

Fantz, R., and Nevis, S. (1967). Pattern préferences and perceptual-cognitive development in early infancy. *Merrill-Palmer Q. Behav. Dev.* 13:77–107.

Friedlander, B. Z. (1971). Listening, language and the auditory environment: Automated evaluation and intervention, in J. Hellmuth (Ed.), *Exceptional Infant*, vol. 2. New York: Brunner/Mazel.

Gesell, A., and Amatruda, C. (1964). *Developmental Diagnosis*. New York: Harper & Row.

Hardy, W. G. (1960). *Language Acquisition* (Monograph). Stanford: Institute on Childhood Aphasia, Stanford University Press.

Ingram, D. (1976). Current issues in child phonology, in D. Morehead and A. Morehead (Eds.), *Normal and Deficient Child Language*. Baltimore: University Park Press.

Kohlberg, L., and Turiel, E. (1971). Moral development and moral education, in G. Lesser (Ed.), *Psychology and the Educational Process*. Chicago: Scott Foresman.

Kramer, Y., and Rosenblum, L. (1970). Responses to frustration in one-year-old infants. *Psychosom. Med.* 32:243–257.

Lenneberg, E. H. (1967). *The Biological Foundations of Language*. New York: Wiley.

MacNamara, J. (1972). Cognitive basis of language learning in infants. *Psychol. Rev.* 79:1–13.

Morely, M. (1965). *The Development and Disorders of Speech in Childhood*. Baltimore: Williams & Wilkins.

Piaget, J. (1926). *The Language and Thought of the Child*. New York: Harcourt Brace.

Piaget, J. (1932). *The Moral Judgment of the Child*. London: Kegan Paul.

Piaget, J. (1937). *The Construction of Reality in the Child.* New York: Basic Books, 1954.

Pikler, E. (1971). Learning of motor skills on the basis of self-induced movements, in J. Hellmuth (Ed.), *Exceptional Infant,* vol. 1. New York: Brunner/Mazel.

Rheingold, H. L. (1966). The development of social behavior in the human infant, in H. Stevenson (Ed.), *Concept of Development.* Monograph of the Society for Research in Child Development, No. 31.

Ricciuti, H. (1968). Social and emotional behavior in infancy. *Merrill-Palmer Q. Behav. Dev.* 14:82–100.

Sameroff, A. (1975). Early influences on development: Fact or fancy. *Merrill-Palmer Q. Behav. Dev.* 21:267–294.

Sameroff, A., and Chandler, M. (1975). Reproductive risk and the continuum of caretaking casuality, in F. D. Horowitz, *et al.* (Eds.), *Review of Child Development Research,* vol. 4. Chicago: University of Chicago Press.

Schilder, P. (1938). *Image and Appearance of Human Body.* London: Paul, French and Trubner.

Shirley, M. M. (1931). *Postural and Locomotor Development.* Minneapolis: Minnesota University Press.

Simmel, M. L. (1966). Developmental aspects of the body scheme. *Child Dev.* 37:83–95.

Sroufe, L., Waters, E., and Matas, L. (1974). Contentual determinants of infants' affective response, in M. Lewis and L. Rosenblum (Eds.), *The Origins of Fear.* New York: Wiley.

Sroufe, L., and Wunsch, J. (1972). The Development of Laughter in the First Year of Life. *Child Dev.* 43:1326–1344.

Todd, G., and Palmer, B. (1968). Social reinforcement of infant babbling. *Child Dev.* 39:591–596.

Vygotsky, L. S. (1962). *Thought and Language.* Cambridge, Mass.: MIT Press.

Wolff, P. H. (1966). The causes, controls and organization of behavior in neonates. *Psychol. Issues* Vol. 5, No. 1.

Chapter 3

Arlow, J. A., and Brenner, C. (1964). *Psychoanalytic Concepts and the Structural Theory.* New York: International Universities Press.

Baldwin, A. (1968). Social-learning theory of child development, in A. L. Baldwin (Ed.), *Theories of Child Development.* New York: Wiley.

Bandura, A., and Walters, R. H. (1963). *Social Learning and Personality Development.* New York: Holt, Rinehart and Winston.

Bowlby, J. (1946). *Forty-four Juvenile Thieves: Their Characters and Home Life.* London: Bailere, Tindal and Cox.

Dollard, J., and Miller, N. E. (1950). *Personality and Psychotherapy, An Analysis in Terms of Learning, Thinking and Culture.* New York: McGraw-Hill.

Erikson, E. H. (1963). *Childhood and Society* (2nd ed.) New York: Norton.

Eysenck, H. J. (1960). *The Structure of Human Personality.* London: Methuen.

Flavell, J. H. (1963). *The Developmental Psychology of Jean Piaget.* New York: Van Nostrand.

Freud, A. (1946). *The Ego and the Mechanisms of Defense.* New York: International Universities Press.

Freud, A. (1946). *The Psycho-Analytic Treatment of Children.* London: Mago.

Freud, A. (1965). *Normality and Pathology in Childhood.* New York: International Universities Press.

Freud, S. (1900). *The Interpretation of Dreams,* Standard Edition, vols. 4 and 5. London: The Hogarth Press, 1953.

Freud, S. (1923). *The Ego and the Id,* Standard Edition. London: The Hogarth Press, 1961.

Freud, S. (1940). An Outline of Psychoanalysis, in *The Complete Psychoanalytical Works of Sigmund Freud* Standard Edition, vol. 23. London: The Hogarth Press, 1964.

Hartmann, H. (1939). *Ego Psychology and the Problem of Adaptation.* New York: International Universities Press.

Hartmann, H. (1950). Psychoanalysis and developmental psychology. *Psychoanal. Study Child* 5:7–17.

Heider, F. (1958). *The Psychology of Interpersonal Relations.* New York: Wiley.

Inhelder, B., and Piaget, J. (1958). *The Growth of Logical Thinking from Childhood to Adolescence.* New York: Basic Books.

Kris, E. (1950). Notes on the development and on some current problems of psychoanalytic child psychology. *Psychoanal. Study Child* 5:24–46.

Mahler, M. S. (1967). On human symbiosis and the vicissitudes of the individuation. *J. Am. Psychoanal. Assoc.* 15:710–762.

Modgil, S. (1974). *Piagetian Research: A Handbook of Recent Studies.* New York: Humanities Press.

Pavlov, I. P. (1927). *Conditioned Reflexes.* London: Oxford University Press.

Piaget, J. (1954). *The Construction of Reality in the Child.* New York: Basic Books.

Piaget, J. (1963). *The Origins of Intelligence in Children.* New York: Norton.

Piaget, J. (1972). Intellectual evolution from adolescence to adulthood. *Human Dev.* 15:1–12.

Rapaport, D. (1960). The structure of psychoanalytic theory, in *Psychological Issues,* vol. 2, No. 2, Monograph 6. New York: International Universities Press.

Skinner, B. F. (1969). *Contingencies of Reinforcement: A Theoretical Analysis.* New York: Appleton-Century-Crofts.

Chapter 4

Abrams, S., and Neubauer, P. B. (1975). *Object Orientedness: The Person or the Thing.* Presented at the meeting of the Psychoanalytic Association of New York.

Ackerman, N. W. (1968). The role of the family in the emergence of child disorders, in E. Miller (Ed.), *Foundation of Child Psychiatry.* New York: Pergamon Press.

Alpert, A., Neubauer, P. W., and Weil, A. P. (1956). Unusual variation in drive endowment. *Psychoanal. Study Child* 11:125.

Bergman, P., and Escalona, S. (1949). Unusual sensitivities in very young child. *Psychoanal. Study Child* 3(4):33.

Berlin, I. N. (1969). Resistance to change in mental health professionals. *Am. J. Orthopsychiatry* 39:109–115.

Biller, H. (1970). Father absence and the personality development of the male child. *Dev. Psychol.* 2:181–201.

Birch, H. G. (1972). Malnutrition, learning and intelligence. *Am. J. Public Health* 62:773–784.

Bohman, M. (1972). A study of adopted children, their background, environment and adjustment. *Acta Paediatr. Scand.* 61:90–97.

Bowlby, J. (1951). *Maternal Care and Mental Health.* Geneva: World Health Organization.

Bowlby, J. (1969). *Attachment and Loss, vol. 1: Attachment*. London: The Hogarth Press.

Bridger, W. H., and Reiser, M. F. (1959). Psychophysiologic studies of the neonate. *Psychosom. Med.* 21:265.

Brown, G. W., and Birley, J. L. T. (1968). Crises and life changes and the onset of schizophrenia. *J. Health Soc. Behav.* 9:203–214.

Carey, W. B. (1972b). Night awakening and temperament in infancy. *J. Pediatr.* 84:756–758.

Carey, W. B. (1974). Clinical application of infant temperament measurements. *J. Pediatr.* 81:823–828.

Cattell, R. B. (1950). *Personality: A Systematic and Factual Study*. New York: McGraw-Hill.

Chess, S., and Hassibi, M. (1970). Behavior deviations in mentally retarded children. *J. Am. Acad. Child Psychiatry* 9:282–297.

Chess, S., and Korn, S. (1970). Temperament and behavior disorders in mentally retarded children. *Arch. Gen. Psychiatry* 23:122.

Chess, S., Korn, S., and Fernandez, P. (1971). *Psychiatric Disorders of Children with Congenital Rubella*. New York: Brunner/Mazel.

Chess, S., Thomas, A. *et al.* (1967). Behavioral problems revisited: Findings of an anthrospective study. *J. Acad. Child Psychiatry* 6:2.

Chess, S., Thomas, A., and Cameron, M. (1976). Temperament: Its significance for school adjustment and academic achievement. *New York University Educ. Rev.* 7.24–29.

Clark, K. B. (1970). *Fifteen Years of Deliberate Speed*. New York: Saturday Review.

Cohler, B. J., Grunehaum, H. *et al.* (1975). Perceived life-stress and psychopathology among mothers of young children. *Am. J. Orthopsychiatry* 45:58–73.

Cole, M., and Bruner, J. S. (1971). Cultural differences and inferences about psychological processes. *Am. Psychologist* 26:867–876.

Coles, R. (1968). Northern children under desegregation. *J. Study Interpersonal Processes* 31:1–15.

Cravioto, J. DeLicardie, E. R., and Birch, H. G. (1966). Nutrition, growth and neurointegrative development: An experimental and ecologic study. *J. Pediatr.* 38 (2, Part II, Supplement): 319–372.

Carvioto, J., and Robles, B. (1965). Evolution of adaptive and motor behavior during rehabilitation from kwashiorkor. *Am. J. Orthopsychiatry* 35:449–464.

Daly, R. (1970). Chromosome aberrations in 50 patients with idiopathic mental retardation and in 50 control subjects. *Pediatrics* 77:444–453.

Deutsch, M. (1969). Happenings on the way back to the forum: Social science I.Q. and race differences revisited. *Harv. Educ. Rev.* 39:523–557.

Dobbing, J. (1968). The effects of experimental undernutrition on development of the nervous system, in N. S. Scrimshaw and J. E. Gordon (Eds.), *Malnutrition, Learning and Behavior*. Cambridge, Mass.: MIT Press.

Dohrenwend, B. S. (1973). Life events as stressors: A methodological inquiry. *J. Health Soc. Behav.* 14:167–175.

Drillien, C. (1970). The small-for-date infant. *Etiology and Prognosis in Pediatric Clinics of North America*, 17:983–1001.

Elmer, E., and Gregg, G. S. (1967). Developmental characteristics of abused children. *Pediatrics* 40:596–602.

Escalona, S., and Gorman, H. (1953). Emotional development in the first year of life, in *Problems of Infancy and Childhood*. New York: Josiah Macy, Jr. Foundation, p. 11.

Evans, S. L., Reinhart, J. B., and Succop, R. A. (1972). Failure to thrive: A study of 45 children and their families. *J. Am. Acad. Child Psychiatry* 11:440–457.

Fish, B. (1957). The detection of schizophrenia in infancy: A preliminary report. *J. Nerv. Ment. Dis.* 125:1–24.

Framo, J. (1970). Symptoms from a family transactional viewpoint. *Family Therapy in Transaction: Int. Psychiat. Clinic* 7:119–131.

Freud, S. (1950). Analysis, terminable and interminable, in *Collected Papers*, vol. 5. London: The Hogarth Press, p. 316.

Fries, M., and Woolf, P. (1953). Some hypotheses on the role of the congenital activity type in personality development. *Psychoanal. Study Child* 8:48.

Frisch, R. E. (1971). Does malnutrition cause permanent mental retardation in human beings? *Psychiatr. Neurol. Neurochir.* 74:463–479.

Garbino, J. (1976). A preliminary study of some ecological correlates of child abuse: The impact of socioeconomic stress on mothers. *Child Dev.* 47:178–185.

Gelles, R. (1973). Child abuse as psychopathology: A sociological critic and reformulation. *Am. J. Orthopsychiatry* 43:611–621.

Gesell, A., and Ames, L. B. (1937). Early evidences of individuality in the human infant. *J. Gen. Psychol.* 47:339.

Glidewell, J. C. (1968). Behavior symptoms and degree of sickness, in S. B. Sells (Ed.), *The Definition and Measurement of Mental Health*. Washington: U.S. Department of Health, Education and Welfare, National Center for Health Statistics.

Goodman, J. D., Silberstein, R. M. and Mandell, W. (1963). Adopted children brought to child psychiatric clinic. *Arch. Gen. Psychol.* 9:451–456.

Gottfried, A. W. (1973). Intellectual consequences of perinatal anoxia. *Psychol. Bull.* 80:231–242.

Graham, F., Ernhart, C. B., *et al.* (1961). Development three years after perinatal anoxia and other potentially damaging newborn experience. *Psychol. Monogr.* Vol. 76, No. 522.

Graham, P., Rutter, N., *et al.* (1973). Temperamental characteristics as predictors of behavior disorders in children. *Am. J. Orthopsychiatry* 43:328–339.

Grey-Walter, W. (1953). Electroencephalographic development of children, in J. M. Tanner and B. Inhelder (Eds.), *Discussion on Child Development*, vol. 1. New York: International Universities Press, pp. 132–60.

Grossman, H. J., and Greenberg, N. Y. (1957). Psychosomatic differentiation in infancy. *Psychosom. Med.* 19:293.

Guilford, J. P. (1959). *Personality*. New York: McGraw-Hill.

Harvald, B., and Hauge, M. (1965). Hereditary factors elucidated by twin studies, in J. V. Neel, M. S. Shaw, and J. Schull (Eds.), *Genetics and the Epidemiology of Chronic Diseases*. Washington: U.S. Department of Health, Education, and Welfare.

Henderson, L. J. (1913). *The Fitness of the Environment*. New York: Macmillan.

Hertzig, M. E. (1974). Neurologic findings in prematurely born children at school age, in D. Ricks, A. Thomas, and M. Roff (Eds.), *Life History Research in Psychopathology*, vol. 3. Minneapolis: University of Minnesota Press.

Hertzig, M. E., Birch, H. G., Thomas, A., and Mendez, O. A. (1968). Class and ethnic differences in the responsiveness of preschool children to cognitive demands. Monograph of the Society for Research in Child Development 33:1–69.

Herzog, E., and Sudia, C. (1968). Fatherless homes: A review of research. *Children*, Sept.–Oct., pp. 177–182.

Holmes, G., Miller, J., and Smith, E. (1968). Neonatal bilirubinemia in production of long term neurological deficits. *Am. J. Dis. Children* 116:37–43.

Kagan, J. (1971). *Change and Continuity in Infancy*. New York: Wiley, p. 11.

Kallmann, F. (1953). *Heredity in Health and Mental Disorders*. New York: Norton.

Katz, I. (1969). A critique of personality approaches to negro performance with research suggestions. *J. Soc. Issues* 25:13–28.

Kempe, G. H., Silverman, F., *et al.* (1962). The battered child syndrome. *J. Am. Med. Assoc.* 181:17–24.

Klein, R. E., Gilberto, O., *et al.* (1969). Performance of malnourished in comparison with adequately nourished children (Guatemala). Paper given at Annual Meeting of the American Association for the Advancement of Science, Boston, Mass., Dec. 30, 1969.

Kogelschatz, J. L., Adams, P. L., *et al.* (1972). Family styles of fatherless households, *J. Am. Acad. Child Psychiatry* 11:365–383.

Lawton, J. J., and Gross, S. F. (1964). Review of psychiatric literature on adopted children. *Arch. Gen. Psychiatry* 11:635–644.

Marcus, J., Thomas, A., and Chess, S. (1969). Behavioral individuality in kibbutz children. *Isr. Ann. Psychiatry Relat. Discip.* 7(1):43–54.

McDermott, J. F. (1968). Parental divorce in early childhood. *Am. J. Psychiatry* 124:1424–1432.

McDermott, J. F., Harrison, S., *et al.* (1965). Social class and mental illness in children: Observations of blue collar workers. *Am. J. Orthopsychiatry* 35:500–508.

McDermott, J. F., Harrison, S., *et al.* (1967). Social class and mental illness in children: The diagnosis of organicity and mental retardation. *J. Am. Acad. Child Psychiatry* 6:309–320.

McKusick, V. A. (1966). *Mendelian Inheritance in Man: Catalogs of Autosomal Dominant and X-Linked Phenotypes.* Baltimore: Johns Hopkins Press.

Mead, M. (1962). A cultural anthropologist's approach to maternal deprivation, in *Deprivation of Maternal Care.* Geneva: World Health Organization.

Mednick, S., and Schulsinger, F. (1968). Premorbid characteristics related to breakdown in children with schizophrenic mothers, in D. Rosenthal and S. Ketty (Eds.), *The Transmission of Schizophrenia.* New York: Pergamon Press.

Meili, R. (1959). A longitudinal study of personality development, in L. Jessner and E. Pavenstedt (Eds.), *Dynamic Psychopathology in Childhood.* New York: Grune & Stratton, pp. 106–123. (This is a summary of a monograph report, *Anfange der Charakterentwicklung.* Bern: Hans Hunber, 1957).

Meyers, J. K., Lindenthal, J. J., *et al.* (1972). Life events and mental status: A longitudinal study. *J. Health Soc. Behav.* 13:398–406.

Minkowski, A., and Larroche, J. (1966). Development of nervous system in early life, in F. Falkner, (Ed.), *Human Development.* Philadelphia: Saunders.

Mirsky, I. A. (1953). Psychoanalysis and the biological sciences, in F. Alexander and H. Ross (Eds.), *Twenty Years of Psychoanalysis.* New York: Norton, pp. 155–176.

Murphy, L. B. and Moriarty, A. E. (1976). *Vulnerability, Coping and Growth.* New Haven: Yale University Press.

Mussen, P., Maldonado, Z., and Beytagh, L. (1969). Industrialization, child rearing practices and children's personality. *J. Exp. Psychol.* 580:115:

Pasamanick, B. (1968). Epidemiologic investigations of some prenatal factors in the production of neuropsychiatric disorders, in S. B. Sells (Ed.), *The Definition and Measurement of Mental Health.* Washington: U.S. Department of Health, Education and Welfare, National Center for Health Statistics.

Pasamanick, B., and Knobloch, H. (1966). Retrospective studies on the epidemiology of reproductive causality: Old and new. *Merrill-Palmer Q. Behav. Dev.* 12:7–29.

Pavlov, I. P. (1927). *Conditioned reflexes: An investigation of the physiological activity of the cerebral cortex* (Trans. and Ed., G. V. Anrep). London: Oxford University Press.

Resnick, P. J. (1969). Child murder by parents: A psychiatric review of filicide. *Am. J. Psychiatry* 126:325–334.

Richmond, J. B., and Lustman, S. L. (1955). Autonomic function in the neonate. *Psychosom. Med.* 17:269.

Rabkin, J. G., and Struening, E. L. (1976). Life events, stress and illness. *Science* 194:1013.

Rodman, H. (1968). Family and social pathology in the ghetto. *Science* 161:756–762.

Rollins, N., and Blackwell, A. (1973). Some roles children play in their families. *J. Am. Acad. Child Psychiatry* 12:511–530.

Rosenthal, D. (1970). *Genetic Theory and Abnormal Behavior*. New York: McGraw-Hill Series in Psychology.

Rosenthal, D., and Kety, S. S. (Eds.) (1968). *The Transmission of Schizophrenia*. New York: Pergamon Press.

Rosenthal, D., Wender, P., et al. (1975). Parent-child relationships and psychopathological disorders in the child. *Arch. Gen. Psychiatry* 32:466–476.

Rubin, R. A., Rosenblatt, C., et al. (1973). Psychological and educational sequelae of prematurity. *J. Pediatr.* 52:352–363.

Rutter, M. (1972). *Maternal Deprivation Reassessed*. London: Penguin Books.

Sameroff, A. J. (1975). Early influences on development: Fact or fancy. *Merrill-Palmer Q. Behav. Dev.* 21:267–294.

Schaffer, H. R. (1971). *The Growth of Sociability*. London: Penguin Books.

Schaffer, H. R., and Emerson, P. E. (1964). The development of social attachments in infancy. Monograph of the Society for Research in Child Development, Vol. 29, No. 94.

Schachter, F. F., and Apgar, V. (1959). Perinatal asphyxia and psychological signs of brain damage in childhood. *Pediatrics* 24:1016–1025.

Schechter, F., Carlson, P., et al. (1964). Emotional problems in adoptee. *Arch. Gen. Psychiatry* 10:109–118.

Scholom, A. H. (1975). The Relationship of Infant and Parent Temperament to the Prediction of Child Adjustment. Doctoral dissertation, Michigan State University.

Schultz, C., and Aurbach, H. (1971). The usefulness of cumulative deprivation as an explanation of educational deficiencies. *Merrill-Palmer Q. Behav. Dev.* 17:27–40.

Scrimshaw, N. S. (1969). Early malnutrition and central nervous system function. *Merrill-Palmer Q. Behav. Dev.* 15:375–378.

Selye, H. (1950). The physiology and pathology of exposure to stress. *Acta Montreal*.

Shirley, M. M. (1931). *The First Two Years: A Study of Twenty-five Babies*. Minneapolis: University of Minnesota Press. [Reprinted in 1971.]

Smart, R. G., and Bateman, K. (1968). The chromosomal and teratogenic effects of lysergic acid diethylamide: A review of current literature. *Can. Med. Assoc. J.* 99:805–810.

Sobel, E. (1961). Infant mortality and malformations in children of schizophrenic women: Preliminary data and suggested research. *Psychiatr. Q.* 35:60–65.

Sollenberger, R. T. (1968). Chinese-American child rearing practices and juvenile delinquency. *J. Soc. Psychol.* 74:13–23.

Stoch, M., and Smythe, P. (1963). Does undernutrition during infancy inhibit brain growth and intellectual development? *Arch. Dis. Childh.* 38:546–552.

Szasz, T. (1961). *The Myth of Mental Illness*. New York: Harper & Row.

Thomas, A., and Chess, S. (1972). Development in middle childhood. *Psychiatry* 4:331–341.

Thomas, A., and Chess, S. (1976). Evolution of behavior disorders into adolescence. *Am. J. Psychiatry* 133:5.

Thomas, A., and Chess, S. (1977). *Temperament and Development*. New York: Brunner/Mazel.

Thomas, A., Chess, S., et al. (1963). *Behavioral Individuality in Early Childhood*. New York: New York University Press.

Thomas, A., Chess, S., and Birch, H. (1968). *Temperament and Behavior Disorders in Children.* New York: New York University Press.

Thomas, A., Chess, S., Sillen, J., and Mendez, O. (1974). Cross-cultural study of behavior in children with special vulnerabilities to stress, in D. F. Ricks, A. Thomas, and M. Roff (Eds.), *Life History Research in Psychopathology*, vol. 3. Minneapolis: University of Minnesota Press, pp. 53–67.

Thorpe, L. P. (1960). *The Psychology of Mental Health* (2nd ed.). New York: Ronald Press.

Torgersen, A. M. (1973). Temperamental Differences in Infants: Their Cause as Shown Through Twin Studies. Doctoral dissertation, University of Oslo, Norway.

Tousseing, P. W. (1962). Thoughts regarding the etiology of psychological difficulties in adopted children. *Child Welfare* 41:59–62.

Wallerstein, J. S., and Kelly, J. B. (1975). The effects of parental divorce: Experiences of the preschool child. *J. Am. Acad. Child Psychiatry* 14:600–616.

Weiner, G. (1968). Scholastic achievement at age 12–13 of the prematurely born infants. *J. Spec. Educ.* 2:237–241.

Wender, P., Rosenthal, D., *et al.* (1974). Crossfostering: A research strategy for clarifying the role of genetic and experiential factors in the etiology of schizophrenia. *Arch. Gen. Psychiatry* 30:121–128.

Westman, J., Cline, D., *et al.* (1970). Role of child psychiatry in divorce. *Arch. Gen. Psychiatry* 23:416–420.

Whiting, B., and Edwards, C. P. (1973). Cross-cultural analysis of sex differences in the behavior of children aged 3–11. *J. Soc. Psychol.* 91:171–188.

Whitten, C. F., Pettit, M. G., *et al.* (1969). Evidence that growth failure from maternal deprivation is secondary to undereating. *J. Am. Med. Assoc.* 209:1675–1682.

Williams, R. V. (1956). *Biochemical Individuality.* New York: Wiley.

Winnick, M. (1969). Malnutrition and brain development. *Pediatrics* 74:667–679.

Wolkind, H. (1944) Sex differences in the aetiology of antisocial disorders in children in long term residential care. *Br. J. Psychiatry* 125:45.

Yamazaki, J. N. (1966). A review of the literature on the radiation dosage required to cause manifest central nervous system disturbances from *in utero* and postnatal exposure. *Pediatrics* 37:877–897.

Zigler, E. (1970). Social class and the socializing process. *Review of Educational Research* 40:87–110.

Chapter 5

Ackerly, W. C. (1964). Latency age children who threaten or attempt to kill themselves. *J. of Am. Acad. Child Psychiatry* 6:242–261.

Annell, A. L. (Ed.) (1972). *Depressive States in Childhood and Adolescence.* New York: Halsted Press.

Bender, L. (1953). *Aggression, Hostility and Anxiety in Children.* Springfield, Ill.: Charles C Thomas.

Bender, L. (1959). Children and adolescents who have killed. *Am. Psychol.* 116:510–513.

Bender, L. (1972). Aggression in Children, in S. Frazier (Ed.), *Aggression.* Baltimore: William & Wilkins, 1974.

Bowlby, J. (1944). Forty-four juvenile thieves: Their characters and home life. *Int. J. Psychoanal.* 25:19–53.

Cloward, R., and Ohlin, L. (1960). *Delinquency and Opportunity.* Glencoe, Ill.: Free Press.

Cohen, A. K. (1955). *Delinquent Boys: The Culture of the Gang.* Glencoe, Ill.: Free Press.

Connell, P. H. (1965). Suicidal Attempts in Childhood and Adolescence, in J. H. Howells (Ed.), *Modern Perspective in Child Psychiatry*. New York: Brunner/Mazel.

Cytryn, L. and McKnew, D. H. (1974). Factors influencing the changing clinical expression of the depressive process in children. *Am. J. Psychiatry* 131:879–881.

Delinquency Prediction: A Progress Report (1961). New York: New York City Youth Board.

Ferracutti, F., and Dinitz, S. (1972). Cross-cultural aspects of delinquent and criminal behavior, in S. Frazier (Ed.), *Aggression*. Baltimore: Williams & Wilkins, 1974.

Finch, S. (1962). The psychiatrist and juvenile delinquency. *J. Am. Acad. Child Psychiatry* 1:619–635.

Glaser, K. (1967). Masked depression in children and adolescents. *Am. J. Psychiatry* 21: 565–574.

Glueck, S., and Glueck, E. T. (1950). *Unraveling Juvenile Delinquency*. New York: Commonwealth Fund.

Glueck, S., and Glueck, E. (1968). *Delinquents and Nondelinquents in Perspective*. Cambridge, Mass.: Harvard University Press.

Hewitt, L. S., and Jenkins, R. L. (1946). *Fundamental Patterns of Maladjustment: The Dynamics of Their Origin*. Springfield, Ill.: Charles C Thomas.

Kvaraceus, W. C. (1961). Forecasting juvenile delinquency: A three year experiment. *Exceptional Child* 27:429–435.

Makkay, E. S. (1962). Some problems in the differential diagnosis of the antisocial character disorders in latency. *J. Am. Acad. Child Psychiatry* 1:414–430.

Malmquist, C. P. (1971). Depressions in childhood and adolescence. *N. Engl. J. Med.* 284:887–893, 955–961.

Mattsson, A., Seese, L. R., and Hawkins, J. W. (1969). Suicidal behavior as child psychiatric emergency. *Arch. Gen. Psychiatry* 20:100–109.

McRae, K., and Lowe, S. (1968). Aggressive behavior in the pre-school child. *Pediatrics* 72:821–828.

Miller, W. (1959). Lower class culture as a generating milieu of gang delinquency. *J. Soc. Issues* 14:5–19.

Poznanski, E., Krahenbuhl, V. and Zrull, J. (1976). Child depression: A longitudinal perspective. *J. Am. Acad. Child Psychiatry* 15:491–501.

Poznanski, E., and Zrull, J. P. (1970). Child depression: Clinical characteristics of overtly depressed children. *Arch. Gen. Psychiatry* 23:8–15.

Quay, H. C. (Ed.) (1965). *Juvenile Delinquency: Research and Theory*. New York: Van Nostrand.

Redl, F., and Wineman, D. (1952). *Controls from Within: Techniques for the Treatment of the Aggressive Child*. Glencoe, Ill.: Free Press.

Robins, L. N. (1966). *Deviant Child Grown Up: A Sociological and Psychiatric Study of Sociopathic Personality*. Baltimore: Williams & Wilkins.

Shaffer, D. (1974). Suicide in childhood and early adolescence. *J. Child Psychol. Psychiatry* 15:275–291.

Siegel, A. E. (1972). Televised violence: Recent research on its effects, in S. Frazier (Ed.), *Aggression*. Baltimore: Williams & Wilkins, 1974.

Spitz, R. A., and Wolf, K. M. (1946). Anaclitic depression: An inquiry into the genesis of psychiatric condition in early childhood. *Psychoanal. Study Child* 2:314–342.

Szurek, S. A. and Johnson, A. M. (1969). The genesis of antisocial acting out, in S. A. Szurek and I. N. Berlin (Eds.), *The Antisocial Child: His Family and His Community*. Palo Alto, Calif.: Science & Behavior Books.

Toolan, J. M. (1962). Suicide and suicidal attempts in children and adolescents. *Am. J. Psychiatry* 118:719–724.

Toolan, J. M. (1971). Depression in adolescents, in J. H. Howells (Ed.), *Modern Perspective in Adolescent Psychiatry*. New York: Brunner/Mazel, pp. 359–378.

Van Amerongen, S. T. (1963). Permission, promotion, and provocation of antisocial behavior. *J. Am. Acad. Child Psychiatry* 2:99–117.

Vandersall, T. A., and Wiener, J. M. (1970). Children who set fires. *Arch. Gen Psychiatry* 22:63–71.

Yarrow, L., and Goodwin, M. (1973). The immediate impact of separation: Reaction of infants to a change in mother figures, in J. Stone, H. T. Smith, and L. B. Murphy (Eds.), *The Competent Infant*. New York: Basic Books, pp. 1032–1040.

Chapter 6

Aird, R. B., and Yamamoto, T. (1966). Behavior disorders of childhood. *Electroenceph. Clinic. Neurophysiol.* 21:148–156.

Ames, L. B., Metraux, R. W. *et al.* (Eds.) (1974). *Child Rorschach Responses: Developmental Trends from 2 to 10 years*. New York: Brunner/Mazel.

Anastasia, A. (1968). *Psychological Testing* (3rd ed.). New York: Macmillan.

Bayley, N. (1958). Value and limitations of infant testing. *Children* 5:165–196.

Bellak, T. (1950). The Children's Apperception Test (C.A.T.), in A. I. Rabin and M. R. Haworth (Eds.), *The Projective Techniques with Children*. New York: Grune & Stratton.

Bender, L. (1938). *Visual Motor Gestalt Test and its Clinical Use*. Monograph Series, No. 3. Menasha, Wisconsin: George Banta Publishing Co.

Bender, L. (1952). *Child Psychiatric Techniques*. Springfield, Ill.: Charles C Thomas.

Bender, L. (1958). Problems in conceptualization and communication in children with developmental alexia. *Proc. Am. Psychopathological Assoc.* 46:155–176.

Burns, R. C., and Kaufman, S. H. (1972). *Action, Styles and Symbols in Kinetic Family Drawing*. New York: Brunner/Mazel.

Capute, A. J., Niedermyer, E. F., and Richardson, F. (1968). The electroencephalogram in children with minimal cerebral dysfunction. *Pediatrics* 41:1104–1114.

Carter, S., and Gold, A. D. (1972). The nervous system: Diagnosis of neurologic diseases, in Barnett and Einhorn (Eds.), *Pediatrics* (15th ed). New York: Appleton-Century-Crofts.

Chapman, L. J., and Chapman, J. P. (1973). *Disordered Thought in Schizophrenia*. New Jersey: Century Psychology Series, Prentice-Hall.

Chein, I. (1945). On the nature of intelligence. *J. Gen. Psychol.* 32:111–126.

Cohen, D. J. (1976). The diagnostic process in child psychiatry. *Psychiatr. Ann.* 6:29–35.

Corah, N. L., and Pantera, R. E. (1965). Effects of perinatal anoxia after seven years. *Psychol. Monog.* Vol. 79, No. 596.

Dodge, P. R. (1964). Neurologic history and examination, in T. W. Farmer (Ed.), *Pediatric Neurology*. New York: Harper & Row.

Doll, E. A. (1953). *The Measurement of Social Competence*. U.S. Educational Test Bureau, Educational Publishers.

DuBois, P. H. (1970). *A History of Psychological Testing*. Boston: Allyn and Bacon.

Fenton, G. (1974). The straightforward EEG in psychiatric practice. *R. Soc. Med.* 67:911–918.

Fink, M., and Bender, M. B. (1953). Perception of simultaneous tactile stimuli in normal children. *Neurology* 3:27–34.

Fish, J., and Larr, C. (1972). A decade of change in drawings by black children. *Am. J. Psychiatry* 129:421–426.

Freud, A. (1965). *Normality and Pathology in Childhood*. New York: International Universities Press.
Frostig, M. (1963). Visual perception in the brain damaged child. *Am. J. Orthopsychiatry* 33:665.
Goldfarb, W. (1974). *Growth and Change of Schizophrenic Children in Longitudinal Study*. New York: Halsted.
Goodenough, F. L. (1926). *Measurement of Intelligence by Drawings*. New York: Harcourt.
Goodman, J., and Sours, J. (1967). *The Child Mental Status Examination*. New York: Basic Books.
Halpern, F. (1960). The Rorschach test with children, in A. I. Rabin and M. R. Haworth (Eds.), *Projective Techniques with Children*. New York: Grune & Stratton.
Harris, D. B. (1963). *Children's Drawings as Measures of Intellectual Maturity*. New York: Harcourt.
Hertz, M. R. (1960). The Rorschach in adolescence, in A. I. Rabin and M. R. Haworth (Eds.), *The Projective Techniques with Children*. New York: Grune & Stratton.
Hughes, J. R., and Park, G. E. (1968). The EEG in dyslexia, in P. Kellaway and I. S. Petersen (Eds.), *Functional Aspects of EEG Foci in Children—Clinical Data and Longitudinal studies in Clinical Electroencephalography of Children*. New York: Grune & Stratton.
Kennard, M. (1960). Value of equivocal signs in neurological diagnosis. *Neurology* 10:753–764.
Kools, J. A., and Tweedie, D. (1975). Development of praxis in children. *Percep. Motor Skills* 40:11–19.
Koppitz, E. M. (1964). *Bender Gestalt Test for Young Children*. New York: Grune & Stratton.
Koppitz, E. M. (1968). *Psychological Evaluation of Children's Human Figure Drawings*. New York: Grune & Stratton.
Lairy, G. C., and Harrison, A. (1968). In P. Kellaway and I. S. Peterson (Eds.), *Functional Aspects of EEG Foci in Children—Clinical Data and Longitudinal Studies in Clinical Electroencephalography of Children*. New York: Grune & Stratton.
Lewis, M., and McGurk, H. (1972). Evaluation of infant intelligence scores—true or false. *Science* 178:174–176.
Machover, K. (1953). Human figure drawings of children. *J. Projective Tech.* 17:85–91.
McClelland, D. C. (1973). Testing for competence rather than for "intelligence." *American Psychologists*, Vol. 28, No. 1.
Moriarty, A. E. (1966). *Constancy and I. Q. Change: A Clinical View of Relationship between Tested Intelligence and Personality*. Springfield, Ill.: Charles C Thomas.
Paine, R. S. (1962). Minimal chronic brain syndrome in children. *Dev. Med. Child Neurol.* 4:21–27.
Rapaport, D., Gill, M., and Schafer, R. (1968). *Diagnostic Psychological Testing* (rev. ed. by R. R. Holt). New York: International Universities Press.
Shetty, R. (1973). Some neurologic, electrophysiologic and biochemical correlates of the hyperkinetic syndrome. *Pediatr. Ann.* 2:29–34.
Silver, L. B. (1976). The playroom diagnostic evaluation of children with neurologically based learning disabilities. *J. Am. Acad. Child Psychiatry* 15:240–256.
Simmons, J. E. (1974). *Psychiatric Examination of Children* (2nd ed.). Philadelphia: Lea and Febiger.
Spearman, C. (1923). *The Nature of Intelligence and the Principle of Cognition*. London: Macmillan.
Suinn, R. M., and Oskamp S. (1969). *The Predictive Validity of Projective Measures*. Springfield, Ill.: Charles C Thomas.

Terman, L. M., and Oden, M. (1959). *Genetic Studies of Genius*, vols. 1–5. Stanford: Stanford University Press.

Tolor, A. and Schulberg, H. (1963). *An Evolution of the Bender–Gestalt Test*. Springfield, Ill.: Charles C Thomas.

Trojaborg, W. (1968). Changes of spike foci in children, in P. Kellaway and I. S. Petersen (Eds.), *Functional Aspects of EEG Foci in Children—Clinical Data and Longitudinal Studies in Clinical Electroencephalography of Children*. New York: Grune & Stratton.

Wepman, J. M. (1958). *Auditory Discrimination Test Manual of Direction* (preliminary ed.). New York: Roland Press.

Wikler, A., Dixon, J., and Parker, J. (1970). Brain function in problem children and controls, psychometric, neurological and electroencephalographic comparisons. *Am. J. Psychiatry* 127:634–646.

Chapter 7

Cameron, K. (1957). Symptom classification in child psychiatry. *Rev. Psychiatr. Infant.* 25(Facsimile 6):241–245.

Cameron, K. (1958). Diagnostic categories in child psychiatry. *Br. J. Med. Psychol.* 28(Part 1):67–71.

Chess, S. (1969). *An Introduction to Child Psychiatry* (2nd ed.). New York: Grune & Stratton.

Chess, S. (1971). Classification of Psychiatric Disorders of Childhood and Adolescence. Paper presented at the World Psychiatric Association, Mexico City, Nov. 1971.

Diagnostic and Statistical Manual of Mental Disorders (DSM II) (2nd ed.) (1968). Washington: The American Psychiatric Association.

International Statistical Classification of Diseases, Injuries and Causes of Death (8th revision) (1965). Geneva: World Health Organization.

Kanner, L. (1948). *Child Psychiatry* (2nd ed.). Springfield, Ill.: Charles C Thomas, pp. 205–206.

Psychopathological Disorders in Childhood: Theoretical Considerations and a Proposed Classification (1966). New York: Group for the Advancement of Psychiatry.

Rutter, M., Lebovici, S., Eisenberg, L., Sneznevskij, A. V., Sadoun, R., Brooke, E., and Lin, T-Y. (1969). A tri-axial classification of mental disorders in childhood. *J. Child Psychol. Psychiatry* 10:41–61.

Rutter, M., Shaffer, D., and Shepard, M. (1973). An evaluation of the proposal for a multi-axial classification of child psychiatric disorders. *Psychol. Med.* 3.2:244–250.

Spitzer, R. L., Sheehy, M., and Endicott, J. (1977). *DSM III: Guiding Principles in Psychiatric Diagnosis*, S. H. Rakoff, Stanur, and Kedwarel (Eds.). Chicago: American Psychiatric Association.

Veith, I. (1957). Psychiatric nosology: From Hippocrates to Kraepelin. *Am. J. Psychiatry* 114:385–389.

Chapter 8

Aisenberg, R. B., Wolff, P. H., and Rosenthal, D. (1973). Psychological impact of cardiac catheterization. *Pediatrics* 51:1051–1059.

Bernstein, N. R., Sanger, S., and Fras, I. (1969). The functions of the child psychiatrist in the management of severely burned children. *J. Am. Acad. Child Psychiatry* 8:620–636.

Futterman, E. H. (1975). Studies of family adaptational responses to a specific threat, in E. J. Anthony (Ed.), *Explorations in Child Psychiatry*. New York: Plenum Press.

Galdston, R., and Gamble, W. J. (1969). On borrowed time: Observations on children with implanted pacemakers and their families. *Am. J. Psychiatry* 126:104–108.

Mattsson, A., and Gross, S. (1966). Adaptational and defensive behavior in young hemophiliacs and their parents. *Am. J. Psychiatry* 122:1349–1356.

Newman, C. J. (1976). Children of disaster: Clinical observation at Buffalo Creek. *Am. J. Psychiatry* 133:306–312.

Richmond, J. B., and Waisman, H. A. (1955). Psychological aspects of management of children with malignant diseases. *Am. J. Dis. Child.* 89:42–47.

Spinetta, J. J. (1974). The dying child's awareness of death: A review. *Psychol. Bull.* 81:256–260.

Chapter 9

Anders, T. F., and Weinstein, P. (1972). Sleep and its disorders in infants and children: A review. *J. Pediatr.* 50:311–324.

Anthony, E. J. (1957). An experimental approach to the psychopathology of childhood: Encopresis. *Br. J. Med. Psychol.* 30:156–162, 172–174.

Bender, L. (1954). *A Dynamic Psychopathology of Childhood*. Springfield, Ill.: Charles C Thomas.

Bender, L., and Blau, A. (1937). Reactions of children to sexual relations with adults. *Am. J. Orthopsychiatry* 7:520.

Bender, L., and Blau, A. (1952). Follow-up report on children who had atypical sexual experience. *Am. J. Orthopsychiatry* 22:825.

Bieber, I. (1966). Sadism and masochism, in S. Arieti (Ed.), *American Handbook of Psychiatry*, vol. 3. New York: Basic Books.

Birns, B. (1976). The emergence and socialization of sex differences in the earliest years. *Merrill-Palmer Q. Behav. Dev.* 22:229–254.

Bruch, H. (1963). Disturbed communication in eating disorders. *Am. J. Orthopsychiatry* 33:99–104.

Cooper, M. (1957). *Pica*. Springfield, Ill.: Charles C Thomas.

Foulkes, D., Larson, J., Swanson, E. M., and Rordin, M. (1969). Two studies of childhood dreaming. *Am. J. Orthopsychiatry* 39:627–643.

Freud, S. (1905). *Three essays on the theory of sexuality*, Standard Edition, vol. 7. London: The Hogarth Press.

Gerard, M. (1939). Enuresis: A study in etiology. *Am. J. Orthopsychiatry* 9:48–58.

Gesell, A., and Amatruda, C. S. (1940). *Developmental Diagnosis* (3rd ed.). New York: Harper Medical, 1974.

Halpern, W. (1977). The treatment of encopretic children. *J. Am. Acad. Child Psychiatry* 16:478–499.

Hammer, S. L., and Campbell, M. M., *et al.* (1972). An interdisciplinary study of adolescent obesity. *J. Pediatr.* 80:373–383.

Hampson, J. L., and Hampson, J. G. (1961). The ontogenesis of sexual behavior in man, in N. C. Young (Ed.), *Sex and Internal Secretions*, vol. 2, Baltimore: Williams & Wilkins.

Kagan, J. (1964). Acquisition and significance of sex typing and sex-role identity, in M. L. Hoffman and L. W. Hoffman (Eds.), *Review of Child Development Research*, vol. 1. New York: Russell Sage Foundation.

Kanner, L. (1972). *Child Psychiatry* (4th ed.). Springfield, Ill.: Charles C Thomas.

Kales, A. (Ed.) (1969). *Sleep—Physiology and Pathology: A Symposium.* Philadelphia: Lippincott.

Knittle, J. (1972). Obesity in childhood: A problem in adipose tissue cellular development. *J. Pediatr.* 81:1048–1059.

Kremer, M., and Rifkin, A. (1969). The early development of homosexuality: A study of adolescent lesbians. *Am. J. Psychiatry* 126:129–134.

Litin, E., Griffin, M., and Johnson, A. M. (1956). Parental influence in unusual sexual behavior in children. *Psychoanal. Q.* 25:37–55.

Lovibond, S. H. (1964). *Conditioning and Enuresis.* New York: Macmillan.

Lucas, A. R., Duncan, J. W., and Piens, V. (1976). The treatment of anorexia nervosa. *Am. J. Psychiatry* 133:1034–1038.

Mayer, J. (1966). Some aspects of the problem of regulation of food intake and obesity. *N. Eng. J. Med.* 274:610–616, 663–673, 722, 731.

Money, J., and Dalery, I. (1976). Iatrogenic homosexuality. *J. Homosexuality* 1:357–371.

Newman, L. E. (1976). Treatment for the parents of feminine boys. *Am. J. Psychiatry* 133:683–687.

Offer, D., and Offer, J. (1971). Four issues in the developmental psychology of adolescents, in J. G. Howells (Ed.), *Modern Perspectives in Adolescent Psychiatry.* New York: Brunner/Mazel.

Oppel, W., Harper, P., and Rider, R. (1968). Social, pathological and neurological factors associated with nocturnal enuresis. *J. Pediatr.* 42:627–641.

Prugh, G. P., Wermer, H., and Lord, J. (1954). On significance of the anal phase in pediatrics and child psychiatry: Workshop, in G. E. Gardiner (Ed.), *Case Studies in Childhood Emotional Disabilities.* New York: American Orthopsychiatric Association.

Ragins, N., and Schacter, J. (1971). A study of sleep behavior in two year old children. *J. Am. Acad. Child Psychiatry* 10:217–235.

Ramsey, C. V. (1943). The sexual development of boys. *Am. J. Psychol.* 56:217–233.

Robins, L. N. (1966). *Deviant Children Grown Up.* Baltimore: Williams & Wilkins.

Rutter, M. (1970). Sex differences in children's response to family stress, in E. J. Anthony and C. Koupernik (Eds.), *The Child in His Family.* London: Wiley, p. 165.

Rutter, M. (1971). Normal sexual development. *J. Child Psychol. Psychiatry* 11:259–283.

Schofield, M. (1971). Normal sexuality in adolescence, in J. G. Howells (Ed.), *Modern Perspectives in Adolescent Psychiatry.* New York: Brunner/Mazel.

Sears, R. R., Maccoby, E. E., and Levin, H. (1957). *Patterns of Child Rearing.* New York: Harper & Row.

Silverman, J. A. (1974). Anorexia nervosa: Clinical observation in a successful treatment plan. *J. Pediatr.* 84(1):66–73.

Stoller, R. J. (1968). Male childhood transexualism. *J. Am. Acad. Child Psychiatry* 7(2):193–209.

Warren, W. (1968). A study of anorexia nervosa in young girls. *J. Child Psychol. Psychiatry* 9:27–40.

Wulff, M. (1946). Fetishism and object choice in early childhood. *Psychoanal. Q.* 12:450.

Zarcone, V. (1973). Narcolepsy. *N. Eng. J. Med.* 228:1156–1166.

Chapter 10

Alexander, F. (1950). *Psychosomatic Medicine: Its Principles and Applications.* New York: Norton.

Block J. (1968). Further considerations of psychosomatic predisposing factors in allergy. *Psychosom. Med.* 30:202–208.

Block, J., Harvey, E., Jennings, P., and Simpson, E. (1966). Clinicians conceptions of the asthmatogenic mother. *Arch. Gen. Psychiatry* 15:610.

Dubo, S., McLean, J., Ching, A., Wright, H., Kauffman, P., and Sheldon, J. (1961). A study of relationship between family situation, bronchial asthma and personal adjustment in children. *J. Pediatr.* 59:404–414.

Fitzelle, G. (1959). Personality factors and certain attitudes toward child rearing among parents of asthmatic children. *Psychosom. Med.* 21:208–217.

Hahn, W. (1966). Autonomic responses of asthmatic children. *Psychosom. Med.* 28:323–332.

Miller, H., and Baruch, D. W. (1957). The emotional problems of childhood and their relation to asthma. *Am. J. Dis. Child.* 93:242–245.

Minuchin, S., Baker, L., *et al.* (1975). A conceptual model of psychosomatic illness in children. *Arch. Gen. Psychiatry* 32:1031–1040.

Owen, F., and Williams, G. (1961). Patterns of respiratory disturbance in asthmatic children evoked by the stimulus of the mother's voice. *Am. J. Dis. Child.* 102:133–134.

Purcell, K. (1963). Distinction between sub-groups of asthmatic children: Children's perceptions of events associated with asthma. *J. Pediatr.* 31:486–494.

Purcell, K., Bernstein, L., and Bukantz, S. (1961). A preliminary comparison of rapidly remitting and persistently steroid-dependent, asthmatic children. *Psychosom. Med.* 23:305–310.

Rutter, M. (1970). Discussion, in E. H. Hare and J. K. Wing (Eds.), *Psychiatric Epidemiology*. London: Oxford University Press, pp. 202–208.

Sperling, M. (1968). Asthma in children: An evaluation of concepts and therapies. *J. Am. Acad. Child Psychiatry* 7:44–58.

Sternbach, R. (1966). *Principles of Psychophysiology*. New York: Academic Press.

Chapter 11

Adams, M., and Glasner, J. (1954). Emotional involvements in some form of mutism. *J. Speech Hear. Dis.*, 19:56–69.

Adams, P. L. (1973). *Obsessive Children: A Sociopsychiatric Study*. New York: Brunner/Mazel.

Anthony, E. J. (1967). Psychiatric disorders of childhood, psychoneurotic disorders, in A. M. Freedman and H. I. Kaplan (Eds.), *Comprehensive Text Book of Psychiatry*. New York: Williams & Wilkins, pp. 1387–1406.

Argas, S. (1959). The relationship of school phobia to childhood depression. *A. J. Psychiatry* 116:533–539.

Berecz, J. (1968). Phobias of childhood, etiology and treatment. *Psychol. Bull.* 70:694–720.

Coolidge, J. C., Brodie, R. D., and Feeney, B. A. (1964). A 10 year follow-up study of 66 school phobic children. *Am. J. Orthopsychiatry* 34:675–695.

Eisenberg, L. (1958). School phobia, diagnosis, genesis and clinical management. *Pediatr. Clin. N. Am.* 5:645–666.

Elson, A., Pearson, C., *et al.* (1964). Follow-up study of childhood elective mutism. *Arch. Gen. Psychiatry* 13:182–187.

English, O. S., and Pearson, G. H. (1937). *Common Neurosis of Children and Adults*. New York: Norton.

Eysenck, H. J., and Rachman, S. (1965). *The Causes and Cures of Neurosis*. San Diego: Robert R. Knapp.

Freud, A. (1965). *Normality and Pathology in Childhood.* New York: International Universities Press.

Frommer, E. A. (1967). Treatment of childhood depression with antidepressant drugs. *Br. Med. J.* 1:117–136.

Frommes, I. A. (1968). Depressive illness in childhood. *Br. J. Psychiatry,* Special Supplement, pp. 2–117.

Halpern, W. I., Hammond, J. *et al.* (1971). A therapeutic approach to speech phobia *J. Am. Acad. Child Psychiatry* 10:94–107.

Janet, P. (1876). La notion de personalité. *Rev. Sci.,* Vol. 11.

Kahn, J. H., and Nursten, J. P. (1962). School phobias: Refusal, a comprehensive view of school phobia and other failures of school attendance. *Am. J. Orthopsychiatry* 32:707–718.

Kanner, L. (1972). *Child Psychiatry* (4th ed.). Springfield, Ill.: Charles C Thomas.

Langford, S. W. (1937). Anxiety attacks in children. *Am. J. Orthopsychiatry* 7:210–218.

Lapouse, R., and Monk, N. (1959). Fears and worries in a representative sample of children. *Am. J. Orthopsychiatry* 29:803–818.

Looff, D. H. (1970). Psychophysiological and conversion reaction, selective incidence in verbal and nonverbal families. *J. Am. Acad. Child Psychiatry* 9:318–331.

MacFarlane, J. W., Allen, L., and Honzik, M. (1954). *A Developmental Study of the Behavior Problems of Normal Children.* Berkeley. University of California Press.

Poznanski, E. O. (1973). Children with excessive fears. *Am. J. Orthopsychiatry* 43:428–438.

Proctor, J. I (1958). Hysteria in childhood. *Am. J. Orthopsychiatry* 28:394–407.

Rachman, S., and Costello, C. (1961). The etiology and treatment of children's phobias: A review, in S. Harrison and J. McDermott (Eds.), *Childhood Psychopathology.* New York: International Universities Press.

Rock, N. L. (1971). Conversion reactions in childhood: A clinical study on childhood neurosis. *J. Am. Acad. Child Psychiatry* 10:65–93.

Waldron, S. (1976). The significance of childhood neurosis for adult mental health: A follow-up study. *Am. J. Psychiatry* 133:532–538.

Watson, J. B., and Vorgan, J. J. B. (1917). Emotional reactions and psychological experimentation. *Am. J. Psychol.* 28:163–174.

Weiss, M., and Burke, A. G. (1967). A 5 to 10 year follow-up of hospitalized school phobic children and adolescents. *Am. J. Orthopsychiatry* 37:294–295.

Wolpe, J. (1963). Systematic desensitization of phobias. *Am. J. Psychiatry* 119:1062–1068.

Wright, T. L. (1968). A clinical study of children who refuse to talk in school. *J. Am. Acad. Child Psychiatry* 7:603–617.

Zeigler, D. K. (1967). Neurological disease and hysteria, the differential diagnosis. *Int. J. Neuropsychiatry* 3:388–396.

Chapter 12

Akerley, M. S. (1975). The invulnerable parent. *J. Autism Child. Schizophrenia* 5:275–280.

Annell, A. L. (1969). Lithium in the treatment of children and adolescents. *Acta Psychiatr. Scand. Suppl.* 270:19–33.

Anthony, E. J. (1969). A clinical evaluation of children with psychotic parents. *Am. J. Psychiatry* 126:177–184.

Anthony, J., and Scott, P. (1960). Manic–depressive psychosis in childhood. *J. Child Psychol. Psychiatry* 1:53–72.

Bartak, L., Rutter, M., and Cox, A. (1975). A comparative study of infantile autism and specific developmental receptive language disorder, I: The children. *Br. Jr. Psychiatry* 126:127–144.

Bender, L. (1947). Childhood schizophrenia: A clinical study of one hundred schizophrenic children. *Am. J. Orthopsychiatry* 17:40–50.

Bender, L. (1966). The concept of plasticity in childhood schizophrenia, in P. H. Hoch and J. Zubin (Eds.), *Psychopathology of Schizophrenia*. New York: Grune & Stratton.

Bender, L., and Freedman, A. (1952). A study in the first three years in the maturation of schizophrenic children. *Q. J. Child Behav.* 4:245–272.

Bleuler, E. (1950). *Dementia Praecox, or The Group of Schizophrenias*. New York: International Universities Press.

Campbell, M. (1973). Biological interventions in psychoses of childhood. *J. Autism Child. Schizophrenia.* 3.:347–373.

Chess, S. (1971). Autism in children with congenital rubella. *J. Autism Child. Schizophrenia* 1:33–47.

Churchill, D. W. (1969). Psychotic children and behavior manifestation. *Am. J. Psychiatry* 125:1585–1590.

Cohen, D. J., Caparulo, B., and Shaywitz, B. (1976). Primary childhood aphasia and childhood autism: Clinical, biological and conceptual observations. *J. Acad. Child Psychiatry* 15:604–645.

Creak, M. (1961). Schizophrenic syndrome in childhood: Progress report of a working party. *Cerebral Palsy Bull.* 3:501.

Creak, M. (1968). Childhood psychosis: A review of 100 cases. *Br. J. Psychiatry.* 109:84.

DeMyer, M. (1975). Research in infantile autism: A strategy and its results. *Biol. Psychiatr.* 10:433–452.

DeSanctis, S. (1973). On some varieties of dementia praecox, in S. A. Szurek and I. N. Berlin (Eds.), *Clinical Studies in Childhood Psychoses*. New York: Brunner/Mazel.

Desmond, M. M., Wilson, G. S. et al. (1970). The early growth and development of infants with congenital rubella. *Adv. Teratol.* 4:40–63.

Eisenberg, L. (1957). The course of childhood schizophrenia. *Arch. Neurol. Psychiatr.* 78: 69–83.

Feinstein, S. C. (1973). Diagnostic and therapeutic aspect of manic–depressive illness in early childhood. *Early Child Dev. Care* 3:1–12.

Fish, B. (1960). Involvement of central nervous system in infants with schizophrenia. *Arch. Neurol.* 2:115.

Fish, B. (1971). Contributions of developmental research to a theory of schizophrenia, in J. Hellmuth (Ed.), *Exceptional Infant, vol. 2: Studies in Abnormalities*. New York: Brunner/Mazel.

Gittelman, M., and Birch, H. (1967). Childhood schizophrenia: Intellect, neurologic status, perinatal risk, prognosis and family pathology. *Arch. Gen. Psychiatry* 17:16–25.

Goldfarb, W. (1961). *Childhood Schizophrenia*. Cambridge, Mass.: Harvard University Press, The Commonwealth Fund.

Heller, T. (1973). Reported by Kanner, L. *Childhood Psychosis: Initial Studies and New Insights*. New York: Halsted Press.

Kallmann, F. J. (1950). The genetics of psychosis: An analysis of 1,232 index families. *Am. J. Human Genet.* 2:385–390.

Kanner, L. (1943). Autistic disturbances of affective contact. *Nervous Child* 2:217–250.

Kanner, L. (1949). Problems of nosology and psychodynamics in early infantile autism, in *Childhood Psychosis: Initial Studies and New Insights*. Washington: V. H. Winston & Sons, 1973.

Kanner, L., and Eisenberg, L. (1956). Early infantile autism, 1943–1955. *Am. J. Orthopsychiatry* 26:556–566.

Kanner, L. (1972). *Child Psychiatry* (4th ed.). Springfield, Ill.: Charles C Thomas.

Kennard, M. A. (1959). The E.E.G. in psychological disorders: A review. *Psychosom. Med.* 15:95.

Knobloch, H., and Pasamanick, B. (1962). Mental subnormality. *N. Eng. J. Med.* 266:1045–1051.

Lotter, V. (1966). Epidemiology of autistic conditions in young children, I: Prevalence. *Soc. Psychiatry* 1:124–137.

Mahler, M. S. (1952). On child psychosis and schizophrenia: Austistic and symbiotic infantile psychosis, in *The Psychoanalytic Study of the Child*, vol. 7. New York: International Universities Press.

Mahler, M. S., Ross, J. R., and De Fries, Z. (1949). Clinical studies in benign and malignant cases of childhood psychosis (Schizophrenia-Like). *Am. J. Orthopsychiatry* 19:295–304.

Matthysse, S. W., and Kidd, K. K. (1976). Estimating the genetic contribution to schizophrenia. *Am. J. Psychiatry* 133:185–191.

McDermott, J. F., Harrisson, S. I., *et al.*, (1967). Social class and mental illness in children: The question of childhood psychosis. *Am. J. Orthopsychiatry* 37:548–557.

Miller, R. T. (1974). Childhood schizophrenia: A review of selected literature. *Int. J. Ment. Health* 3:3–46.

Ornitz, E. M. and Ritvo, E. R., (1976). Syndrome of autism: A clinical review. *Am. J. Psychiatry* 133:609–662.

Piggot, L. R., and Simson, C. B. (1975). Changing diagnosis of childhood psychosis. *J. Autism Child. Schizophrenia* 5:239–245.

Pollack, M., *et al.* (1966). Pre- and perinatal complications and "childhood schizophrenia": A comparison of five controlled studies. *J. Child Psychol. Psychiatry Allied Discip.* 7:235–242.

Rank, B. (1949). Adaptation of the psychoanalytic technique for the treatment of young children with atypical development. *Am. J. Orthopsychiatry* 19:130–139.

Rimland, B. (1964). *Infantile Autism*. The Century Psychology Series. New York: Meredith.

Ritvo, E. R., Cantwell, D. *et al.* (1971). Social class factors in autism. *J. Autism Child. Schizophrenia* 1:297–310.

Rutter, M. (1966). Prognosis: Psychotic children in adolescence and early adult life, in J. K. Wing (Ed.), *Early Childhood Autism: Clinical, Educational and Social Aspects*. Oxford: Pergamon Press.

Rutter, M. (1967). Schooling and the autistic child. *Special Education* 56:19–24.

Rutter, M. (Ed.) (1971). *Infantile Autism: Concepts, Characteristics and Treatment*. Edinburgh: Churchill Livingstone.

Rutter, M. (1972). Childhood schizophrenia reconsidered. *J. Autism Child. Schizophrenia* 2:315–337.

Rutter, M., Greenfield, D., and Lockyer, L. (1967). A five to fifteen year follow-up study of infantile psychosis: II. Social and behavioral outcome. *Br. J. Psychiatry* 113:1183–1199.

Schopler, E., and Loftin, J. (1969). Thought disorders in parents of psychotic children: A function of test anxiety. *Arch. Gen. Psychiatry* 20:174–181.

Szurek, S. A. (1973). Attachment and psychotic detachment, in S. A. Szurek and I. N. Berlin (Eds.), *Clinical Studies in Childhood Psychoses*. New York: Brunner/Mazel.

Treffert, D. A. (1970). Epidemiology of infantile autism. *Arch. Gen. Psychiatry* 22:431–438.

Waxler, N. C., and Mishler, E. G. (1971). Parental interaction with schizophrenic children and well siblings. *Arch. Gen. Psychiatry* 25:223–231.

Chapter 13

Baumeister, A. (Ed.) (1967). *Mental Retardation: Appraisal, Education, Rehabilitation*. Chicago: Aldine.

Begab, M. J., and Richardson, S. A. (Eds.) (1975). *The Mentally Retarded and Society: A Social Science Perspective*. Baltimore: University Park Press.

Crandall, B. (1977). Genetic disorders and mental retardation. *J. Am. Acad. Child Psychiatry* 16:88–108.

Grossman, H. J. (Ed.) (1973). *Manual on Terminology and Classification in Mental Retardation*. Washington: American Association on Mental Deficiency, Special Publication, No. 2.

Inhelder, B. (1968). *The Diagnosis of Reasoning in the Mentally Retarded*. New York: John Day.

Koh, R., and Dobson, J. C. (Eds.) (1976). *The Mentally Retarded Child and his Family*. New York: Brunner/Mazel.

Luria, A. R. (1963). *The Mentally Retarded Child*. New York: Pergamon Press.

Menolascino, F. J. (1969). Emotional disturbance in mentally retarded children. *Am. J. Psychiatry* 126:168–176.

Mercer, J. R. (1976). Sociocultural factors in educational labeling, in M. J. Begab and S. A. Richardson (Eds.), *The Mentally Retarded and Society*. Baltimore: University Park Press.

Milgram, N. A. (1973). Language and cognition in mental retardation, in D. K. Routh (Ed.), *The Experimental Psychology of Mental Retardation*. Chicago: Aldine.

O'Connor, H., and Hermelin, B. (1961). Visual and stereognostic shape recognition in normal children and mongol- and non-mongol imbeciles. *Am. J. Ment. Defic.* 68:85–90.

Penrose, L. S. (1963). *The Biology of Mental Defect*. New York: Grune & Stratton.

Philips, I., and Williams, N. (1975). Psychopathology of mental retardation: A study of 100 mentally retarded children. *Am. J. Psychiatry* 132:1265–1271.

Ross, G., and Ross, W. (1973). Conditioning in mental retardation, in D. K. Routh (Ed.), *The Experimental Psychology of Mental Retardation*. Chicago: Aldine.

Routh, D. K. (Ed.) (1973). *The Experimental Psychology of Mental Retardation*. Chicago: Aldine.

Rutter, M. (1971). The description and classification of infantile autism, in D. Churchill, G. Alpern, and M. DeMyer (Eds.), *Infantile Autism*. Springfield, Ill.: Charles C Thomas.

Spitz, H. H. (1963). Field theory in mental deficiency, in N. R. Ellis (Ed.), *Handbook of Mental Deficiency*. New York: McGraw-Hill.

Szymanski, L. (1977). Psychiatric diagnostic evaluation of mentally retarded individuals. *J. Am. Acad. Child Psychiatry* 16:67–87.

Wood, N. E. (1960). *Communication Problems and Their Effect on the Learning Potential of the Mentally Retarded Child*. Washington: U.S. Office of Education, CRP #184.

Zeaman, D., and House, B. J. (1963). The role of attention in retardate discrimination learning, in N. R. Ellis (Ed.), *Handbook of Mental Deficiency: Psychological Theory and Research*. New York: McGraw-Hill.

Zigler, E. (1973). Rigidity and social reinforcement effects in the performance of institutionalized and noninstitutionalized normal and retarded children. *J. Personality* 31:258–269.

Zigler, E., and Balla, D. (1977). Personality factors in the performance of the retarded: Implications for clinical assessment. *J. Am. Acad. Child Psychiatry* 16:19–37.

Zigler, E., Hodgden, L., and Stevenson, H. (1968). The effect of support on the performance of normal and feebleminded children. *J. Personality* 26:106–122.

Chapter 14

Bender, L. (1957). Specific reading disability as a maturational lag. *Bull. Orton Society* 7: 155–176.

Critchley, M. (1970). *The Dyslexic Child*. Springfield, Ill.: Charles C Thomas.

Cruickshank, W. M. (1977). Myths and realities in learning disabilities. *J. Learn. Disabilities* 10:51–58.

De Hirsch, K. (1974). Learning disabilities: An overview. *Bull. N.Y. Acad. Med.* 50:459–479.

Gruber, E. (1962). Reading disability, binocular coordination and ophthalmograph. *Arch. Ophthalmol.* 67:280–288.

Mackworth, J. E. (1973). Some models of the reading process: Learner and skilled readers, in S. Sapir and A. Nitzburg (Eds.), *Children with Learning Problems*. New York: Brunner/Mazel.

Orton, S. T. (1937). *Reading, Writing and Speech Problems in Children*. New York: Norton.

Rabinovitch, R. D. (1959). Reading and learning disabilities, in S. Arieti (Ed.), *American Handbook of Psychiatry*, vol. 1. New York: Basic Books.

Silver, A., and Hagin, R. (1964). Specific reading disability: Follow-up studies. *Am. J. Orthopsychiatry* 34:95–102.

Thompson, L. (1973). Learning disabilities: An overview. *Am. J. Psychiatry* 130:393–399.

Torgensen, J. K. (1977). The role of non-specific factors in the task performance of learning disabled children: A theoretical assessment. *J. Learn. Disabilities* 10:27–34.

Witelson, S. F. (1977). Developmental dyslexia: Two right hemispheres and none left. *Science* 195:309–314.

Chapter 15

Bartak, L., Rutter, M., and Cox, A. (1975). A comparative study of infantile autism and specific developmental receptive language disorder, I: The children. *Br. J. Psychiatry* 126:127 144.

Beech, H., and Fransella, F. (1968). *Research and Experiments in Stuttering*. Oxford: Pergamon Press.

Coriat, I. H. (1928). Stammering: A psychoanalytic interpretation. *Nervous and Mental Disease*. Monograph, No. 47. New York.

de Ajuriaguerra, J., Jaeggi, A., Guignard, F., Kocher, F., Maquard, M., Roth, S., and Schmid, E. (1976). The development and prognosis of dysphasia in children, in D. Morehead and A. Morehead (Eds.), *Normal and Deficient Child Language*. Baltimore: University Park Press.

Eisenson, J. (1971). Speech defects: Nature, causes and psychological concomitants, in S. Cruickshank (Ed.), *Psychology of Exceptional Children and Youth* (3rd ed.) Englewood Cliffs, N.J.: Prentice-Hall.

Hardy, W. (1960). *Institute on Childhood Aphasia*. Monograph. Stanford: Stanford University Press.

Head, H. (1926). *Aphasia and Kindred Disorders of Speech*. London: Cambridge University Press.

Ingram, T. (1969). Developmental disorders of speech, in P. Vincken and G. Bruyn (Eds.), *Handbook of Clinical Neurology*, vol. 4. Amsterdam: North-Holland.

Johnson, W., Brown, S., Curtis, J., Edney, J., and Keaster, J. (1948). *Speech Handicapped School Children*. New York: Harper & Row.

Karlin, I. W. (1950). Stuttering: The problem today. *J. Am. Med. Assoc.* 143:732:736.

Orton, S. T. (1937). *Reading, Writing and Speech Problems in Children*. New York: Norton.

Ryan, B. P. (1974). *Programmed Therapy for Stuttering in Children and Adults.* Springfield, Ill.: Charles C Thomas.
Shames, G. (1968). Dysfluency and stuttering. *Pediatr. Clinic N. Am.* 15:691.
Simon, N. (1975). Echolalic speech in childhood autism. *Arch. Gen. Psychiatry* 32:1439–1448.

Chapter 16

Aird, R. B. (1968). Clinical syndromes of the limbic system. *Int. J. Neurol.* 6(3–4):346–352.
Aird, R. B., and Yamamoto, T. (1966). Behavior disorders of childhood, electroencephalograph. *Clin. Neurophysiol.* 21:148–156.
Cooper, J. E. (1965). Epilepsy in a longitudinal survey of 5000 children. *Br. Med. J.* 1:1020.
de la Burdé, D., and Choate, M. S. (1975). Early asymptomatic lead exposure and development at school age. *J. Pediatr.* 87(4):638–642.
Flor-Henry, P. (1969). Schizophrenic-like reactions and affective psychoses associated with temporal lobe epilepsy. *Am. J. Psychiatry* 126(3): 25–35.
Graham, P., and Rutter, M. (1968). Organic brain dysfunction and child psychiatric disorder. *Br. Med. J.* 3:697–700.
Herrington, R. N. (1969). The personality in temporal lobe epilepsy, in "Current Problems in Neuropsychiatry." *Br. J. Psychiatry*, Special Publication, No. 4, pp. 1315–1320.
Menolascino, F. J. (1969). Emotional disturbances in mentally retarded children. *Am. J. Psychiatry* 126(2):168–176.
Nuffield, E. J. A. (1961). Neurophysiology and behavior disorders in epileptic children. *J. Ment. Sci.* 107:438–458.
Ounsted, C. (1966). *Biological Factors in Temporal Lobe Epilepsy.* London: Heinemann.
Pond, D. A. (1961). Psychiatric aspects of epileptic and brain damaged children. *Br. Med. J.* 2:1454–1459.
Pond, D. A. (1969). Temporal lobe epilepsy in children *Br. J. Psychiatry*, Special Publication, No. 4, pp. 1377–1384.
Shaffer, D. (1973). Psychiatric aspects of brain injury in childhood: A review. *Dev. Med. Child Neurol.* 15,2:211–220.
Voeller, K. K. S., and Rothenberg, M. B. (1973). Psychosocial aspects of management of seizures in children. *Pediatrics* 51:1072–1082.

Chapter 17

Birch, H. (Ed.) (1963). *Brain Damage in Children.* Baltimore: Williams & Wilkins.
Birch, H. G. and Walker, H. A. (1966). A preceptual and perceptual-motor dissociation: Studies in schizophrenia and brain-damaged psychotic children. *Arch. Gen. Psychiatry* 14:113–118.
Bradley, C. (1937). The behavior of children receiving Benzedrine. *Am. J. Psychiatry* 94:577–585.
Clements, S. (1966). *Minimal Brain Dysfunction in Children.* Monograph No. 3. Washington: U.S. Department of Health, Education and Welfare.
Grinspoon, L., and Singer, S. (1973). Amphetamines in the treatment of hyperkinetic children. *Harv. Educ. Rev.* 43:515–555.
Hartcollis, P. (1968). The syndrome of minimal brain dysfunction in young adult patients. *Bull. Menninger Clinic* 32:102–114.
Mendelson, W., Johnson, D., and Stewart, M. (1971). Hyperactive children as teenagers: A follow-up study. *J. Nerv. Ment. Dis.* 153:273–279.

Menkes, M., Rowe, J., and Menkes, J. A. (1967). Twenty-five year follow-up study on the hyperkinetic child with minimal brain dysfunction. *Pediatrics* 39:393–400.

Morris, H., Jr., Escoll, P., and Wexler, R. (1965). Aggressive behavior disorders of childhood: A follow-up study. *Am. J. Psychiatry* 112:991–997.

Quitkin, F., and Klein, D. (1969). Two behavioral syndromes in young adults related to possible brain dysfunction. *J. Psychiatr. Res.* 7:131–142.

Safer, D. J., Allen, R. P., and Barr, E. (1975). Growth rebound after termination of stimulant drugs. *J. Pediatr.* 86:113–116.

Statterfield, J., Cantwell, D. P. *et al.* (1972). Physiological studies of the hyperkinetic child. *Am. J. Psychiatry* 128:1418–1424.

Chapter 18

Baumeister, A., and Rollings, J. (1976). Self-injurious behavior, in N. Ellis (Ed.), *International Review of Research in Mental Retardation*, vol. 8. New York: Academic Press.

Chess, S. (1970). Emotional problems in mentally retarded children, in F. J. Menolascino (Ed.), *Psychiatric Approaches to Mental Retardation*. New York: Basic Books.

DeLissovoy, V. (1961). Head banging in early childhood: A study of incidence. *J. Pediatr.* 58.803–805.

Green, A. (1967). Self-mutilation in schizophrenic children. *Arch. Gen. Psychiatry* 17:234–244.

Greenberg, H. R., and Sarner, C. A. (1965). Trichotillomania: Symptom and syndrome. *Arch. Gen. Psychiatry* 12:482–489.

Kanner, L. (1972). *Child Psychiatry* (4th ed.). Springfield, Ill.: Charles C Thomas.

Kelman, D. (1965). Gilles de la Tourette's disease in children: A review of the literature. *J. Child Psychiatry Psychol.* 6:219–226.

Lapouse, R., and Monk, M. (1958). An epidemiologic study of behavior characteristics in children. *Am. J. Pub. Health* 48:1134–1144.

Mahler, M. S. (1949). A psychoanalytic evaluation of tics in psychopathology of children. *Psychoanal. Study Child* 3(4):279–310.

Manningo, F. V., and Delgado, R. A. (1969). Trichotillomania in children: A review. *Am. J. Psychiatry* 26:505–511.

Pasamanick, B. and Kawi, A. (1956). A study of the association of prenatal and paranatal factors with the development of tics in children: A preliminary investigation. *J. Pediatr.* 48:596–601.

Torup, E. (1962). A follow-up study of children with tics. *Acta Paediatr.* 51:261–268.

Woodrow, K. M. (1974). Gilles de la Tourette's disease: A review. *Am. J. Psychiatry* 131:100–103.

Zausmer, D. (1954). Treatment of tics in children. *Arch. Dis. Child.* 29:537–542.

Chapter 19

Adelson, E., and Fraiberg, S. (1974). Gross motor development in infants blind from birth. *Child Dev.* 45:114–126.

Altshuler, K. Z. (1974). The social and psychological development of the deaf child: Problems, their treatment and prevention. *Am. Ann. Deaf* 119:365–376.

Berlinsky, S. (1952). Measurement of the intelligence and personality of the deaf: A review of the literature. *J. Speech Hear. Disorders* 17:39–54.

Bowe, F. (1974). Deafness and mental retardation, in J. D. Schein (Ed.), *Education and Rehabilitation of Deaf Persons with Other Disabilities*. New York: Deafness Training and Research Center, New York University School of Education.

Brothers, R. J. (1973). Arithmetic computation: Achievement of visually handicapped students in public schools. *Exceptional Children* 39:575–576.

Chess, S. (1971). Autism in children with congenital rubella. *J. Autism Child. Schizophrenia* 1:33–47.

Chess, S. (1974a). *Final Report, Behavior and Learning of School-Age Rubella Children*, Project No. MC-R-360184-03-0. Washington: U.S. Department of Health, Education and Welfare.

Chess, S. (1974b). The influence of defect on development in children with congenital rubella. *Merrill-Palmer Q. Behav. Dev.* 24:225–274.

Chess, S., Korn, S., and Fernandez, P. (1971). *Psychiatric Disorders of Children with Congenital Rubella*. New York: Brunner/Mazel.

Cruickshank, W. N. (1953). The multiply handicapped cerebral palsied child. *Exceptional Children* 20:16–22.

Elonen, A. S., and Zwarenstyne, S. B. (1963). Michigan's summer program for multiple-handicapped blind children. *Outlook for the Blind* 57(3):77–82.

Facts About Blindness (1972). New York: American Foundation for the Blind.

Ficocielo, C. The total child approach to educating deaf–blind children, in L. Milgrom and R. McCartin (Eds.), *The Deaf–Blind Child: Determining a Direction*. Seattle: University of Washington.

Fraiberg, S. (1971). Intervention in infancy: A program for blind infants. *J. Acad. Child Psychiatry* 10:381–405.

Fraiberg, S., and Freedman, D. A. (1964). Studies in the ego development of the congenitally blind child. *Psychoanal. Study Child* 19:113–169.

Freedman, D. A. (1971). Congenital and perinatal sensory deprivation in early development. *Am. J. Psychiatry* 127:115–121.

Freeman, R. D. (1967). Emotional reactions of handicapped children. *Rehabilitation Literature* 28:274–281.

Freeman, R. D. (1970). Psychiatric problems in adolescents with cerebral palsy. *Dev. Med. Child Neurol.* 12:64–70.

Furth, H. G. (1971). Linguistic deficiency and thinking: Research with deaf subjects 1964–1969. *Psychol. Bull.* 76:58–72.

Goldberg, B., Lobb, H., and Kroll, H. (1975). Psychiatric problems of the deaf. *Can. Psychiatr. Assoc. J.* 20:75–83.

Gouin Décarie, T. (1969). A study of the mental and emotional development of the Thalidomide child, in B. M. Moss (Ed.), *Determinants of Infant Behavior*, vol 4. London: Methuen.

Healey, W., and Karp-Nortman, D. (1975). *The Hearing Impaired Mentally Retarded: Recommendations for Action*. Washington: Division of Developmental Disabilities of Rehabilitation Services Administration, U.S. Department of Health, Education and Welfare.

Jensema, C., and Trybus, R. J. (1974). *Reported Emotional/Behavioral Problems among Hearing Impaired Children in Special Educational Programs: United States, 1972–73*. E Series R, No. 1. Washington: Office of Demographic Studies, Gallaudet College.

Lemkau, P. U. (1961). The influence of handicapping conditions on child development. *Children* 8:43–47.

Lesser, S. R., and Easser, B. R. (1972). Personality differences in the perceptually handicapped. *J. Am. Acad. Child Psychiatry* 11:458–466.

Little, W. J. (1858). On the influence of abnormal parturition. Reprinted in the *Cerebral Palsy Bulletin*, 1958, 1:5–36, from *Lancet*, Nov. 13.

Marah, G. G., and Munset, T. L. (1974). Evidence of the early impairment of verbal intelligence in Duchenne Muscular Dystrophy. *Arch. Dis. Child.* 49:118–122.

Mayer, J. (1966). Difficulties in handling the "human element" in the psychological evaluation of blind children. *The New Outlook for the Blind* 60:273–278.

McFie, J., and Robertson, J. (1973). Psychological test results of children with thalidomide deformities. *Dev. Med.* 15:719–727.

Meadow, E. P. (1968). Early manual communication in relation to the deaf child's intellectual, social, and communicative functioning. *Am. Ann. Deaf* 113:29–41.

Meyer, E. (1953). Psychological and emotional problems of deaf children. *Am. Ann. Deaf* 98:472–477.

Minde, K., Hackett, J. D., Killon, D., and Silver, S. (1972). How they grow up: 41 physically handicapped children and their families. *Am. J. Psychiatry* 128:104–109.

Mindel, E., and Vernon, M. (1971). *They Grow in Silence.* Silver Springs, Md.: National Association of the Deaf.

Myklebust, H. R. (1958). The deaf child with other handicaps. *Am. Ann. Deaf* 103:496–509.

Myklebust, H. R. (1971). *The Psychology of Deafness.* New York: Grune & Stratton.

National Association for Visually Handicapped. *Vital and Health Statistics, June 1973.* Rockville, Maryland: U.S. Department of Health, Education, & Welfare, Series 11, No. 115.

Norris, M. (1956). What affects blind children's development. *Children,* Vol. 3, No. 4.

Norris, M., Spaulding, P., and Brodie, F. (1957). *Blindness in Children.* Chicago: University of Chicago Press.

Pless, I. B., and Roghmann, K. J. (1971). Chronic illness and its consequences: Observations based on three epidemiological surveys. *J. Pediatr.* 79:351–359.

Rainer, J. D., Altshuler, K., Kallman, F., and Demming, W. (Eds.) (1963) *Family and Mental Health Problems in a Deaf Population.* New York: State Psychiatric Institute.

Rainer, J. D., and Altshuler, K. (Eds.) (1967). *Psychiatry and the Deaf.* Washington: U.S. Department of Health, Education and Welfare.

Rapoport, J. L. (1969). A case of congenital sensory neuropathy diagnosed in infancy. *J. Child Psychol. Psychiat.* 10:63–68.

Robinson, R. D. (1973). The frequency of other handicaps in children with cerebral palsy. *Dev. Med. Child Neurol.* 15:305–312.

Rosenstein, J. (1961). Perception, cognition and language in deaf children. *Exceptional Children* 27:276–284.

Rutter, M. (1972). *Maternal Deprivation Reassessed.* Baltimore: Penguin Books.

Schein, J. D. (1968). *The Deaf Community.* Washington: Gallaudet Press.

Schein, J. D., and Bushnaq, S. (1962). Higher education for the deaf in the United States: A retrospective investigation. *Am. Ann. Deaf* 107:416–420.

Schlesinger, H. S., and Meadow, K. D. (1972). *Sound and Sign: Childhood Deafness and Mental Health.* Berkeley: University of California Press.

Suppes, P. (1974). A survey of cognition in handicapped children. *Rev. Educ. Res.* 44: 95–129.

Vernon, M. (1967). The relationship of language to the thinking process. *Arch. Gen. Psychiatry* 16:325–333.

Vernon, M. (1969a). *Multiply Handicapped Deaf Children* (Research Monograph). Washington: Council for Exceptional Children.

Vernon, M. (1969b). Sociological and psychological factors associated with hearing loss. *J. Speech Hear. Res.* 12:541–563.

Vernon, M., and Brown, D. W. (1964). A guide to psychological tests and testing procedures in the evaluation of deaf and hard-of-hearing children. *J. Speech Hear. Disord.* 29:414–423.

Who is the visually handicapped child? (1973). New York: American Foundation for the Blind, p. 12.

Williams, C. E. (1968). Behavior disorders in handicapped children. *Dev. Med. Child Neurol.* 10:736–740.

Wolff, P. H. (1970). Critical periods in human cognitive Development. *Hospital Practice*, November.

Wright, D. (1971). *Deafness.* New York: Stein & Day.

Chapter 20

Getzels, J. W. (1962). *Creativity and Intelligence: Explorations with Gifted Students.* New York: Wiley.

Hollingworth, L. S. (1926). *Gifted Children: Their Nature and Nurture.* New York: Macmillan.

Hollingworth, L. S. (1942). *Children above 180 I.Q.* Yonkers-on-Hudson, N.Y.: World Book Company.

Terman, M., L., and Oden, M. (1959). *Genetic Studies of Genius*, vols. 1–5. Stanford: Stanford University Press.

Torrance, E. P. (1964). Education and creativity, in C. W. Taylor (Ed.), *Creativity, Progress and Potential.* New York: McGraw-Hill.

Witty, P. (Ed.) (1951). *The Gifted Child.* Boston: D.C. Health.

Chapter 21

Ausubel, D. P. (1957). *Theory and Problems of Adolescent Development.* New York: Grune & Stratton.

Benedict, R. (1949). Continuities and discontinuities in cultural conditioning, in S. I. Harrison and J. F. McDermott (Eds.), *Childhood Psychopathology.* New York: International Universities Press.

Caplan, G., and Lebovici, S. (Eds.) (1969). *Adolescence: Psychological Perspectives.* New York: Basic Books.

Chess, S., Thomas, A., and Cameron, M. (1976). Sexual attitudes in a middle class adolescent population. *Am. J. Orthopsychiatry* 46:689–701.

Fleming, C. M. (1963). *Adolescence.* Bungay, Suffolk, England: Richard Clay.

Howells, J. G. (Ed.). (1971). *Modern Perspectives in Adolescent Psychiatry.* New York: Brunner/Mazel.

Hudgens, R. W. (1974). *Psychiatric Disorders in Adolescents.* Baltimore: Williams & Wilkins.

Lewin, K. (1939). In, Seidman, J. M. (Ed.) (1960), *The Adolescent: A Book of Readings* (rev. ed.). New York: Holt-Dryden.

Masterson, J. F. (1964). *Psychiatric Dilemma of Adolescence.* Boston: Little, Brown.

Masterson, J. F. (1968). The psychiatric significance of adolescent turmoil. *Am. J. Psychiatry* 124:107–112.

Offer, D. (1969). *The Psychological World of the Teenager: A Study of Normal Adolescent Boys.* New York: Basic Books.

Offer, D., and Offer, J. (1971). Four issues in the developmental psychology of adolescents, in J. G. Howells (Ed.), *Modern Perspectives in Adolescent Psychiatry.* Edinburgh: Olver and Boyd.

Offer, D., Marcus, D. and Offer, J. L. (1970). A longitudinal study of normal adolescent boys. *Am. J. Psychiatry* 126:917–924.

Thomas, A., and Chess, S. (1976). Evolution of behavior disorders into adolescence. *Am. J. Psychiatry* 133:539–542.

Weiner, I. B., and Del Gaudio, A. C. (1976). Psychopathology in adolescents. *Arch. Gen. Psychiatry* 33:187–197.

Chapter 22

Abramovitz, C. (1976). The effectiveness of group psychotherapy with children. *Arch. Gen. Psychiatry* 33:320–330.

Achenbach, T. M. (1974). Issues in the treatment of psychopathology, in *Developmental Psychopathology*. New York: Ronald Press.

Akerman, N. (1963). Family diagnosis and therapy. *Current Psychiatric Therapies* 3: 205–211.

Allen, F. (1962). Child psychotherapy, in J. Masserman (Ed.), *Current Psychiatric Therapies*, vol. 2. New York: Grune & Stratton.

Anthony, J. E. (1964). Varieties and vicissitudes of the therapeutic situation in the treatment of children, in *Proceeding of the 6th International Congress of Psychotherapy*. Basel: S. Krager.

Atkins, T. E., and Rose, J. A. (1962). Emergency referrals for institutional admission. *Am. J. Orthopsychiatry* 32:347–348.

Bandura, A. (1969). *Principles of Behavior and Modification*. New York: Holt, Rinehart & Winston.

Bandura, A., and Walters, R. H. (1963). *Social Learning and Personality Development*. New York: Holt, Rinehart & Winston.

Beck, L., Langford, W. S. *et al.* (1975). Childhood chemotherapy and later drug abuse and growth curve: A follow up study of 30 adolescents. *Am. J. Psychiatry* 132:436–437.

Bettelheim, B. (1966). Training the child-care worker in a residential center. *Am. J. Orthopsychiatry* 36:694–705.

Beumont, P. J., *et al.* (1974). The effects of phenothiazines on endocrine functions, I: Patients with inappropriate lactation and amenorrhea. *Br. J. Psychiatry* 124:413–419.

Campbell, M. (1973). Biological interventions in psychosis of childhood. *J. Autism Child. Schizophrenia* 3:347–373.

Carek, D. J. (1972). *Principles of Child Psychotherapy* Springfield, Ill.: Charles C Thomas.

Carek, D. J. (1974). Integrative techniques of child psychiatry, in J. Masserman (Ed.), *Current Psychiatric Therapies*. New York: Grune & Stratton.

Churchill, D. W. (1969). Psychotic children and behavior modification. *Am. J. Psychiatry* 125:1585–1589.

Conners, C. K. (1971). Psychological effects of stimulant drugs in children with minimal brain dysfunction. *Pediatrics* 49(5):702–708.

Eisenberg, L. (1972). The clinical use of stimulant drugs in children. *Pediatrics* 49(5):709–715.

Erikson, E. (1963). *Childhood and Society* New York: Norton.

Fish, B. (1966). Drug treatment of children, in N. Kline, and H. Lehmann (Eds.), *Psychopharmacology*. Boston: Little, Brown.

Fish, B. (1971). The "one child, one drug" myth of stimulants in hyperkinesis: Importance of diagnostic categories in evaluating treatment. *Arch. Gen. Psychiatry* 24:193–203.

Fisher, S. (Ed.) (1959). *Child Research in Psychopharmacology*. Springfield, Ill.: Charles C Thomas.

Frank, J. D. (1968). Methods of assessing the results of psychotherapy, in R. Porter (Ed.), *The Role of Learning in Psychotherapy*. New Jersey: Ciba Foundation.

Freeman, R. T. (1967). The home visit in child psychiatry: Its usefulness in diagnosis and training. *J. Am. Acad. Child Psychiatry* 6:276–294.

Freud, A. (1964). Some recent developments in child analysis. *Proceeding of the 6th International Congress of Psychotherapy.*

Frommer, E. (1968). Depressive illness in childhood, in A. Coppen and A. Walk (Eds.), Recent developments in affective disorders. *Br. J. Psychiatry,* Special Publication, No. 2, pp. 117–136.

Gair, D. S., and Solomon, A. D. (1962). Diagnostic aspects of psychiatric hospitalization of children. *Am. J. Orthopsychiatry* 32:445–462.

Gallagher, J. (1962). Educational methods with brain-damaged children, in J. Masserman (Ed.), *Current Psychiatric Therapies,* vol. 2. New York: Grune & Stratton.

Ginott, H. G. (1961). *Group Psychotherapy with Children.* New York: McGraw-Hill.

Grinspoon, L., and Singer, S. (1973). Amphetamines in the treatment of hyperkinetic children. *Harv. Educ. Rev.* 43:515–555.

Haley, J. (1970). Family therapy. *Int. J. Psychiatry* 9:233–242.

Hassibi, M. (1976). Children in crisis, in Glick *et al.,* (Eds.). *Psychiatric Emergencies.* New York: Grune & Stratton.

Haworth, M. R. (Ed.) (1964). *Child Psychotherapy: Practice and Theory.* New York: Basic Books.

Klein, M. (1932). *The Psychoanalysis of Children.* London: The Hogarth Press.

Laufer, M. W., Denhoff, E., and Solomons, G. (1957). Hyperkinetic impulse disorder in children's behavior problems. *Psychosom. Med.* 19:38–49.

Lennard, H. L. and Bernstein, A. (1960). *The Anatomy of Psychotherapy: Systems of Communication and Expectation.* New York: Columbia University Press.

Levitt, E. E. (1971). Research in psychotherapy with children, in A. E. Bergin and S. L. Garfield (Eds.), *Handbook of Psychotherapy and Behavior Change. An Empirical Analysis.* New York: Wiley.

Marks, I. M. (1976). The current status of behavioral psychotherapy, theory and practice. *Am. J. Psychiatry* 133:253–261.

McAndrew, J. B., Case, Q., and Treffert, D. A. (1972). Effects of prolonged phenothiazine intake in psychotic and other hospitalized children. *J. Autism Child. Schizophrenia* 2:75–91.

McDermott, J. F., and Char, W. F. (1974). The undeclared war between child and family therapy. *J. Am. Acad. Child Psychiatry* 13:422–436.

Montalvo, B., and Pavlin, S. (1966). Faulty staff communication in a residential treatment center. *Am. J. Orthopsychiatry* 36:706–711.

Moustakas, C. (1973). *Children in Play Therapy.* New York: Jason Aronson.

Piaget, J. (1962). *Play, Dreams and Imitation in Childhood.* New York: Norton.

Rachman, S., and Costello, G. G. (1961). The etiology and treatment of children's phobias: A review. *Am. J. Psychiatry* 118:235–240.

Reusch, J. (1973). *The Therapeutic Communication.* New York: Norton.

Rosenthal, A. J., and Levine, S. V. (1971). Brief psychotherapy with children: Process of therapy. *Am. J. Psychiatry* 128:2.

Rosenthal, P. A., Mosteller, J., *et al.* (1974). Family therapy with multiproblem, multichildren families in a court clinic setting. *J. Am. Acad. Child Psychiatry* 13:126–142.

Schaefer H., and Martin, P. L. (1969). *Behavioral Therapy* (2nd ed.). New York: McGraw-Hill.

Shephered, M., Oppenheim, B., and Mitchell, S. (1971). *Childhood Behavior and Mental Health.* New York: Grune & Stratton.

Sonis, M. (1967). Residential treatment, in A. M. Freedman and H. F. Kaplan (Eds.), *Comprehensive Textbook of Psychiatry.* Baltimore: Williams & Wilkins.

Speck, R. V. (1964). Family therapy in the home. *Journal of Marriage and Family* 26: 72–76.

Speers, R. W., and Lansing, C. (1965). *Group Therapy in Childhood Psychosis.* Chapel Hill: University of North Carolina Press.

Ullmann, L. P., and Kasner, L. (Eds.) (1965). *Case Studies in Behavior Modification.* New York: Holt, Rinehart and Winston.

Waizer, J., Hoffman, S. P., *et al.* (1974). Outpatient treatment of hyperactive school children with Impiramine. *Am. J. Psychiatry* 131(5):587–91.

Wherry, J. S., and Wollersheim, J. P. (1967). Behavior therapy with children: A broad overview *J. Am. Acad. Child Psychiatry,* 6:346–370.

Winnicott, D. W. (1971). A case of anti-social behaviour, in J. G. Howells (Ed.), *Modern Perspectives in Child Psychiatry.* New York: Brunner/Mazel.

Wolpe, J. (1958). *Psychotherapy by Reciprocal Inhibition.* Stanford: Stanford University Press.

Zilbach, J. J., Bergel, E., and Gass, C. (1972). Role of the young child in family therapy, in C. J. Sager and H. Kaplan (Eds.), *Progress in Group and Family Therapy.* New York: Brunner/Mazel.

Chapter 23

Belmont, I., and Birch, H. G. (1974). The effect of supplemental intervention on children with low reading-readiness scores. *J. Spec. Educ.* 8(1):81–89.

Berlin, I. N. (1975). *Advocacy for Child Mental Health.* New York: Brunner/Mazel.

Blank, M. (1970). Implicit assumptions underlying preschool intervention programs. *J. Social Issues* 26:15–34.

Crandall, B. F. (1977). Genetic disorders and mental retardation. *J. Am. Acad. Child Psychiatry* 16:88–108.

Mellsop, G. W. (1972). Psychiatric patients seen as children and adults: Childhood predictors of adult illness. *J. Child Psychol. Psychiatry* 13:91–101.

Pichel, J. I. (1974). Long term follow-up study of sixty adolescent psychiatric outpatients. *Am. J. Psychiatry* 131:140–144.

Robins, L. N. (1966). *Deviant Children Grown Up.* Baltimore: Williams & Wilkins.

Roff, M. (1972). A two-factor approach to juvenile delinquency and the later histories of juvenile delinquents, in M. Roff, *et al.* (Eds.), *Life History Research in Psychopathology,* vol. 2. Minneapolis: The University of Minnesota Press.

Rutter, M. L. (1972). Relationship between child and adult psychiatric disorders. *Acta Psychiatr. Scand.* 48:3–21.

Stein, Z. A., and Sussjr, M. W. (1971). Changes over time in the incidence and prevalence of mental retardation, in J. Hellmuth (Ed.), *Exceptional Infant, vol. 2: Studies in Abnormalities.* New York: Brunner/Mazel.

Chapter 24

Allinsmith, W., and Goethols, G. (1962). *The Role of Schools in Mental Health.* New York: Basic Books.

Altman, M. (1972). A child psychiatrist steps into the classroom. *J. Am. Acad. Child Psychiatry* 11:231–242.

Bazelon, D. L. (1974). The problem child—Whose problem? *J. Am. Acad. Child Psychiatry* 13:193–201.

Bower, E. (1969). *Early Identification of Emotionally Handicapped Children in School.* Springfield, Ill.: Charles C Thomas.

Caplan, G. (Ed.) (1961). *Prevention of Mental Disorders in Children.* New York: Basic Books.

Chess, S., and Lyman, M. (1969). A psychiatric unit in a general hospital pediatric clinic. *Am. J. Orthopsychiatry* 39:1.

Forman, M. A., and Hetznecker, W. (1972). Varieties and vagaries of school consultation. *J. Am. Acad. Child Psychiatry* 11:694–704.

Hetznecker, W., and Forman, M. A. (1971). Community child psychiatry: Evolution and direction. *Am. J. Orthopsychiatry* 41:350–370.

La Vietes, R., and Chess, S. (1969). A training program in school psychiatry. *J. Am. Acad. Child Psychiatry* 8:84–96.

Lawrence, M. M. (1971). *The Mental Health Teams in the Schools.* New York: Behavioral Publications.

Panzetta, A. P. (1971). *Community Mental Health: Myth and Reality.* Philadelphia: Lea & Febiger.

Rafferty, F. T. (1975). Community mental health centers and the criteria of quantity and universality of services for children. *J. Am. Acad. Child Psychiatry* 14:5–17.

Chapter 25

Bazelon, D. L. (1974). "The problem child"—Whose problem? *J. Am. Acad. Child Psychiatry* 13:193–201.

Benedeck, E. (1972). Child custody laws: Their psychiatric implications. *Am. J. Psychiatry* 129:326–328.

Benedeck, E. P., and Benedek, R. S. (1972). New child custody laws: Making them do what they say. *Am. J. Orthopsychiatry* 42:825–834.

Derdyn, A. P. (1975). Child custody consultation. *Am. J. Orthopsychiatry* 45:791–801.

Derdyn, A. P. (1976a). Child custody contests in historical perspective. *Am. J. Psychiatry* 133:1369–1376.

Derdyn, A. P. (1976b). A consideration of legal issues in child custody contests. *Arch. Gen. Psychiatry* 33:165–178.

Farer, L. G. (1969). Rights of children: The legal vacuum. *Am. Bar Assoc. J.* 55:1151–1156.

Ginsberg, L. H. (1973). An examination of the civil rights of mentally ill children. *Child Welfare* 52:14–25.

A Guide to New York's Child Protection System. Legislative Document, 1974, No. 27.

Juvenile Justice Confounded: Pretentions and Realities of Treatment Services (1972). New York: Committee on Mental Health Services Inside and Outside the Family Court in the City of New York.

Kahn, A. J. (1953). *A Court for Children.* New York: Columbia University Press.

Katz, B. F. (1975). Children, privacy, and nontherapeutic experimentation. *Am. J. Orthopsychiatry* 45:802–812.

Katz, S. N. (1976). The changing legal status of foster parents. *Children Today* 5:11–13.

McDermott, J. F., Char, W. F. J., et al. (1973). The concept of child advocacy. *Am. J. Psychiatry* 130:1203–1206.

Murdock, C. W. (1973). Civil rights of the mentally retarded—Some critical issues. *Family Law Quarterly* 7:1–4.

New York State Association for Retarded Children v. *Carey* (1975). *Mental Retardation and the Law.* (June 1975). Washington: U.S. Department of Health, Education and Welfare.

Nir, Y., and Cutler, R. (1973). Therapeutic utilization of the juvenile court. *Am. J. Psychiatry* 130:1112–1117.

Peck, H., and Horowitz, J. (1958). *A New Pattern for Mental Health Services in a Children's Court.* Springfield, Ill.: Charles C Thomas.

Shoor, M., and Speed, M. H. (1969). Seven years of psychiatric consultation in a juvenile probation department. *Psychiatr. Q.* 43:147–163.

Index